INSIGHTS

FACTS AND STORIES BEHIND
TRIGEMINAL NEURALGIA

LESLEY SHANNON

INSIGHTS

FACTS AND STORIES BEHIND
TRIGEMINAL NEURALGIA

Joanna M. Zakrzewska, M.D., FDSRCS, FFDRCSI

Professor of pain in relation to oral medicine, Honorary Consultant
Clinical and Diagnostic Oral Sciences Dental Institute
Barts and the London Queen Mary's School of Medicine and
Dentistry, London, UK

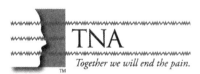

Together we will end the pain.

TRIGEMINAL NEURALGIA ASSOCIATION
Gainesville, Florida

Printed by Whitehall Printing Company, Naples, Florida
10 9 8 7 6 5 4 3

Grateful acknowledgement is made for permission to use the cover graphic:
Oregon Health and Science University
Andy Rekito, department of Neurological Surgery

Chapter Illustrators:
Malcolm Willett - medical cartoonist
Helen McParland BDS, FDSRCS

Published by

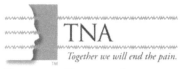

Together we will end the pain.
TRIGEMINAL NEURALGIA ASSOCIATION
925 Northwest 56th Terrace, Suite C, Gainesville, FL 32605

ISBN: 978-0-9672393-4-7

CONTENTS

FOREWORD

We are taught that *success* is a journey, not a destination. In the case of Trigeminal Neuralgia Association (TNA), that journey began in 1990, when Claire Patterson, a visionary TN sufferer, addressed the need for a patient oriented association that could provide information, comfort and support for those afflicted by this excruciatingly painful disease which is often misdiagnosed and inappropriately treated. Supported by Dr. Peter Jannetta, famed proponent of microvascular decompression surgery as a response to TN, Claire built a national association that now brings TN and related conditions more and more into the light of day. With support groups all over the US and correspondent organizations elsewhere, a website that hosts more daily visitors than Disney World, a program of national and regional conferences that attract increasing attendance, and publications that provide up to date information on all aspects of facial pain, TNA's continuing journey assures new patients the expectation of speedier access to both diagnosis and appropriate treatment.

Education of patients, lay public as well as healthcare workers is essential if awareness of this devastating condition is to be increased. This book is unique in that it represents a collaboration between healthcare professionals and patients showing how both can contribute to the production of a text that is based on scientific facts and supported by patients' experiences. Through TNA, Professor Joanna Zakrzewska, or Dr. Zak as she likes to be called, was able to gather the individual stories of patients with TN and related conditions that are at the heart of this work. This was no mean achievement but something that TNA could facilitate based on its growing database of patients and the willingness of patients to share their stories, recognizing that TNA can make a difference in helping to end the pain. This book complements *"Striking Back!"*, as it uses a different approach and is written in lay language by a healthcare professional. As such, it is an important addition to TNA's list of publications and an important resource to all in combating facial pain.

It is not surprising that Dr. Zak chose to use patients' stories for this book as a little of her history will demonstrate. Having graduated from both medicine and dentistry and specialized in Oral Medicine she gained a personal chair for her extensive national and international research in the field of facial pain. She is the only overseas member of TNA's Medical Advisory Board and Chairman of the Medical Advisory Board of TNA UK, which she co-founded. Referred to as a pioneer in patient care by the British Medical Association, she is a strong advocate for evidenced based medicine and high quality clinical research. With nearly two decades of clinical work in this area she sees more patients with trigeminal neuralgia a year than most clinicians see in a lifetime and this puts her in the unique position of being able to speak from vast experience. Anyone who has heard her speak at a TNA National Conference will know of her fierce and steadfast support for patients' rights and the need for patients to be listened to. We are proud that she chose TNA to be her publisher and that she approached the task with great enthusiasm giving up her spare time to write what we think is an important advance in understanding facial pain and how to confront it. We are also proud to call Joanna our friend and a fellow voyager on our journey.

The journey continues. In recent years, a dramatic increase in research on the physiology of neuropathic pain has been undertaken and the advent of functional neuroimaging has demonstrated alterations in brain activity associated with neuropathic pain. The prospect of developing new therapies for treating and, perhaps, curing neuropathic facial pain, such as TN and related conditions, thus becomes a more attainable goal and TNA has begun to support select research projects. These include grants to begin an epidemiology study and the study of the impact of Botox on facial pain.

While support of these initiatives is important, the need remains for a comprehensive *Trigeminal Neuralgia and Related Facial Pain Research Program*. In May 2005, TNA established the *Facial Pain Research Institute* to foster such a program. As a result, the *Facial Pain Research Institute* has entered into a collaborative arrangement with the McKnight Brain Institute of the University of Florida, in Gainesville, Florida, where TNA's National Office is now located. Through this collaboration, the McKnight Brain Institute will conduct research and develop new treatments for thousands of people who suffer from debilitating neuropathic facial pain disorders. TN, as readers may know, is universally considered to be the most painful affliction known to medical practice and, while not fatal, has been called the "suicide disease."

Without a cure, medications and surgeries have proven effective in alleviating the pain only for some patients. Other patients are either unresponsive, build a resistance to the treatments or experience undesirable side effects. For this reason, it is imperative that we fast track TN research and bring relief to the thousands of people who suffer in pain every day.

The *Trigeminal Neuralgia and Related Facial Pain Research Program* will do just that by leveraging the state-of-the-art facilities at the McKnight Brain Institute, creating a new professorship, attracting leading researchers from around the world, and maintaining a research support team, with the goal of understanding the causes of facial pain disorders and developing treatments to end the pain. The partnership between *TNA's Facial Pain Research Institute* and the McKnight Brain Institute is a transformational event and crucial to the advancement of research and treatment of chronic facial pain.

This book by Dr. Zak will bring understanding and encouragement to those who suffer from facial pain. Their journey is our journey until we can eradicate the unacceptable face of pain. To do this, TNA must develop resources, financial as well as human, to continue its journey and fuel the *Trigeminal Neuralgia and Related Facial Pain Research Program*, while assuring patients of continued access to TNA's many other programs. The fine work which this book represents will inspire many in their personal journey. We hope that many will be inspired to support TNA's own journey and hasten the day when, together, we can end the pain!

Roger Levy
Chairman, Board of Directors
Trigeminal Neuralgia Association
1-800-923-3608   www.endthepain.org

INTRODUCTION

"It was March 8, 1995, my daughter's birthday and I left the school shortly after the bell. A student graciously handed me a package of M & M (candies) in thanks for some extra help, as I went out of the door. With a warm feeling of being appreciated, I tore open the package as soon as I entered my car. Out of the parking lot, heading south on a brilliantly sunny day, I tossed a few candies into my mouth. Upon biting down, the most excruciating, hot, electrical shock penetrated my left eye. With my eyes welled up with tears, I struggled to concentrate on the road. Immediately I arrived home I called my dentist. Luckily he assured me that there was no dental problem. … several days went by with no pain and I convinced myself it was just some freakish incident. One that I hoped I would never experience again. A week later, while teaching, the horrible shocks returned …..."

This vivid excerpt from a description of a sufferer's first attack of trigeminal neuralgia sets the scene for this book.

Welcome to our story of trigeminal neuralgia be you a sufferer, a spouse or relative, a healthcare provider or a lay person who wants to understand more and help. This book provides information that is of equal importance to the patient and the non specialist health care provider. It provides a level playing field for patients and health care professionals to move on within the limits of our current knowledge. One of the most dramatic changes in 21st century medical practice is in the relationship between physician and patient. This needs to be on an equal partnership, which means that both groups have the same access and share the same information. The health care professional becomes the manager of the knowledge and helps the patient interpret it so that decision-making is a shared function, although the ultimate decision remains with the patient.

Our whole lives are made up of stories and some of our earliest memories are of stories told to us by our parents or loved ones. These stories all have a beginning, a series of events that gradually unfold and an ending. They draw us in, absorb our attention and so engage us as I hope you already have been by this opening story. Not only do we live by narrative but we also suffer by narrative. Stories in medicine do more than facilitate conversation, they probe the depths of an illness and they allow for greater understanding of patients, of healthcare providers and of ourselves, thereby leading to changes in our perceptions.

I want to tell you a story because I want you to get caught up in it since it matters to me that you can understand why you need to become involved. Together we will be stronger in our response to this severe facial pain and be able to make a difference that will change our lives. As the narrator, I have selected what to tell and what to omit but what you, the reader, finds inside depends on you. As the poet Ben Orki (1998) says in his "*Ode to the Book*"

> "*A book's power is the mirror of your mental might.*
> *A mirror wherein the world dreams.*
> *The freest country. The only place*
> *with an open border*
> *and infinite interior space.*
> *This miraculous touch from heart to eye,*
> *this binding of love that can make us whole.*"

Hundreds of patients have contributed to this book through the stories they have shared with me, during consultations, during patient meetings, and in written material that so many sufferers have sent in from round the world. I have also had access to drawings, paintings and sculptures to enhance the story telling.

Trigeminal neuralgia sufferers! I have learned from you. I have felt the inner hurt, fear, despair, loneliness, loss of integrity and hope expressed in the stories I have been privileged to hear and read. I hope this book shows you that I have listened and tried to answer the questions you have asked.

To those of you who do not have trigeminal neuralgia I hope after reading the text and responding to the illustrations you will have learned something of what sufferers of trigeminal neuralgia go through even when they appear to be indistinguishable in a crowd. We can all offer empathy and help, either in caring for these patients or by supporting much needed research in this area.

This is the story of our joint effort to learn about trigeminal neuralgia and to shift our perceptions about it. For the sufferer the pain may still be there but it will be experienced differently. It is possible that the deeper understanding gained from reading this book will lead to a reduction in suffering. This is a book of hope and support.

My previous book on "*Assessment and Management of Orofacial Pain*" was based on scientific facts, which we call evidence based medicine. It has been argued that narrative and a sophisticated evidence based medicine approach cannot co-exist. Science seeks knowledge and tries to discover the truth about diseases. Clinical practice, or the art of medicine, tries to discover how the patients' illness threatens the personhood of each individual.

Eric Cassell argues in his book on *"The Nature of Suffering"* that medicine has devoted a disproportionate amount of time on science alone and undervalued subjective but often value laden and impossible to measure facts. Medicine has failed to attend to human suffering, which is essential if the art of clinical practice is to advance alongside scientific knowledge.

This book represents an attempt, to combine art and science, since I believe this is a powerful way of getting across the message that more research is needed before the Trigeminal Neuralgia Association's theme *"together we will end this pain"* can become a reality.

Every patient with trigeminal neuralgia would like to hold their doctor in an arm lock and not let go until they have been freed from the terror of the pain. But the doctor is also afraid of this arm lock as he/she cannot provide a cure for everyone. I want you to understand it from this perspective so we can all diminish our fear of this pain which makes the suffering worse.

This is not a book you need to read from cover to cover in one session. It is one to swallow and digest slowly, to keep by the bedside and return to. You can delve into it at any point, once you see how it is organised.

Each chapter begins with a sufferer's narrative, which introduces the topic for the chapter or presents the particular problem that will be addressed. In addition, Michael Pasternak, President of TNA US, sent me reams of questions that are used in each chapter to make the text more readable and to make it easier to find information.

Many of the scientific statements are also, supported by quotes from patients. Each chapter includes a series of tables called **Key Facts**, as well as a summary, which can be used to assess the contents of each chapter. Other tables provide practical information for patients or more technical data.

I have tried to point out, as far as possible, where the information is based on good- quality evidence and where it has not been substantiated by scientific investigations. There also is a section on areas of potential future research, which highlights the questions that need to be addressed.

A reading list of key books, chapters or papers, which provide the evidence for the statements made, as well as Internet sites is provided at the end of each chapter. More detailed references may be found in our book, **"Assessment and Management of Orofacial Pain"**.

Throughout the book we will follow the story of Mrs, G. (based on a couple of my patients) who will serve as a roadmap as she makes her journey through her condition, stopping off at times or going down the wrong route at others. Her stories will provide you with the human element needed to develop a deeper understanding.

Medical words and phrases, especially those related to the diagnosis and treatment of trigeminal neuralgia, are defined in a glossary at the end of the book. I am very grateful to George Weigel, co-author of **Striking Back! The Trigeminal Neuralgia and Face Pain Handbook**, for allowing me to use his glossary as a starting point. Other special references include an appendix in Chapter 5 that lists medications commonly used in the US and UK.

A book such as this cannot be written without collaboration from many individuals and I think it is true to say that this is a truly international, multidisciplinary effort. I believe the cartoons drawn by Malcolm Willett enhance the book more than any words. Malcolm knew nothing about trigeminal neuralgia when I first approached him for help. He read the book and then worked very hard to match up each chapter with an appropriate cartoon. Not only has he captured the essence of this condition but his cartoons show that humour can lighten the burden of this disease. Helen MacParland, a dentist working in my facial pain clinic, herself offered to help draw the technical pictures to help interpret the words. I have also benefited from illustrations given to me by Professor Hugh Coakham, a neurosurgeon with whom I have been working for a number of years, my PhD Student Mr T.P.Jorns, and a colleague in Thailand Assistant Professor Stuart McEachen not only provided me with some images but also taught me how to use the software to edit pictures. Rosa Sepple, an artist patient of mine, has painted several pictures on the theme of trigeminal neuralgia and I have included a couple of these in the book.

The drafts were read by a range of patients. Claire Patterson, Founder of TNA US read each chapter and supplied especially useful information for the chapter on support groups. If not for her this book would never have been written as it was her enormous efforts that persuaded me to come to a TNA US conference and to then accept the challenge of facilitating the setting up of the UK group. Joanna Gardner, another sufferer, on the executive board of the UK TNA, working on the remote Island of Mull diligently returned chapters not only tracked but full of wise comments. Jillie Abbott, who has been setting up UK regional groups provided feedback on the chapter on support groups. Finally Arline Phillips, in a remarkably short time went through the completed book twice and once again provided invaluable input.

This book would not have been possible without the enormous input I have had from patients from both sides of the Atlantic and down under. Not only did they come to focus group meetings and allow us to tape record the meetings but also provided a vast amount of written material. Beth Heitman, at the time support group co-ordinator, at TNA US appealed to patients to send in their stories by Email. She then co-ordinated the emails and sent them to me both electronically and digitally. I hope the list on page XVII of the book includes everyone who contributed. I am grateful to the leaders of the national support groups in the UK, Carole Straker and in Australia, Irene Wood for their input and access to their members. Jane Boles, executive director at the TNA US headquarters acted as co-ordinator and patiently acknowledged all the emails that came flooding in with corrections and pictures. At the head was Michael Pasternak, President of TNA US with his list of questions and regular phone calls to check on progress. I am grateful to all at Whitehall Printing Company for their work on the book especially Myron Hirsch.

Writing such a book always places an enormous toll on the family who inevitably are affected. I am particularly grateful to them as I promised them I would not be writing another book after I finished the last one barely three years ago. My daughter Krystyna's artistic talent provided me with a sounding board for all the illustrations and it was a brain storming session with her that finally decided on the title. My son, Konrad, provided technical IT support and my husband showed remarkably forbearance with the hours I spent in front of the computer. All my daily chores were taken over by an ever helpful Maria Maslanka who cooked remarkable meals for all the family to enjoy.

My grateful thanks go to all, including those I may have forgotten to mention and I hope that this book through its distribution round the world will help in reducing the suffering that trigeminal neuralgia brings to all.

"Those who have suffered much are like those who know many languages; they have learned to understand and to be understood by all"
Mad Swetchine.

CONTRIBUTORS

This is a list which I hope is comprehensive, of all patients and supporters in the US, UK and Australia who provided information for the book by attending focus groups, sending emails, letters, writing poems or painting. Even if I did not use something from everyone's contribution the whole gave me incredible insight into the suffering that people with trigeminal neuralgia go through. My apologies to anyone I have omitted or whose name does not appear correct.

Abbot, Jillie
Adachi, Darryl
Allen, Krystal
Allen, Krystal
Althea-Spence, Valerie
Ashby, Rhonda
Baehr, Jim
Bagwell, Anna
Bailey, Doris
Bailey, Janet
Bala, Peggy
Beck, Jean
Betty, Cory
Betty, Doss
Biszantz , Terah
Bloomfield, Bennett
Boon, Jan W
Boudreaux, Mitzie
Brace, Carrie E
Bruten, Janet
Buck, Margaret
Buekseb, Neal
Cahill, Jr Edward A.
Calhoun, Brad
Calow, Janet
Caneclides, Lafata

Carmody, Deb
Caroll, Lee J
Clough, Jennifer
Cook, Regina
Cornwell, John
Cuzzivoglio, Sher
Denmark, Nancy
Drharcourt
Easterday, Shanon
Ezell, Cynthia
Faeth, Dave
Fetterly, Jane
Foster, Joan
Friesenhahn, Lynn
Fritch, John
Funtsie, Judy
Gardner, Joanna
Gardner, Karen
Gillard, Neill
Gliozzi, Emilia
Goerish, Gloria
Gustavson, Fran
Haber, Hilary
Hancock, M
Hare, William
Harmer, Rohn

Harned, J R Edwin
Heitman, Beth
Hercher Therese
Hewitz, June
Hogan, Kathleen
Hrouda, Joe
Hughes, Jaylene
Jenniges, Maggie
Judy
Katy
Katz, Sherri
Keltie, Norma
Keltie, Norma
Lasley, Cynthia
Lawhern, Richard
Lewis, Jana
Luscinski, Shirley
Lynch, Carole
Madden, Jack
Madden, Jack
Martina
McAuley, Joe
McCann, NancyLou
McKenna, Linda
Minnick, Betty
Murai, R
Mytn, Simon
Oslund, Marge
Pannapacker, Donna
Peck, Alton
Peg
Porter, Helen
Potter, Pat
Price ,Betty
Purchase, Ruthi
Redmann, Laurie
Reisch, L
Renuka
Reynosa, Vivian
Ruther, Peggy

Sepple, Rosa
Sharon
Shaw, Laura J
Simon, Laurie
Smith, Gavin
Smith, Milton Orin
Stacey, Loretta
Stapler , Bob
Stephen, Lissa
Straker, Carole
Stratton, Joan
Taff, Windy
Taylor Kristy
Terry, Val
Tim Guith
Tippett, Ben
Tull, Joyce
Unruh, Rodney
Walton, Mollie
Weaver, Bill
Weigel, George
White, Charles
Whitesides, Cathie
Whiting, Jerry
Williams, Suzanne I
Witham, Patricia
Wood , Irene

INSIGHTS

FACTS AND STORIES BEHIND
TRIGEMINAL NEURALGIA

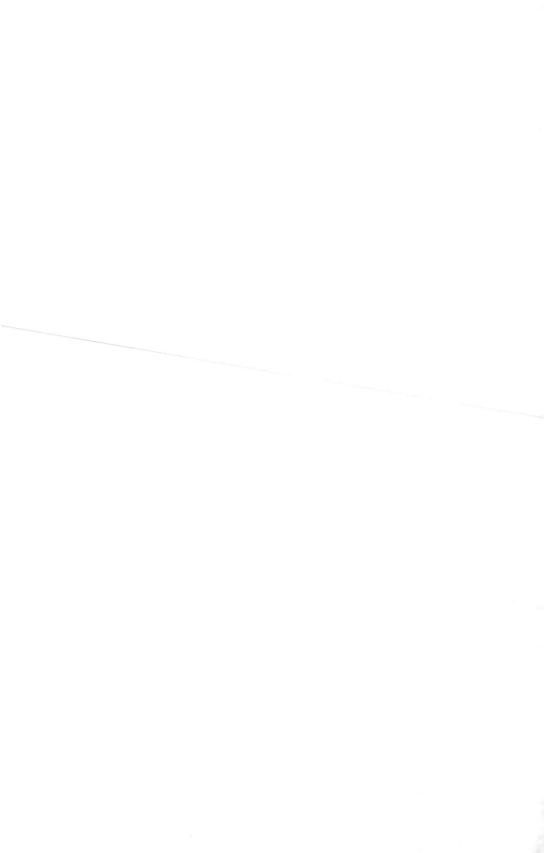

CHAPTER 1

PRESENTATION AND DIAGNOSIS OF TRIGEMINAL NEURALGIA

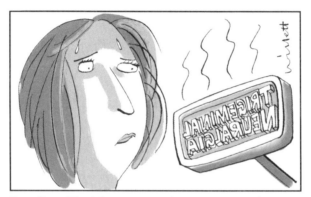

Branding: Obtaining a correct diagnosis is crucial, since this will dictate future management.

"I was standing in the shower with the hot water spraying on my face. It was a fast, jarring jolt of lightning pain on the left side of my face. For the next couple of weeks I was immobile. All activities and interest stopped. My time was spent waiting apprehensively for the next gruesome jab of staggering pain to hit my face. I dreaded waking up to start another day of electrical-like pains." .....

Betty Price describes her pain experience in a poem:

Oh the horror of this pain
The ice pick stabs again
The quickness of the pain
Has come and gone again.
Sometimes it lasts forever
And I think that I might die
At other times it is a burning
Sometimes just a twitch
My face may sometimes quiver
This you hope no one will see
It may feel like Novacaine
That is beginning to wear off
What a weird feeling!
There has been no shot at all
Now it is time to
Brush those teeth
Here comes great fear again
So I bow my head and pray my prayer...
God take this pain from me.

The International Association for the Study of Pain defines trigeminal neuralgia as "a sudden, usually unilateral, severe, brief, stabbing, recurrent pain in the distribution of one or more branches of the fifth cranial nerve." This definition provides a description of the condition, but the suffering it causes can only be expressed by the sufferers themselves: "*unbearable pain, screaming pain, lightning bolt, electric shock, electric explosion, sword and fire, suffering, misery, hell, horrific, horror, a lost day, unknown future, trapped, discouragement, despair, death.*" These are words that were chosen in response to the question, "When you think of trigeminal neuralgia, what do you think of?" (presented at the Trigeminal Neuralgia Association conference 2004).

Trigeminal neuralgia is currently the only facial pain that really benefits from major surgical procedures; hence an accurate diagnosis is essential.

Those of you with trigeminal neuralgia will be able to make an immediate diagnosis from the story/poem I have just quoted. But why does it sometimes take such a long time to obtain an accurate diagnosis? As this patient writes, "*After five years of pain, endless doctors, dentists and endodontists, an emergency doctor walks in, talks to me for three minutes and tells me I am a classic case of trigeminal neuralgia."* As in everything, a prepared mind finds what it is looking for.

1. HOW DO WE DIAGNOSE TRIGEMINAL NEURALGIA?

The diagnosis of trigeminal neuralgia is currently made solely on the story the patient tells. In medical jargon – the history. This is the case with many other diseases. Despite our new technologies, it has been estimated that a thorough medical history results in correct diagnosis in 75 % of cases, while physical examination contributes 12 % to the diagnosis, and investigations or tests only 11 %. However, health care professionals' confidence in the diagnosis is much higher if supported by objective test results. In trigeminal neuralgia, we currently have no highly reliable tests and so have to rely exclusively on the history.

What do we mean by history taking?

History taking is a fine art that has to be learned and perfected during a health care professional's lifetime. To be successful, it must be patient-centered. Not only does the doctor need to encourage the patient to tell a good story; he or she needs to become involved in it, respond to it and then also be a compelling storyteller. History taking involves more than just good communication; it attempts to systematically unravel a patient's symptom, look for associations and suggest a likely diagnosis. Skilled history takers will carefully explore the chief complaint that the patient presents with, and will ask questions around it. They will delve deeper for underlying issues, clarify the findings with the patient, sometimes repeating the same question in a different way and then re-telling the story to the patient to see if it has been understood correctly.

History taking is not just finding out about the disease itself, but crucially determining the impact of the illness on the patients and all those they are in contact with. It includes eliciting patients' explanations of their illnesses and encouraging patients to express their emotions. Each patient's experience of pain is unique, so the physician must pay attention to the sufferers' motivation, values, desires, thoughts and feelings, as well as the way they experience the pain.

Physicians who establish empathy with their patients, support patients' feelings and emotions, show respect for their patients' viewpoints, are nonjudgmental and strive for a partnership, are the ones who can build a positive relationship. This builds up the trust between doctor and patient and leads the patient to feel understood and cared for and helps create a longlasting therapeutic relationship.

There is emerging evidence that patient satisfaction with care relies heavily on these aspects: ensuring patients' history is taken fully, fears and worries are addressed and reasons are given for what is done or not done. Our own analysis in our facial pain clinic showed that 127 patients described the main treatment goals as follows: *"to understand my condition better, be reassured that it is not a sign of more serious disease, and improve communication with doctors about my condition."*

This process involves not just listening, but also observing, since the nonverbal clues may be stronger than the verbal ones. Illustrations in this book help to get across certain messages faster than the narrative.

Unfortunately, modern technology, with its ability in many instances to make an accurate diagnosis, has meant that many doctors have not acquired the art of history taking. How many doctors can say that as juniors they were observed and given an appraisal exclusively of their competence in history taking? Medical schools have taken this on board and all are now specifically teaching and assessing communication skills. History taking involves more than just finding out about the pain.

The whole process should include the factors shown in the Table 1 below.

Table 1

WHAT HISTORY TAKING SHOULD ESTABLISH
• General pain history as presented by the patient, including prior treatments
• Any other problems in the mouth, face or head that may be related, e.g. hearing loss
• Medical history, including other illnesses
• Drug use, including all those currently and previously taken for the pain, those taken for other conditions and reactions to them
• Dental history, including fillings, root canal treatments, extractions
• Short psychiatric history to determine presence of depression, anxiety, fear
• Feelings about illness
• Family history to see if other members have the same pain
• Social history, including who can help and what activities need to be done
• Quality of life, including effect of pain on their environment and social life
• Health beliefs and expectations

A patient should feel that at the end of the consultation, the following questions have been addressed:

- What do you think caused your pain?
- Why do you think it started when it did? What else was happening in your life at the time?
- What do you think your chronic pain does to you (your body, and equally importantly your emotional reactions)? How do you think this pain works?
- How severe is your pain? Will it have a short or long course?
- What type of treatment do you think you should receive?
- What results do you hope to receive from this treatment?
- What are the chief problems (at work, at home, with friends) your continued pain has caused you?

How to ensure successful history taking?

When going to the doctor, it is likely that a patient may have one or more of these concerns:

- Will I be able to tell my story or will I be in too much pain?
- Will I tell it accurately?
- Will the doctor understand and believe me?
- Will I get treatment that will cure my pain?

To reduce this anxiety, it is useful to reflect before going to the doctor on the story that needs to be told. Writing down things is a useful way of doing this. I try to direct patients' thoughts by sending out a two page leaflet listing the questions that will be asked. It is based on the American Pain Society leaflet and is shown in Table 2 below.

Table 2

PAIN ASSESSMENT

health care providers use the word assessment to describe questions they ask to learn more about you and your pain. When you come to the facial pain clinic, the doctor will ask about your pain and pain relief. The better you describe the pain, how it affects your life and activities, and what works to relieve it, the easier it will be for you to get help. Since there are no specific tests to make a diagnosis of facial pain, we have to rely on what you tell us and on the questionnaires you complete. It may be helpful if you read through this before your appointment with the doctor and think about the answers to these questions.

Continued...

...Continued

Where does it hurt? Does the pain move from one place to another?

Tell the doctor exactly how the pain feels. Does it feel like it's on the inside of your mouth or face? Or does it seem like it is on the outside? Point to the places that hurt. Show the doctor where the pain moves if it travels from one place to another. Use a drawing of the outline of a face to show the places where it hurts. Be sure to show all of the places that hurt, not just the spot that hurts the most.

Do you have more than one spot where it hurts?

You may have more than one kind of pain - some caused by the disease or disorder, some by the treatments, and some unrelated - a stress headache, for instance. It is important to describe each kind of pain in detail.

When does the pain happen? How long does it last? Does the pain come and go? Or is it there all the time? Is this pain new? Have you ever had this pain before? When does it begin? When does it end?

Describing pain this way helps others know more about the pain.

Does the pain keep you from doing all you want to do?

Pain may stop people from moving, eating, working, playing, or getting around. Sometimes pain interferes with thinking and concentration. Pain can interfere with being close to other people. Describing how pain limits your life will help your doctor set goals with you for dealing with pain.

Does pain interrupt your sleep? Does it change your mood? Affect your appetite?

When pain interferes with sleep, mood, or appetite, it can affect all parts of life. A first goal for treatment is to ensure a good night's sleep. When you are well rested, you have more energy to try to get well, to talk with others, to enjoy life, and to do the things that are important to you. Pain can also cause you to feel grumpy or sad, especially when it lasts a long time. Pain can change the way you eat and cause you to gain or lose weight. Pain that won't go away can change the way you feel about yourself and others. Explaining how pain affects you can help others understand more about your pain and how to make it better.

What do you think causes the pain?

Your doctor needs to know what you think is happening and causing your pain. Doctors will look for the cause of the pain. But even if the cause is not found, pain can be treated.

What makes the pain better? What makes it worse?

People try things to relieve pain. Some work well; others may not work at all. Sometimes pain occurs when you eat or open your mouth wide. Sometimes staying in one position eases the pain. Telling your doctor about these things can help him or her control your pain more quickly.

What have you tried to relieve the pain?

Different kinds of pain respond to different treatment. You may already have found things that work well to relieve the pain. You may have tried relaxation, meditation, heat, cold, or mild exercise. These may all relieve some kinds of pain. If so, your doctor will want to include these actions in your treatment plan.

You also might have tried things, such as certain medicines, that did not relieve the pain. Your doctor needs to know this in order to avoid delays in finding just the right treatment for you.

Continued...

...*Continued*

Your doctor also needs to know all of the over-the-counter medications you take and what medicines have been prescribed for you by another doctor or nurse practitioner. Some medicines can't be taken together. Some medicines with different names contain the same chemicals and could be harmful if too much is taken.

What medicines are you taking for pain right now?

Describe all the medicines you have tried for pain in the last two or three days. Be prepared to list all other medicines as well. List the name, amount of medicine, time the medicine was taken, amount of relief, and any side effects.

How are you currently taking medications to relieve pain?

Sometimes medications that have not worked before might be effective if taken in a different way. Describe exactly how and when you are taking medicines now. Your doctor needs to know if the way you are taking medicine is different from the instructions on the bottle.

Describe how long the medicine takes to work. How long does pain relief last? Does all of the pain go away after you take the medicine? Does the pain return before the next dose is due?

Answers to these questions make it easier to come up with a plan that works to relieve your pain.

Do you have any side effects from medicines you are taking? Do you have any allergies?

Medicines for severe pain tend to cause side effects. These could include feeling drowsy, unable to walk straight, not being able to think clearly. Talk about other side effects that cause problems some may be avoidable. Discuss your allergies to medicines and other things. Describe how the allergy showed itself and when you first noticed it.

Do you have any worries about taking medicines for pain relief?

Many people worry about taking medicines for pain relief. They worry about addiction and other side effects. Addiction rarely occurs in people taking medicines for the relief of pain. Your doctor needs to know how you feel about this. The doctor should explain that it is not a problem. Ask questions about other worries you may have.

How much relief would allow you to get around better? What is your goal for pain relief? What are your other concerns?

You may be asked to set a goal for pain relief. The goal may be based on the ratings scale (for example, 2 on a scale of 0 to 10). Or, your goal may focus on activities you would like to carry out (eating without pain, being able to work). The aim of the treatment plan is to meet the goals you set for pain relief. You may also want reassurance that the pain is not a sign of something serious.

Tell the doctor a little about yourself, your childhood, work, leisure activities, the people you live with.

The doctor will ask you some questions about your life, since this information helps the doctor understand how the pain may have arisen and how people around you respond to it. It will also help in trying to set some goals to work toward.

Modified from the American Pain Foundation
Facial Pain Clinic, Barts and London NHS Trust
July 2004

It is useful to think through what the treatment goals are for the sufferer. In the appendix is an example of a treatment goals questionnaire that I use routinely with all my patients to ensure that I have elicited all the patients' concerns.

The patient must feel comfortable with the doctor, and emotions such as expressed by this patient should not arise: *"Every doctor I saw made me feel as if I was crazy. There were some who would just sit and look at me and I still do not know what they were hoping to figure out by staring me down. Many more had me feeling that I was alone in this — that there was nothing out there that would ever help me. I was going to spend every day of my life in this tortured state."* There are others who find a "doctor who actually believed me." What patients need is *"a doctor who will listen to you, work with you and is willing to learn with you."*

All patients have a right to be understood and this may mean that the consultation may need to be offered in a different language. Patients should alert the doctor to this so that interpreters or advocates can be brought in, since they are likely to be more useful than a relative or friend in translating.

It is well recognized that patients only remember part of a consultation and that the worse the news being given, the less the patient remembers. The patient may recall as little as 15 % of the information. I encourage patients to bring in partners who can serve as a second pair of ears and can contribute their story to the consultation, often providing a very useful perspective. Everyone tells a story differently.

If a patient is in severe pain at the time of consultation, it may be very difficult to provide a history, not just because talking brings on the pain but also because it is difficult to concentrate on anything while suffering from severe pain. If the area of pain can be identified, i.e. has a trigger point, it may be useful for the doctor to give the patient a local anesthetic such as is given by dentists. In most instances, this should provide relief for an hour or two and enable a more meaningful consultation to take place.

For the physician taking the history, it is important that a patient be given time to explain the problem, especially in the opening stages. It has been shown that physicians interrupt a patient's opening statement within 30 seconds and yet most patients, if allowed to continue uninterrupted, will only speak for 2.5 minutes, with an average of 90 seconds in the primary care sector. In observed consultations, it was found that only 23 % of patients were allowed to complete their opening statement.

Recently one of my patients provided me with the following opening statement, *"A shooting pain in front and behind my ear made worse by swallowing."* I immediately made the diagnosis of glossopharyngeal neuralgia, even though the letter of referral said the patient had temporomandibular pain.

As every senior doctor will teach his junior staff, "Listen to the patient and he will tell you the diagnosis."

History taking requires time. Hence the more prepared the patient is, the less time is lost. Doctors also should acknowledge that they need some time with patients in pain and so may need to book longer or supplementary appointments. The consultation at which the diagnosis is being made is the appointment that requires more time than any other. Potentially, it will dictate the future course of a patient's life.

Once a patient has acquired a diagnosis or label, it is difficult to change. It channels everything in one direction and, if incorrect, can have severe implications. A recent "story" from the TNA US office tells of a young person diagnosed as having trigeminal neuralgia in an emergency room. The patient was put on carbamazepine, but a few days later his dentist found a large dental abscess which, when treated, resulted in pain relief. The British Pain Society has suggested that the first consultation in the secondary care sector should be at least 45 minutes.

Platt et al (2001) summarize good history taking in this sentence: "The two most useful physician qualities may be curiosity and patience – curiosity to ask questions such as "tell me about yourself," and patience to wait for the answer."

Why are patients asked to complete questionnaires?

Questionnaires complement the work of a physician and help with the history taking, since they provide the physician with information that there is insufficient time to collect during the consultation, and which is organized in a standard format. They can be crucial in the making of a diagnosis, providing data on factors that affect the pain and providing more objective evidence of the quality of life of a patient with pain.

Pain is such a personal, subjective phenomenon that it cannot be tested with any investigation at present, and it is very difficult to map language onto pain. Further details and examples of questionnaires are given in Chapter 4.

Does a physical examination provide further evidence for the diagnosis?

It is important to observe patients during the consultation, since certain behaviors can help to reinforce the history. These include factors such as guarding of the face, covering the face with a scarf when it is windy outside, or just not moving the face if at all possible. With experience, pain can be "seen." As one sufferer stated, *When I ask my husband how he knows that I am in pain, he says he can see it in my eyes."* Some patients with trigeminal neuralgia may experience some swelling or redness of the face during a pain attack. However, a patient who is found to have redness of the eye, tearing and a stuffy nose on one side, together with severe restlessness, will probably be suffering from cluster headaches and not trigeminal neuralgia.

A careful dental examination is important to exclude dental causes of pain, which can and do coexist.

A neurological examination is important, especially of what are called the cranial nerves (see Chapter 3). If the trigeminal neuralgia is due to a tumor or multiple sclerosis, then the functioning of these specific nerves or even other nerves may be altered. For example, sensation of the face or hearing can be altered if there is a tumor near the trigeminal nerve inside the brain. Multiple sclerosis can also show itself in other parts of the body such as the legs, leading to altered gait and to visual problems.

2. WHAT IS THE PAIN OF TRIGEMINAL NEURALGIA LIKE?

Any patient with trigeminal neuralgia can answer this question better than I, so I will use many of the descriptions patients have given me.

Ryle in 1936 proposed that pain can be described under nine main headings. I will use these in describing this pain, but I begin with the latest scientific description as found in the updated classification of headache and facial pain by the International Headache Society - see Table 3 below.

INTERNATIONAL HEADACHE SOCIETY CRITERIA FOR CLASSICAL TRIGEMINAL NEURALGIA 2004

Description:
*Trigeminal neuralgia is a unilateral disorder characterized by brief electric shock-like pains, abrupt in onset and termination, limited to the distribution of one or more divisions of the trigeminal nerve. Pain is commonly evoked by trivial stimuli, including washing, shaving, smoking, talking and/or brushing the teeth (trigger factors), and frequently occurs spontaneously. Small areas in the **nasolabial fold** and/or chin may be particularly susceptible to the precipitation of pain (trigger areas). The pains usually remit for variable periods.*

Continued...

...Continued

Diagnostic criteria include:

A. Paroxysmal attacks of pain lasting from a fraction of a second to 2 minutes, affecting one or more divisions of the trigeminal nerve and fulfilling criteria B and C

B. Pain has at least one of the following characteristics:
   1. intense, sharp, superficial or stabbing
   2. precipitated from trigger areas or by trigger factors

C. Attacks are stereotyped in the individual patient

D. There is no clinically evident neurological deficit

E. Not attributed to another disorder

Comments:

Classical trigeminal neuralgia usually starts in the second or third divisions, affecting the cheek or the chin. In <5 % of patients, the first division is affected. The pain never crosses to the opposite side, but it may rarely occur bilaterally, in which case a central cause such as multiple sclerosis must be considered. Between paroxysms, the patient is usually asymptomatic, but a dull background pain may persist in some long-standing cases. Following a painful paroxysm, there is usually a refractory period during which pain cannot be triggered. In some cases, a paroxysm may be triggered from somatosensory stimuli outside the trigeminal area, such as a limb, or by other sensory stimulation such as bright lights, loud noises or tastes.

The pain often evokes spasm of the muscle of the face on the affected side (*tic douloureux*).

Although most experts will agree with the above description, the diagnostic criteria have never been validated by well-conducted investigations. What needs to be done is to collect histories from a wide range of patients with facial pain and then see how consistent everyone is in making the same diagnosis. Do these criteria really separate out those with trigeminal neuralgia from those with other causes of pain? There remains considerable controversy about the naming of the potentially different forms, e.g. atypical, classical, secondary, symptomatic. This will be discussed later.

What does it feel like?

There is overall agreement that the pain of trigeminal neuralgia has a very sharp shooting quality associated with it. The following are descriptions given by patients:

* *Ice pick, shocks, live 300-volt current, electric shock-like pains*
* *I actually heard it sizzle on my cheek like if you put your finger in a light bulb*
* *Firings*
* *Lightning jab that would repeat over and over as it got stronger*
* *Hot poker in my cheek*

- *It would feel as if my face was being sliced open from ear to mouth, then as if boiling acid was being poured into the wound*
- *Constant hot knife jabbing volts or stabs in my right cheek area*
- *Sharp electric-like quality*
- *Sometimes a dull ache followed the spikes for 20 minutes or so*
- *Shooting jolts of electricity directly into the raw nerves*
- *While brushing my teeth one morning I got a bolt of lightning exploded in my face. I screamed... the pain was profoundly piercing and pulsating and didn't stop for what seemed like days, when, in fact, it was probably mere seconds. I clutched my mouth, wanting to soften the coming blows. The pain was sharp stabbing, electrical shock-like pains that would last for only seconds; however, there would be a dull sensation after the pain subsided*
- *It is like you have a live wire, and you take the sheeting off the wire and sparks are flying off that. And it is like somebody putting that wire on you; it is excruciating and the most terrible pain you have ever had. It is like having a live wire coming down, down, down and staying there*

Another patient provided a long and poignant account of his pain experience:

"*Imagine for a few moments that every hour of your waking life, you are followed around by a seven-foot-tall demon. The demon tows with him a portable brazier on wheels. It is full of glowing, hot coals. There are several sharp implements heating in the coals: needles, awls, scalpels, and even a fireplace poker. At random moments, the demon reaches into its brazier, withdraws a white-hot implement, and rams it through your cheek, up into your eye, or down into the base of your skull. You are thrown to the ground or against a wall by the pain, quivering in fear, unable even to whimper in protest. Even as the spasm eases, you know that the relief is only because your nerves have been overcome by the pain. It will come back tomorrow if it does not come again today. You know that the demon is never going to go away. It does not care if you are a nice human being. It does not care if you pray hourly. Its only mission in your life is your pain. And it is DEDICATED!*"

Some patients will use descriptions that relate to their professions. These two are from Texan cattle keepers:

"*I use the idea of a cattle prod, I think a lot of us use that one. I say it is like prodding cattle; the pain hits you in your face suddenly just as the prod hits the cattle.*"

"*You touch it and it feels like that electric cattle prod.*"

This one is from a meteorologist:

"I used to say it is like having a cloud above you and being hit in the head by a thunderbolt."

How severe is it?

This patient describes the severity of his pain very well:

"Most people rate their pain level from 0-10. With 10 being the most intense pain that a man could feel or endure, 90% of my pain in the first three years was 3 to 6 level. I experienced level 8-10 pain only 3 to 4 times and then only of short duration. But the level 10 pain doubled me over the ground and I did not have control of my faculties... tears rolled down my cheeks... I could not have chewed or swallowed anything. Imagine toothache, only 10 times worse."

The pain of trigeminal neuralgia can be suicidal and is recognized to be one of the most severe pains that a person can have. In the stories I have been sent, there are two patients who know of a sufferer who committed suicide, and I also know that one of my senior colleagues had a patient who committed suicide some 25 years ago. Many patients express suicidal ideas as these quotes show:

- *"The intensity is unlike anything I could ever imagine; the pain is so strong it steals your mind, it takes over all your thoughts. I prayed for death."*
- *"Wanted to take my own life, but I looked at my husband who was desperately trying to help me fight this, yet feeling so useless and I had to hold on."*
- *"Her quality of life is zero; she is somebody who could be suicidal right now and you can tell by looking at the expression on her face."*
- *"I became very depressed and would spend hours alone in my room in the dark and quiet."*

Few patients share this emotion with their physician and yet this would help physicians understand and empathize better with their trigeminal neuralgia sufferers.

It is well recognized that the severity of pain varies and sometimes this is because of medication. Why this variation occurs remains a mystery.

How does it start?

Some patients will remember their first episode of pain exactly, and often they are dramatic.

Michael Pasternak, president of the Trigeminal Neuralgia Association in the US, remembers it very clearly. The pain hit him so hard that it put him on his knees while he was at a business meeting. He thought it was a terrible ear ache that spread from his ear, to his mouth to his throat. It felt like a lightning bolt, as he gasped for air.

Another patient recalls, *"I had no warnings, I was at a New Year's Eve party and it came like that, and I literally thought I was having a stroke, and I then it went and I forgot about it, and then it came back a few days later, worse and worse and worse."*

Yet another describes *"Eating a sandwich at lunch time and I started getting shock waves but I don't know why."*

This patient's pain also started in relation to eating: *"Then one beautiful Saturday evening, Sept. 8, I had just arrived home after raiding my sister's tomato patch. I popped the first of those beautiful tart tomatoes into my mouth, and I might as well have sunk my teeth into bubbling electric acid. I did not know what was happening, except that an ongoing electric current was somehow switched on inside my mouth, left side of my gum area only, upper and lower. Between the electric currents, I thought dental floss would ameliorate things. Wrong!!! That angered the already angry, waking demons, and, once again, I found myself almost catatonic with fright. I didn't know how to breathe or sleep without bringing pain on. Forget eating or brushing my teeth (I live by myself, so I was mercifully spared the need to explain what was happening to me.) Speaking, at this point, would have been a cruel torment, electric sparks flying with each connection the tongue makes with any part of the mouth."*

Some neurosurgeons have stated that a memorable onset predicts a good outcome from surgery, but there is no evidence for this statement. However, many of the stories that patients have contributed describe a slower onset, e.g.: *"I was relaxing on my dad's rocker eating a bowl of popcorn ...it started as an ache in the upper left teeth so I thought I had something stuck between the gum and tooth. I flossed and there was nothing there. The ache persisted through the weekend and began worsening. There was nothing jolting about it until later."*

And here is a description from a doctor: *"I had been having some bothersome pain to my right molars that felt like a twinge of pain at certain times, especially when I ate or brushed my teeth. Over a period of months, this pain would come and go. It eventually became a sharp jolting stab of pain that would make me grunt out loud and cringe. It felt like an electrical shock emitted to my right upper and lower molars, as well as my right lateral tongue... I knew that often jaw movement, tem-*

perature and pressure change would set it off. Within days, I became unable to eat or talk without significant strain or pain."

Many patients link the onset of pain with an event such as dental treatment, head trauma, infections (especially herpes), or diving.

When does it occur?

Trigeminal neuralgia is paroxysmal and there are periods of complete freedom from pain. The pain comes suddenly and typically lasts for seconds. Many of these can come so close together that it becomes difficult to distinguish them as single bursts. There then comes a period when the nerve becomes refractory to any further stimulus as this patient describes: *"I had to keep chewing as hard and as fast as I could to relieve it."*

The following are very accurate descriptions of the timing of the pain:

- *"Within 30 minutes I had three jolts of pain each lasting 30-45 seconds."*
- *"I was having more than 100 attacks a day. Most of them lasted 20 seconds to 2 minutes each; other times the pain would disappear just as suddenly as it came."*
- *"I was having 20-40 attacks per day. The pain would last only for seconds. The pain would appear about 1 in every 10 days."*
- *"I couldn't even read my kids a bedtime story without having to stop several times in the middle for 30-60 seconds of pain breaks."*

Patients, especially in the early phases of the disease, will then go through a period of absolutely no pain as this patient writes: *"The tic episodes would sometimes completely disappear for as long as six months, then reappear out of nowhere. This pattern went on for four years."*

It remains difficult to determine the frequency and length of pain remission and relapses. It is just this unpredictability that induces such fear in patients. Here are some of their reflections:

- *"There used to be that fear when my turn came to present something - it's going to happen."*
- *"I don't always know if the next day or days I will be feeling well enough to do things."*
- *"We never took trips because if he thought he might have pain, he always wanted to be at home."*
- *"It's terrible when it happens at a very inconvenient time, when you're at work and talking to people, and suddenly you've got this dreadful pain. I've had people look at me and say, are you okay, sit down. They think I'm having a stroke or am drunk."*

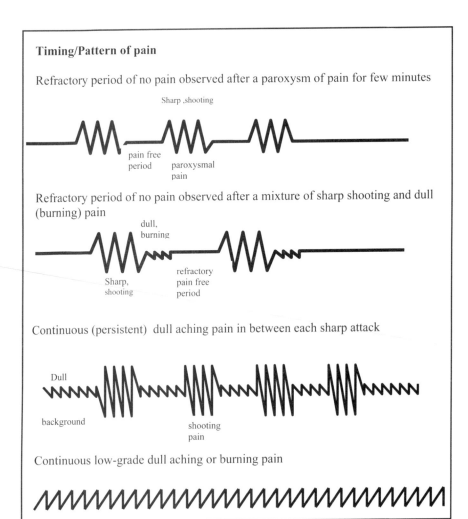

Timing/Pattern of pain

Refractory period of no pain observed after a paroxysm of pain for few minutes

Sharp ,shooting

pain free
period   paroxysmal
             pain

Refractory period of no pain observed after a mixture of sharp shooting and dull (burning) pain

dull,
burning

Sharp,   refractory
shooting   pain free
              period

Continuous (persistent) dull aching pain in between each sharp attack

Dull

background   shooting
                        pain

Continuous low-grade dull aching or burning pain

Timing of pain episodes. These diagrams show a variety of patterns that pain can have, varying from very short stabs of pain with no pain in between as in the top diagram, to a steady pain state with little variation in severity. The top two represent classical trigeminal neuralgia and the third one the atypical form. The last diagram is not trigeminal neuralgia, but some other form of facial pain (drawn by T.P. Jorns).

It has been estimated that 65 % of patients would have the second episode of pain within five years. One or more remissions lasting for six months or longer occur in 50 % of patients. Remissions lasting for over 12 months occur in 25 % of patients. For some patients the remission periods can be very short, and for others they can be long, e.g.:

- *"For about 15 years my pain has come and gone. It would be with me for three months and then be gone for three months."*
- *"My remission is very rapid and it only takes two days to go from excruciating pain to no pain."*
- *"It started as sharp pains that only last a few seconds, and gradually the pain became longer. Sometimes I would have pain striking every few seconds for hours at a time."*

The timing of the pain can change with time, and there is no way in which this can be predicted. Many patients report less or no pain at night during sleep. It remains unclear what the reason for this may be, since one would expect it be present at all times. It could be that the pain severity is not so great as to wake the patient, especially if they have taken medication that makes them sleep. It would be of great interest to hear from spouses as to whether they do observe pain behaviors that fail to wake the pain, but are nevertheless present.

Where is the pain, does it start in a specific spot, does it spread?

The right side of the face is more likely to be affected, and there does not seem to be a link with handedness, age or gender. Many patients will describe particular areas of their face that when touched trigger pain – often called trigger areas. These trigger areas often are at points where the trigeminal nerve emerges from the skull and spreads out on the skin as shown in the diagram below.

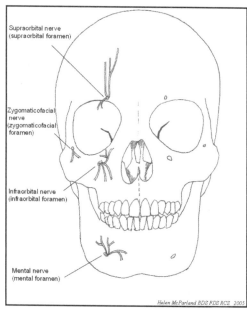

This diagram of the skull shows the major exit points of the trigeminal nerve where the trigeminal nerve comes out onto the surface of the skin. When touched in these points, pain can often be elicited.

Helen McParland BDS FDS RCS 2005

Up to about 4 % of patients may develop bilateral pain (on both sides of the face). It is unlikely that pain will be present on both sides at the same time. The interval between pain starting on the other side of the face is variable and it can be anything from three years to 24 years. Sometimes the pain on the initial side may disappear and only the other side remains active.

Patients with bilateral symptoms did not vary in respect to gender or duration of symptoms, from unilateral cases, but may be younger than most patients with TN. However, there is a higher instance of a family history of **hypertension** and more neurological changes in patients with bilateral pain. There is no data from long-term studies to show how, and if, the number of divisions involved changes with time. Pain of the first division, i.e. around the eye and forehead in isolation, is relatively rare, whereas it is common in patients with cluster headaches.

Does anything make the pain worse or start the pain up?

One of the diagnostic criteria for trigeminal neuralgia is that it is pro-voked by light touch. The stimuli can be mechanical or thermal, although even noise, lights and sweets have been reported as triggering it. Again, I will leave the sufferers to describe it to you:

- *"Everyday functions of talking, yawning, brushing one's teeth, eating, blowing one's nose are punished by deep, mean long stabs of electric current."*
- *"Forget eating or brushing my teeth, speaking at this point would have been cruel torment, electric sparks flying with each connection the tongue makes with any part of the mouth."*
- *"The light breeze from my golden retriever's tail can delight all the world, yet this breeze is a trigger that sets my face on fire."*
- *"Walking into the kitchen and feeling the air blowing out from under the refrigerator can set it off."*
- *"The wind caused me pain, even just touching my mustache gave me pain."*
- *"Temperature changes, drafts, a drop in barometric pressures, stress, fatigue and chewing are other things that trigger my pain."*
- *"No one could hug me. A caress on the cheek or a gust of wind would trigger a terrible pain. Eating and talking would become steadily difficult. I was essentially a prisoner in my own home."*
- *"I had many trigger points that set my trigeminal neuralgia off, licking my lips, touching my face along my jaw around my ear or teeth, brushing my teeth was something I began to fear, forget*

flossing. At times I could not even swallow my own spit. The pain would always be there when I woke up because waking up was a trigger for me."

- *"Touching my lip was no longer the only trigger for the pain; a light wind would do it, so would saying hello when answering the phone. Brushing my teeth was guaranteed agony every morning and evening."*
- *"After a while the pain didn't even seem to be triggered; it just came on by itself as if it had a mind of its own."*

Does anything make the pain better?

There are very few things that help, but trying not to move appears to provide some relief, as this patient points out, *"It helped not to move my face at all, that's why I could sleep at night with it."* Medication provides the only consistent relief.

What other feelings does this pain induce?

Every patient with trigeminal neuralgia will tell you that at times the pain can be suicidal, and this needs to be recorded. A recent study has shown that the following two simple questions are effective in detecting depression: "During the past month have you often been bothered by feeling down, depressed or hopeless?" "During the past month have you often been bothered by having little interest or pleasure in doing things?"

These can be further complemented by questionnaires such as the Beck Depression Inventory or the Hospital Anxiety and Depression Scale. It is important to elicit this symptom, since it is more difficult to manage pain in the presence of depression and it will be present in over one third of patients.

Sufferers may also feel angry, helpless and guilty, and they need to be encouraged to tell the physician about these types of emotions, since the information will lead to better understanding by the physician. Some of the emotions expressed in the next section have never been reported in the medical literature on trigeminal neuralgia.

What are the difficulties of daily living with trigeminal neuralgia?

I asked 30 patients attending the 5th TNA conference in the US to tell me what were their greatest problems of living with trigeminal neuralgia and these were the answers: unpredictability, living minute by minute, uncertainty, anticipation, fear of recurrence, feeling incapacitated, broken, loss or poor quality of life, decreased joy of living, change of lifestyle, lost time, debilitation, non functioning, brushing teeth, medication side effects, isolation, no one understands, frustration of others not understanding, effect on family, compassion.

As one sufferer expressed it, *"It's a war that no one but those of us fighting it can understand."*

The disorder can have a multitude of effects, some of which are discussed below.

Physical effects

Due to the inability to eat, many patients will lose weight. One patient reported he lost 22 pounds in less than a month, while another lost 40 pounds in two months. One patient said she would not waste time eating things like apples, lettuce and other foods that do not contain much calories. Others develop special techniques to eat without stimulating the pain.

Carrying out personal hygiene becomes difficult, as indicated by these patients' comments:

- *"I can't even wash my face sometimes."*
- *"When you're showering, I have a power shower but I have to turn that to one side because there is no way I can have that power. Also, when you're drying your hair, I can only dab with the towel, because of the pain."*
- *"Do you just have to grow a beard?*

Being intimate with a partner is a problem that is not often mentioned and yet is a major disability "I was forced to isolate myself more and more - no one could hug me - a caress on the cheek or a gust of wind could trigger a terrible pain."

Social life is greatly impaired, as indicated by this patient complaint: *"I think it's the feeling that you can't socialize and live what I would call a normal life, not an exceptional life, just a normal life; you just cannot do it."*

Financial effects

Patients who have jobs that involve speaking or using their face find it very difficult to continue working. Here are some of their statements:

- *"This episode started me thinking that I would lose my ability to work, and this is terrifying."*
- *"I am not in a position to return to work."*
- *"I retired about six months before the TN struck. This was a*

blessing because I would not have been able to work at my former job while experiencing TN pain."

- *"It has also impacted my work."*
- *"I have decided not to pursue any more teaching responsibilities, although this is what I had hoped to do after I retire from my current position."*
- *"When you're at work and talking to people, and suddenly you've got this dreadful pain ..... some people get embarrassed."*
- *"I cannot carry as much responsibility as I used to because of how exhausting the pain is."*

Not only will sufferers lose their jobs; they will also use up their finances trying to get the best treatment, and this is a greater problem in countries that do not have free health care. This sufferer describes how she became homeless. *"For more than two months I lived out of one suitcase, a paper bag, which held my laundry, and a big box holding all my medical records. The $237.00 a month I received from welfare wasn't enough to live on, anywhere. I existed from day to day, never knowing where I would be sleeping that night. I used my $237.00 to pay for my medical insurance.*

Not all treatments are covered by insurance. For example, acupuncture therapy may not be covered, but some insurance does pay for chiropractic care.

Psychological effects

"Isolation, depression, fear of increasing pain are just some of the emotions I try to work through."

This sufferer sums up the emotions most frequently expressed by sufferers, both in consultations and in their writings.

Here are some quotes from sufferers about their fears related to the unpredictability of the pain and their ability to cope with it:

- *"The fear never leaves. I know it could come back at any time."*
- *"The pain causes great fear of being out of control, and of course fear of the terrible pain."*
- *"I knew that it would come again soon, and that scared me even more."*
- *"I felt so alone and that there was nobody there to help me."*
- *"I feel very isolated."*

Depression is very common and one patient very graphically compares her emotions to *"a Roller Coaster Ride. They have so many ups and downs with places that go upside down, sideways and tunnels that are so dark that you can't find the light at the end of the tunnel for days at a time. I have a hard time laughing and try everything I can, not to cry and to hide my pain. It is so hard to show my pain. I don't want people to feel bad around me or feel sorry for me. I feel my pain makes them distant … I try to appear cheerful when I am really sad inside… when my depression is up high I can't eat, sleep or think of anything positive."*

One sufferer's statement indicated he was very close to suicide: *"I spent my waking hours trying to overdose, screaming and crying for relief. Emotions? Suicidal at worst, depressed at best."*

Another patient said, *"It is the most hopeless feeling in the world to be in such pain and not be able to do a thing about it."*

As one sufferer expressed it, *"TN sucks enjoyment out of everything in life."*

Another voiced profound anger: *"Even after all these years I still sometimes get angry for having this problem! Sufferers lose their confidence and control of life. It is hell. It is the worst God-awful thing that has ever happened in my life. This pain had taken over my life."*

However, many patients also realize the importance of remaining positive, as expressed in these comments:

- *"I mean, it is very important to have hope that it is not going to be like this for the rest of my life."*
- *"I wanted to keep that positive approach all the time, but I could see how it could drag you down, and you go down and down and down."*
- *"I try so hard to laugh and joke, so I do not cry. I am sick of crying, it is time to laugh and try to find some enjoyment in my life again."*

Effect on family

Although pain is a very personal experience, it affects all those who come in contact with the sufferer. It will affect not just the adults, but also the children in the family as illustrated in these two stories;

1. *"We don't get to do as much as a family. Mom's pain holds us back. That is so hard for me to hear, but it is very true. I do my best to never let it stop us, but at times it gets out of control. My son says it make him sad. Just that one word breaks my heart. Speaking with my oldest daughter, I was surprised to hear she appreciates me more because of TN. That I can live with this painful disorder and still balance all the things needed to run our home. She says it is hard for her to see me in the pain."*

2. *"My children have lived with TN all of their lives. They missed out on many things, like having their mother watch them play baseball, and vacations because I might have an episode as they called them. I never wanted to be too far away from home."*

One patient admits to wishing the pain on her partner so that he would understand her pain better, and in the US I met a couple of trigeminal neuralgia sufferers who are getting married after they met during a support group meeting.

One sufferer recounts her son's reaction to her diagnosis of having trigeminal neuralgia and multiple sclerosis (MS), "Mom, I think they have it backwards-it should be SM for Super Mom." The initial reaction of many relatives is to try to help. One patient said his family sought information on the Internet "to better understand what was happening to me." He also said he had lots of prayers from family and friends.

However, one sufferer observed, *"After a while they get unsympathetic because they get angry because you've still got it."*

There is also the frustration of having to live with a person in pain,as expressed by this sufferer; *"My husband has lived with this since the day we met. He gets very frustrated with me sometimes. He does not understand why it just does not go away with medications and MVD. After 20 years of marriage I can understand his frustrations."*

Some of the frustration is related to lack of understanding and the patient's difficulty in getting across the information. One sufferer lamented, *"How can you make someone understand this? I felt like I was lying about the pain, and I was the one with it!"*

Well-meaning help can also cause problems; *"I have had some relationship-altering arguments with family members over the effects from the pain — about their idea of how I should be treated vs. how I want to be treated."*

A woman patient made this poignant comment, *"My husband reached over to try and calm me and the touch made it even worse and I had to push him away... don't touch me, don't touch me, and he feels rejected."*

Dealing with the community

Although the family may come to understand the sufferer, there is also the wider community that needs to be dealt with as summarized by this sufferer; *"Many friends try to understand and offer support, but many don't understand the pain I feel. They think I have a bad headache or that I should be over this pain by now. Others feel I should seek dif-*

ferent help or other doctors. They feel there should be something to relieve this terrible pain and ask me why I'm not trying to find it, if it is so bad."

There is also the feeling that because there are no visible signs, the pain cannot be severe as expressed by this sufferer.

One patient described the typical dilemma: *"People tell me that I look good and I must be feeling pretty good. They tell me many people are in worse pain than I am or about someone who has a bad headache too."*

The following comments from patients indicate a strong cry for compassionate understanding:

- *"The most frustrating is that you aren't understood or feel as if no one understands how truly painful it is. You wish they could feel the pain for a day so they could understand just a little."*
- *"Many people do not realize that a patient in pain cannot carry out basic activities. They don't know how much energy this pain takes out of you."*
- *"Friends haven't always understood when I don't feel up to talking or doing things because I'm in a lot of pain and can't do any more."*
- *"Many people have never heard of this chronic pain and up to the time I was diagnosed with it, I never knew either, and would probably have been one of those people not understanding."*
- *"I pray that others would become more aware and try to understand. I try to understand that they don't know and are trying to care in their own way too."*

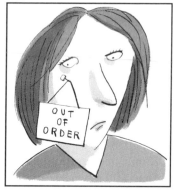

Out of order. Some outward sign of pain could make it easier for a sufferer to communicate about the pain.

This poem probably strikes a cord with many sufferers

Where are all my friends?
Where did they go?
What I've got isn't catching, you know.
I need them now, when I'm feeling so low.

Where are all my friends?
Where did they go?
I'm just a phone call away,
Just to say, I'm thinking of you today.

Where are all my friends?
Where did they go?
I've made new ones, you know
and all my TN friends will never go!

Supporters will often feel helpless and will express it like this: "You just can't do anything for them." Many sufferers are very appreciative of the support they get, and it is important that they let their supporters know this.

One grateful patient shared the following: *"I was blessed. During this time the only constant was my friends. I had such wonderful friends. They took turns letting me stay in their homes, cancelled frequent flyer miles so I could make the trips to Pittsburgh, fed me and made sure I had a roof over my head and food. Although most of them feel extremely helpless at times, they have always been there as well and without my family and friends I would not have made it this far."*

Keeping a sense of one's identity is not easy, as this sufferer points out: *"I'd rather they just see me as a person, not as a patient. Makes my close friends very few in number - only those I can trust to see ME first, not my pain. I am a <u>person</u> first after all, a person with pain, not a pain patient with an incidental personality."*

A sense of humor is difficult to maintain, but it can lighten the burden, as described by this sufferer: *"My friends are very supportive, and laugh with me about the things I wear over half of my face when the pain is bad and the weather is cold."*

3. How do patients feel when they obtain their diagnosis?

Obtaining a clear diagnosis for the pain is of crucial importance and is one of the prime reasons why patients seek health care. How this information is given varies widely as sufferers recount:
- *"After the shock of the news, I sat on a bench and cried in disbelief...pull yourself together."*
- *"People get these things....go home and break the news to the family."*
- *"My doctor said, 'I think you've got trigeminal neuralgia and I'm so sorry.'"*
- *"My doctor told me you're not going to die from it, but there'll be times when you'll wish you were dead. Well, that's true."*
- *"Relieved but scared."*

Some doctors are able to make the diagnosis, but know little about trigeminal neuralgia. So they are unable to provide more information. This often happens and makes patients angry, as illustrated in these excerpts from a patient's report:

"I didn't think that my doctor, who I have known for a long time, explained the situation to me. He said, 'I believe you have trigeminal neuralgia,' and I said, I have what? Trigeminal neuralgia. What the heck is that? I'd never heard of it, and he said, 'Don't worry about it, I'll try and take care of it for you.' I said okay, what are we going to do? 'Here, I'll give you a prescription for Tegretol and some other stuff,' and I thought that was going to be it. I'd take the pill and then I'd be fine, but it's not like that at all. As you progress through your disease, you begin to feel alone; you begin to feel angry because somebody did not explain to you what was going to happen to you down the hill."

It remains difficult for the doctor giving the diagnosis to know how much the patient needs to be told at the first visit. On the one hand the doctor may feel it inappropriate to tell the patient about all the surgical options at the first visit, yet for some patients this lack of information can also result in patients feeling fearful. One patient commented, *"I felt fear because none of the doctors were telling me anything and that made me frightened. I needed more information."*

The following story illustrates some of these emotions.
- *"This hit me like a sledge hammer. Not the MS diagnosis, not even the TN diagnosis. But the PROGNOSIS for TN — it was alarming! (There was no good news anywhere in the descriptions of it, none at all. TN just got worse.")*

Reading this in my bed at night, I was filled with dread. No hope was to be found anywhere between the lines, no quantitative translations to relapse times and dates. And what did 'shorter' mean? How does 'more intense' translate? How was 'pain' measured? The worst thing had to do with the rarefied nature of TN: who else would have it? With whom could I share the horror with, or my fears? Who else could I GET information from who knew it from the inside out? Would other sufferers be as hungry as I for information about it, or as desperate to educate themselves about it as I was beginning to feel? Having no answers at that early stage of discovery, but knowing everyone's threshold for pain varies, I comforted myself with the only tool at my disposal: the wise old adage that says: take each day, each month, each year, at a time."

The following are some answers to the question posed during a focus group meeting, "Do you perceive yourself differently now that you have TN?"

- *"Trigeminal neuralgia does changes your identity. Suddenly you see how precious life can be and it makes you reflect on what you are doing."*
- *"It makes you live more for the day and get more out of life as a result."*
- *"I find it difficult to cope with an angry client while going through an attack of pain."*
- *"I am always afraid I will be in the middle of something important when I get an attack."*

4. WHY DOES THE PAIN DIFFER OR BE SIMILAR FOR DIFFERENT PATIENTS?

There are both physiological and psychological factors that influence our perception and experience of pain and result in differences and similarities between patients.

As Patrick Wall writes in his book, **Pain, the Science Of Suffering**, "The public display of pain has the purpose of informing others of the patient's needs, while the private suffering assesses the meaning and consequences of the patient's own miserable state. All pain includes an affective quality that depends on the circumstances of the injury and on the character of the victim."

This concept of pain being a function of both the mind and body has been endorsed by the International Association for the Study of Pain, which defines pain as "an unpleasant sensory and emotional experience associated with actual or potential tissue damage or described in terms of such damage." This definition also stresses that pain is always subjective. The ancient Greeks thought of pain as an emotion, as can be seen in the writings of Hippocrates.

What other factors affect the pain?

Human nature dictates that every person responds individually to pain, but our internal variations are also affected by the attitudes of others around us who impose their expectations of our response. Some of these factors can be controlled by the sufferer and so provide another way of trying to reduce the effect of the pain. The following are some of the factors that may influence our reporting of pain:

1. **Cultural factors** – a popular myth is that people from different cultures experience pain differently. Experiments have not validated this and it appears to be linked more with societal factors, i.e. what is expected from a person by the society in which they live, than with ethnicity. It also relates to perceptions of who may or may not have pain, e.g. "Just because people can't see it, it doesn't mean that you don't truly have something wrong with you."

2. **Context in which the pain occurs** will alter the way we respond to it. If it occurs in the context of war or sport, i.e. while trying to achieve some goal, then pain may not be reported at the time, whereas if it occurs in the medical or dental setting, it is more likely to be reported as such.

3. **Past experiences of pain** are important in that they give us positive or negative memories of what pain was like previously and how successfully it was treated.

4. **Mood State** will have a powerful effect on the way pain is experienced and it is these emotions that need to be assessed at the time of a consultation. Fear, anger, depression, helplessness, anxiety, and negative experiences, such as expressed by the following statements, can hinder recovery. *"I am angry that the doctor tried to say it was in my head, and it took several doctor visits before someone actually put a name to it."* In contrast, this suf-

ferer's response is very positive; "*I think that you should collect pictures of face wear to help us all laugh. Laughter gives back a feeling of control.*"

5. **Gender** – a vast amount of research is being done on whether men or women have higher thresholds for pain. There do appear to be differences, but these could also be related to cultural norms, e.g. men are considered to be tougher and yet women deal with pain more frequently and so may be better at expressing it or at seeking care.

6. **Beliefs about pain** – the meaning of the pain, the ways in which it is interpreted, the expectations about its course and treatment, and beliefs about personal control over it are powerful factors that have been shown to influence pain behavior. This is shown by these statements; "*One good thing is it is not cancer, it won't kill you. You will have days you will feel crummy, but take it from one who knows... keep fighting and don't just give up. God has given me a chance to change my way of life.*" "*Like everyone, we are all subject to disease, pain and suffering.*"

7. **Relationship with the treating clinician** is of crucial importance. It has been shown that the approach of the doctor treating a patient has a powerful effect, and it has been given the name of "**iatroplacebogenesis.**" The following attitude is likely to result in poor responses: "*There is the anger at doctors who don't do their jobs. Yes, they are human, but I need them to take care of me and look into possible future treatments. Why can't they do their best research for me? If I'm a challenging case, why can't they accept the challenge with enthusiasm instead of brushing me off?*" In contrast, this statement is likely to yield a positive effect: "*It is such a HUGE relief to find one who sticks with me and helps by looking into things for me.*"

Psychological Predictors of Chronic Pain

It is now recognized that there are a variety of psychological factors that predispose to continuation of chronic pain and which can explain the different experiences of pain reported by patients. These include the following:

1. Past history of depression or anxiety

2. Fear avoidance behaviors, i.e. resisting attempts to move or use the affected area for fear of damaging it or of exacerbating the pain
3. Current depression, which is very frequently linked with pain
4. Historical or current alcohol and/or substance abuse
5. Poor pain coping skills, including factors such as low beliefs in regard to self-management, tendency to catastrophize about pain, i.e. think of the negative aspects of the pain
6. Life stresses and events as expressed by this sufferer: *"When I get stressed the pain is more frequent, stronger and lasts longer."*
7. Heightened concerned about bodily functions, disease conviction and perception of poor health

5. WHAT DO WE MEAN BY TERMS SUCH AS CLASSICAL, TYPICAL, ATYPICAL, SYMPTOMATIC, IDIOPATHIC, SECONDARY TRIGEMINAL NEURALGIA?

Typical or classical trigeminal neuralgia is the form that conforms to all the descriptions we have used above and one that a group of experts would have no problem with coming to a consensus view about. In his recent classification paper, Burchiel has called this Type 1.

Some sufferers will describe the same classical features, but also describe constant, burning, gnawing pain in the same distribution, e.g. *"throbbing, burning pain. Often feels like something is crawling along my chin."* This is referred to by some as *atypical or non-classical trigeminal neuralgia* whereas Burchiel calls it Type 2 if the constant pain is present for more than 50% of the time.

However, in other patients it is not just the character and timing of the pain that is different; there may be features such as lack of pain-free periods, no trigger points or different location as indicated in this description: *"My right-sided facial pain can best be described as a constant burning sensation akin to having a hot iron put to the skin and then lifted off. It involves all three branches of the trigeminal nerve because I frequently have a deep boring pain, like a screwdriver being stabbed through my right pupil."*

Sufferers may also experience both these types of pain at different times, and Type 1 may change into Type 2. Burchiel has proposed that this change signals progression of the disease and could potentially be related to the level of compression. Research is needed to determine whether this is the case or whether, in fact, these are two different types of trigeminal neuralgia caused by different factors.

It seems logical to suggest that the trigeminal nerve can undergo a wide variety of injuries that can range from complete severance of the nerve to only partial severance. The nerve may only undergo minor damage, which can repair itself, or more severe damage as can occur after an accident that results in it become **atrophic**, i.e. very thin and beyond all repair. Repair may also not be effective and result in the nerve transmitting different signals. Each of these different types of injuries can result in a different pattern of pain.

Many other neuropathic pains such as post-herpetic neuralgia and diabetic neuropathy present with a continuous burning, throbbing type pain that is fairly continuous and also results in local hypersensitivity to light touch. It is common to find that after destructive surgery to the trigeminal nerve, such as radiofrequencycoagulation or a partial sensory rhizotomy, patients will describe a burning, aching type of pain associated with sensory loss. These factors will be discussed in greater detail in Chapter 3.

From an etiological (causation) viewpoint, two more descriptive words are used. *Primary* or *idiopathic* trigeminal neuralgia, the commonest form, is that in which radiological investigations and surgical exploration have excluded multiple sclerosis or other structural abnormalities, and it is thought to be due in the majority of cases to arterial cross-compression of the trigeminal nerve at its exit from the brainstem (see Chapter 3 for details). The terms *secondary* or *symptomatic* trigeminal neuralgia are used for those cases associated with multiple sclerosis and other causes such as tumors and vascular abnormalities, which can be identified on cranial imaging (MRA or MRI scans).

There is no doubt that not everyone fits all criteria as described in the textbooks for the reasons discussed earlier. Now read through the case study on the following page and see if you can decide on the diagnosis.

MRS. G. CASE STUDY

Mrs. S.G. is a 58-year-old housewife who presented with severe facial pain that stopped her eating and talking. This present pain episode had begun three months ago and was gradually becoming more severe.

- *Character*
  - *shooting, sharp, unbearable*
- *Severity*
  - *Moderate to severe*
- *Site, radiation*
  - *Right lower jaw – pain felt both inside the mouth and outside*
- *Duration, periodicity*
  - *individual stabs of pain last for seconds, but these often merge and last several minutes. There are pain-free periods*
- *Provoking factors*
  - *Light touch, eating, talking*
- *Relieving factors*
  - *None; no pain at night during less severe episodes*
- *Associated factors*
  - *Trigger areas*

She gave a history of having had a similar pain one and a half years ago, which had lasted for eight weeks but was not as severe as this episode.

The completed McGill Pain Questionnaire and Brief Pain Inventory

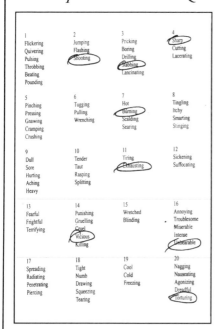

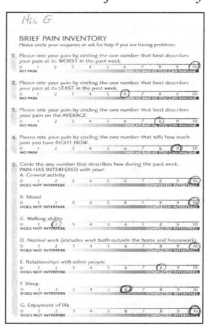

Continued...

> *...Continued*
>
> **Past medical history showed the following:**
> - Surgery for femoral hernia many years ago
> - Hysterectomy for heavy uterine bleeding
> - Varicose veins stripped
> - Three episodes of deep vein thrombosis, one after a fractured ankle and the other two after flying; last episode occurred 10 years ago
>
> **Current medication:**
> Warfarin for 9 years
> Heavy smoker – over 20 a day for 30 years
>
> ---
>
> What is the diagnosis? Are the diagnostic criteria fulfilled? What effect does it have on the patient?
>
> ---
>
> **Discussion**
> The signs and symptoms fulfill the diagnostic criteria for trigeminal neuralgia. The pain is described as being unilateral in the distribution of the trigeminal nerve, very brief, shooting, sharp and stabbing. It is provoked by light touch. There is a history of complete pain relief. The pain has had a powerful effect on the quality of life.

6. IF IT IS NOT TRIGEMINAL NEURALGIA, WHAT IS IT?

The most common causes of orofacial pain are dental ones. Other causes for facial pain are rare and their descriptions, i.e. diagnostic criteria, can be found in the recently updated classification by the International Headache Society (IHS 2004).

Pain in the head and neck is mediated by several nerves (see Chapter 2); the trigeminal nerve, nervus intermedius, glossopharyngeal and vagus nerves and the upper cervical roots *via* the occipital nerves. When these nerves are stimulated by compression, distortion, exposure to cold or other forms of irritation or by a condition of the central pathways, then a stabbing or constant pain can be felt in the area that these nerves supply. These types of pain are called **neuropathic.**

Since it is rare for trigeminal neuralgia to be bilateral, the causes of unilateral orofacial pain only will be discussed. In some cases, the cause is clear, e.g. infection by herpes zoster or a structural abnormality demonstrated by imaging, but in some cases there may be no cause apparent for neuralgic pain and it is these that we will concentrate on. Table 4 on the following pages summarizes the main characteristics of the different types of pain.

Table 4

DIFFERENTIAL DIAGNOSIS OF OROFACIAL PAINS THAT
NO IMMEDIATELY

Condition	Prevalance	Major location & radiation	Timing
Dental			
Pulpal –exposed dentine due to caries, defective restoration, traumatic	Very common	Well localized to a tooth	Can last for 10-20 minutes after sugary stimulus
Fractured or cracked tooth	Fairly common	Localized to one or two teeth, but may be poorly localized difficult to visualise	Very short lasting, seconds intermittent
Pulpal – chronic pulpitis	Common	Poorly localized intraorally	Intermittent, hours
Periodontal – chronic apical periodontitis	Common	Poorly localised, intraoral	Intermittent, minutes to hours
Bony pain- osteomyelitis	Rare	Most often mandible, widespread	Continuous
Denture pain, pressure on mental nerve	Rare	Localised intraoral	Intermittent, daily
Neurological			
Trigeminal neuropathy	Very rare	Trigeminal area but may radiate beyond	Continuous
Glossopharyngeal neuralgia	Very rare	Intraoral in distribution of glossopharyngeal	Each episode last for seconds to 2 mins.
Postherpetic neuralgia	Rare	Most commonly first division of trigeminal	Continuous pain

PRESENT PREDOMINATELY AS UNILATERAL PAINS WITH IDENTIFIABLE CAUSE.

Character/severity	Provoking factors	Associated factors
Sharp, stabbing, throbbing, dull, moderate to severe	Hot, cold or sweet food provoke it, rarely spontaneous	Immediate relief on removal of stimulus
Sharp moderate	Biting, never spontaneous, may be sensitive to heat	Rebound pain, worse after force removed, opposing natural tooth normally present
Mild, dull, throbbing	Occasionally heat	Often large filling present
Mild, dull, throbbing	Large filling	Sinus may be visible, bad taste
Throbbing, severe	Biting on mobile teeth	Temperature, generally unwell, unable to open wide, swelling, may be some numbness, pus, mobile teeth, bony bits
Aching, may be sharp if over mental nerve	Eating with denture	Often redness, ulceration in area of pressure
Dull with sharp exacerbation	Areas of allodynia, light touch	Sensory loss subjective/ objective/progressive, redness and swelling of face may occur
Sharp, stabbing, burning, severe	Swallowing, chewing, talking	No neurological changes
Tingling, severity varies	Tactile allodynia	More than 6 months after acute herpes zoster

Table 4 *continued*

DIFFERENTIAL DIAGNOSIS OF OROFACIAL PAINS THAT
NO IMMEDIATELY

Condition	Prevalance	Major location & radiation	Timing
Vascular			
Cluster headache Episodic pain-free periods, chronic, no remissions	rare	Orbital, supraorbital, temporal	15 –180 minutes to several hours, from 1 every other day to 8/day
SUNCT Shorter-lasting, unilateral neuralgiform, conjunctival injection and tearing	Very rare	Eye and round it, but may radiate to forehead and temple, upper jaw and palate	Each episode last up to 2 mins. Intermittent, several attacks a day and then may remit
Chronic paroxysmal hemicrania	Very rare	Eye, forehead	Pain lasts 2-45 mins, 5-10 daily
Giant cell (temporal) arteritis	Rare	May be bilateral. mostly over temporal artery	Continuous
Temporomandibular disorders, facial arthromyalgia	Relatively common	May be bilateral, around the ear, radiate to neck, temples	Intermittent, may last for hours, may have severe exacerbations
Idiopathic facial pain	Relatively common	May be bilateral or unilateral, can radiate widely beyond trigeminal area, variable location	Intermittent or continuous, often long history of pain
Atypical odontalgia/ phantom tooth	Rare	Intraoral in a tooth or teeth, gingival, moves to another area	Continuous, few minutes to hours

PRESENT PREDOMINATELY AS UNILATERAL PAINS WITH IDENTIFIABLE CAUSE.

Character/severity	Provoking factors	Associated factors
Hot, searing, punctate, severe	Vasodilators e.g. alcohol	Red eye, lacrimation, nasal congestion, runny nose, sweating, small pupil, drooping and/or swelling of eyelid, restlessness
Burning, electrical, stabbing, severe	Neck movements	Red eye, lacrimation, nasal stuffiness, runny nose
Stabbing, throbbing, boring	Head movements, responds to indomethecin	Symptoms as for SUNCT
Aching, throbbing, boring, sharp	Chewing	Jaw claudication (cramp), neck pain, poor appetite, may lose eyesight
Throbbing, sharp or dull aching	Clenching and grinding, opening wide, psychosocial factors, trauma	May be limitation in opening, tenderness of muscles of mastication, altered occlusion, responds to relaxation
Nagging, throbbing, aching, sharp. Wide range of words used and severity mild to moderate	Life events, stress, weather changes, movements	May be change in sensation, facial edema, headaches, other bodily pains, anxiety
Dull, throbbing, may be sharp, mild to moderate	Life events, emotional, teeth hypersensitive to temperature and pressure	Often history of tooth extraction

Dental causes

Most of the common ones are summarized in Table 4.

In recent years a condition called NICO or neuralgia – inducing cavitational osteonecrosis – has been described in the dental literature. Proponents of the condition claim that infections occur in the jawbones that result in the formation of large cavities, which may not be visible on conventional X-rays and which also damage nerves that may be in the area. They suggest that cleaning out these cavities, and treatment with antibiotics, will bring about resolution of the pain. The evidence for the effectiveness of this treatment is lacking, since no randomized controlled trial has been conducted and there are no long-term cohort studies in which independent observers assessed the results. However, Glueck et al have proposed that some patients have a coagulation disorder, which results in impaired venous circulation and venous hypertension of the mandible/maxilla with subsequent development of osteonecrosis (destruction of bone) and hence chronic facial pain. This has been shown in other bones, e.g. hip and long bones and some pilot treatments with coagulation products to repair this defect have been shown to be beneficial.

Patients who have had teeth removed, especially lower wisdom teeth, or have sustained injuries to their face may suffer damage to the nerve supplying that area. As well as experiencing numbness, some will also have pain often described as burning in quality, generally referred to as neuropathic pain.

Other groups postulate that some forms of orofacial pain are of vascular origin and therefore represent a form of facial migraine.

Sinusitis involving the maxillary (over the cheeks), the frontal (forehead) or ethmoidal sinuses (top of the nose) also cause pain, but this is often bilateral and is an acute pain that does not last over three months. It can be due to dental causes, e.g. teeth or bony fragments pushed into the sinus during an extraction.

Chronic idiopathic facial pain and its variants

The commonest non-dental cause of facial pain is idiopathic facial pain, also called atypical facial pain, or chronic orofacial pain. The International Headache Society has recently called it persistent idiopathic facial pain. The term "idiopathic" implies that we still do not really know the cause of this pain, although it is probable that it could be due to nerve injury or damage. It has a much more varied presentation and the diagnostic features listed in the key facts (See Table 5 below) are not highly characteristic. If the pain is located especially around the ear and the temporomandibular joint (jaw joint), then it tends to be called *temporomandibular disorder*. Another variation of this is *atypical odontalgia*, a continuous pain in the teeth or in a tooth socket after extraction in the absence of any identifiable dental cause.

Table 5: Key Facts

DIAGNOSTIC CRITERIA OF PERSISTENT IDIOPATHIC FACIAL PAIN (FORMER NAME ATYPICAL FACIAL PAIN) AS DEFINED BY THE INTERNATIONAL HEADACHE SOCIETY
A. Pain in the face, present daily and persisting for all or most of the day, fulfilling criteria B and C B. Pain is confined at onset to a limited area on one side of the face, and is deep and poorly localized C. Pain is not associated with sensory loss or other physical signs D. Investigations, including X-ray imaging of face and jaws, do not demonstrate any relevant abnormality

Site and radiation: The pain can be unilateral or bilateral, felt inside the mouth only, on the face only or in both locations. The area of the pain can change and it may become more widespread. Around 30% of sufferers describe the pain as being deep, but about 50 % say it is both deep and superficial. The pain radiates widely over the entire face.
Character: The pain is often described as a pressing, drawing, throbbing, pulsing, nagging, aching type of pain, but many sufferers will also describe sharp, stabbing pains.
Duration and periodicity: Many relate the onset of pain to a dental procedure or an injury to the face. Although the pain is often continuous, there can also be periods of remission either during the day or even for weeks.
Severity: The pain can be mild to severe, but in general is less severe than trigeminal neuralgia.
Provoking and relieving factors: There are no clear factors, but stress is often identified.
Associated factors: The main distinguishing factor between trigeminal neuralgia and this form of pain is that it is not provoked by light touch, i.e. eating, touching the face, and talking. Many sufferers also have pain in other parts of the body, e.g. back pain, neck pain, irritable bowel syn-

drome, as well as ringing in the ears (tinnitus) and itchy skin. Accompanying this pain, anxiety and depression may also be elicited and it is difficult to determine whether the depression is due to the pain or whether it was present initially and so led to pain. Many patients will describe the occurrence of life events and stress around the time the pain began.

Many health care professionals consider this pain to be due to psychological factors. I think this is in part because these patients have been extensively tested for psychological changes because no other investigations have been found to be positive. I think all types of chronic pain result in psychological changes, but they have not always been identified due to lack of investigation. There are, for example, very few studies to show the psychological changes that occur in trigeminal neuralgia sufferers, whereas there are several studies reporting on the psychological features of idiopathic facial pain.

Cluster headaches

This is a clearly defined condition that has been well characterized by the International Headache Society and is summarized in the Table 6 key facts below.

Table 6: Key Facts

DIAGNOSTIC CRITERIA FOR CLUSTER HEADACHE AS DEFINED BY INTERNATIONAL HEADACHE SOCIETY

A. At least 5 attacks fulfilling criteria B – D
B. Severe or very severe unilateral orbital, supra-orbital (above the eye), and or temporal (temple) pain lasting 15-180 minutes if untreated
C. Headache is accompanied by at least 1 of the following;
    a. Ipsilateral (same side) conjunctival injection (red eye) and/or lacrimation (weeping or tearing)
    b. Ipsilateral nasal congestion and/or rhinorrhoea (runny nose)
    c. Ispilateral eyelid edema (swelling)
    d. Isilateral forehead and facial swelling
    e. Ipsilateral miosis (small pupil) or ptosis (drooping eyelid)
    f. A sense of restlessness or agitation
D. Attacks have a frequency from 1 every day to 8 per day
E. Not attributable to another disorder

Variants of the classic cluster headache are episodic cluster headaches, in which there are at least two cluster periods lasting 7–365 days and separated by pain-free remission periods of more than 1 month. In the chronic form, there are either no remission periods or periods of less than 1 month.

Glossopharyngeal neuralgia

A pain that has very similar characteristics to trigeminal neuralgia is glossopharyngeal neuralgia. It is described by the IHS as a severe, transient stabbing pain experienced in the ear, base of the tongue, tonsillar fossa or beneath the angle of the jaw. The pain is therefore felt in the distributions of the auricular (ear) and pharyngeal (throat) branches of the vagus nerve, as well as of the glossopharyngeal nerve. It is commonly provoked by swallowing, talking or coughing and may remit and relapse in the fashion of trigeminal neuralgia. The diagnostic criteria are summarized in Table 7 key facts box.

Table 7: Key Facts

DIAGNOSTIC CRITERIA FOR GLOSSOPHARYNGEAL NEURALGIA AS DEFINED BY THE INTERNATIONAL HEADACHE SOCIETY CLASSIFICATION

A. Paroxysmal attacks of facial pain lasting from a fraction of a second to 2 minutes and fulfilling criteria B and C

B. Pain has all of the following characteristics:
   1. unilateral location
   2. distribution within the posterior part of the tongue, tonsillar fossa pharynx (throat) or beneath the angle of the lower jaw and/or in the ear
   3. sharp, stabbing and severe
   4. precipitated by swallowing, chewing, talking, coughing and/or yawning

C. Attacks are stereotyped in the individual patient

D. There is no clinically evident neurological deficit

E. Not attributed to another disorder, which has been ruled out by examination and special investigations

Just as trigeminal neuralgia has a symptomatic form, so there is a symptomatic form of glossopharyngeal neuralgia in which the additional characteristics are aching pain that may persist between paroxysms and sensory impairment that may be found in the distribution of the glossopharyngeal nerve.

Other rare causes of facial pain

These include conditions such as paroxysmal hemicrania, SUNCT – short-lasting unilateral neuralgiform headaches with **conjunctival** injection and tearing, Tolosa-Hunt syndrome, Raeder's paratrigeminal syndrome. These are often known collectively as autonomic trigeminal cephalagias, since they are due to hyperactivity of the trigeminal nerve.

There are also other forms of neuralgia relating to different parts of the head and neck, which have similar symptoms to trigeminal neuralgia, but also include some other characteristic symptoms, e.g. occipital (back of head), geniculate (deep in the ear), superior laryngeal (side of throat). These are all defined in the International Headache Society Classification, which can be downloaded from the society's Web site. They are also described in detail in my book on **Assessment and Management of Orofacial Pain** (see reference list below.)

7. WHY WAS IT SO DIFFICULT TO DIAGNOSE TRIGEMINAL NEURALGIA? IN DEFENSE OF DENTISTS

This quote from a sufferer is familiar to many trigeminal neuralgia sufferers: *"I was angry because my dentist didn't diagnose it. I went to three different dentists; they gave me pain pills, they did a root canal on a tooth that didn't need it."*

If the symptoms are classical, why is trigeminal neuralgia not recognized at the onset? It is likely that the first attack of pain was on one side of the face, top or bottom jaw. It felt very painful and the closest type of pain to this that any patient has experienced before is toothache. Even if the patient had never suffered a toothache, people around would have described their experience. It is therefore likely that the patient assumed that it was a toothache or something similar and so went to see a dentist. The dentist asked a few questions about the pain, tapped some teeth and possibly took some X-rays. After all this, the dentist may have decided that there was a dental problem that could have caused the pain and so proceeded to do some dental treatment. This may or may not have helped the pain. It may have required several visits before the pain settled and it would be reasonable to have assumed it was the dental work and not the natural history of the condition. However, when it comes back again, the patient may then realize that it probably was not due to dental causes.

So why did the patient and the dentist initially miss the diagnosis?

The dentist may have been seeing the patient as an emergency and so had not spent a long time going carefully through the history - he/she may have been assuming that once they looked into the mouth, they would quickly find the cause of the problem. We know it takes time to take a history of pain, since the dentist or doctor needs to know at least nine things about the pain as described earlier in the chapter. Even if a thorough history had been taken, alarm bells would not have necessarily sounded, especially if a dental problem had been found.

The dentist, like the patient, initially went for the most obvious cause for the pain, which was a dental cause. We do this all the time in our lives; common things are common and we go for those before looking for rare things. A practicing dentist in his lifetime will see thousands of patients with dental pain, but only 3 or 4 patients with trigeminal neuralgia.

In my highly specialized practice, I see the opposite — 25 or so new patients with trigeminal neuralgia a year, but only 3-4 patients with dental pain. I will therefore be much more likely to consider the diagnosis than a dentist, in whose mind dental causes top the list of concerns. The dentist was probably taught at dental school about trigeminal neuralgia, but it was possibly a long time ago. The dental student may not have been tested on that knowledge and may never have seen a patient with the condition. The information was forgotten and not retrieved when the trigeminal neuralgia patient came to see the dentist.

It is also important to remember that dental disease is common and that a patient may have trigeminal neuralgia and a dental problem at the same time.

8. WHAT RESEARCH IS NEEDED?

Future researchers need to:
- Validate the diagnostic criteria of trigeminal neuralgia, both the classical and the atypical form.
- Look at the importance of the different characteristics of the pain and whether management of patients would change depending on the major characteristics of the pain.
- Determine what are the best questionnaires to use to diagnosis trigeminal neuralgia and its effect on quality of life, i.e. their specificity, sensitivity and predicative value.

- Evaluate how useful these questionnaires are in assessing the outcome of treatments, i.e. how sensitive are they to change?
- Assess how pain history and examination correlates with MRI findings and operation findings.

SUMMARY

- Trigeminal neuralgia is a sudden, usually unilateral, severe, brief, stabbing, recurrent pain in the distribution of one or more branches of the fifth cranial nerve.
- The diagnosis is made principally through the taking of a patient history with the possible use of questionnaires.
- Trigeminal neuralgia results in considerable effects on psychological and social functioning.
- The experience of trigeminal neuralgia varies in sufferers due to a variety of other factors, some of which can be controlled.
- Classical trigeminal neuralgia is the easiest to diagnose, but not all patients fulfill the criteria, e.g. some have aching dull pain between attacks and this is often termed atypical.
- There are a variety of other causes that result in unilateral sharp pain, the commonest of which are dental pains and idiopathic facial pain.
- Future research needs to confirm the diagnostic criteria of the different forms of trigeminal neuralgia.

Further reading and References

Web sites
Last accessed April 2005

International Headache Society Classification Criteria
http://216.25.100.131/members/Sections/members/login/Temp_Frame
/frameset_26_06_02.htm.

The resourceful patient http://www.resourcefulpatient.org/ is an electronic
book on the role of the doctor and the patient in the 21st century.

On the following Web site, you can perform Prof. Kim Burchiel's
trigeminal neuralgia diagnostic questionnaire:
https://neurosurgery.ohsu.edu/tgndiagnosis/TGNPublic.asp

Books
Greenhalgh T, Hurwitz B (Ed) (1989) **Narrative based medicine** BMJ
Books, London ISBN 0-7279-1223-2

Zakrzewska, JM & Harrison, SD (Ed) (2002) **Assessment and
Management of Orofacial Pain** Elsevier Vol 14 in Series on Pain
Research and Clinical Management London ISBN 0444509844

Report Royal College of Physicians of London. Improving
Communication Between Doctors and Patients. Report of a working
party. 1-38. 1997. London, Royal College of Physicians London

References
Blau JN (1989) Time to Let the Patient Speak. *BMJ* **298**:39.

Drangsholt M and Truelove E (2001) Trigeminal Neuralgia Mistaken
As Temporomandibular Disorder. *J Evid Base Dent Pract* **1**:41-50.

Gask L and Usherwood T (2002) The Consultation. *BMJ* **324**:1567-
1569.

Glueck CJ, McMahon RE, Bouquot JE, Tracy T, Sieve-Smith L and Wang P (1998) A preliminary pilot study of treatment of thrombophilia and hypofibrinolysis and amelioration of the pain of osteonecrosis of the jaws. *Oral Surg Oral Med Oral Pathol Oral Radiol Endod.* **85**:64-73.

Marvel MK, Epstein R M and Beckman H B (2000) Patients, Interrupted? *J Fam Pract* **49**:471.

McAlister FA, Straus S E and Sackett D L (1999) Why We Need Large, Simple Studies of the Clinical Examination: the Problem and a Proposed Solution. CARE-COAD1 Group. Clinical Assessment of the Reliability of the Examination-Chronic Obstructive Airways Disease Group. *Lancet* **354**:1721-1724.

Nurmikko TJ and Eldridge P R (2001) Trigeminal Neuralgia— Pathophysiology, Diagnosis and Current Treatment. *Br J Anaesth* **87**:117-132.

Platt FW, Gaspar DL, Coulehan JL, Fox L, Adler AJ, Weston WW, Smith RC and Stewart M. 2001 "Tell me about yourself": The patient-centered interview. *Ann Intern Med.* **134**:1079-85

Simpson M, Buckman R, Stewart M, Maguire P, Lipkin M, Novack D and Till J (1991) Doctor-Patient Communication: the Toronto Consensus Statement. *BMJ* **303**:1385-1387.

Zakrzewska JM (2002) Diagnosis and Differential Diagnosis of Trigeminal Neuralgia. *Clin J Pain* **18**:14-21.

Zakrzewska JM (2004) Classification issues related to neuropathic trigeminal pain. *J Orofac Pain* **18**: 325-331.

APPENDIX 1

TREATMENT GOALS

Tell us about the benefits you hope for from your treatment. Your answers will be confidential. Twelve possible benefits are listed below. Read each benefit and circle its importance to you, e.g. if 'Returning to work' doesn't apply to you, circle the appropriate response. Be sure to answer all the benefits.

A.	Goal	How important is it to you?
1.	Returning to work, or remaining at work	Very / moderately / slightly / not important
2.	Reducing pain medication	Very / moderately / slightly / not important
3.	To be able to go out for a meal with confidence	Very / moderately / slightly / not important
4.	Feeling less self-conscious in public	Very / moderately / slightly / not important
5.	Understanding my pain problem better	Very / moderately / slightly / not important
6.	Decreasing my tendency to overdo activities	Very / moderately / slightly / not important
7.	Feeling less depressed	Very / moderately / slightly / not important
8.	Being reassured that my pain is not a sign of a more serious disease	Very / moderately / slightly / not important
9.	Improve my ability to socialize	Very / moderately / slightly / not important
10.	Being physically intimate with partner	Very / moderately / slightly / not important
11.	Meeting other people with a similar pain problem	Very / moderately / slightly / not important
12.	Improving communication with doctors about pain	Very / moderately / slightly / not important

CHAPTER 2

ANATOMY OF THE TRIGEMINAL NERVE AND CAUSES OF TRIGEMINAL NEURALGIA

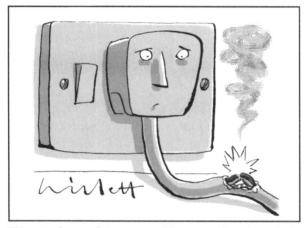

Trigeminal neuralgia is caused by a malfunction of the nervous system.

The following are the responses sufferers gave when asked during a focus group meeting, "What do you think caused your trigeminal neuralgia?"

- *I didn't think there was a cause. I asked my doctor and he said he didn't know what caused it.*
- *I have no idea, but it is something to do with nerve endings.*
- *I have no idea what caused it and neither does my neurologist.*
- *I assumed it comes with age, and settling down, and changing your bone structure and the apertures of the nerves.*

• *The herpes virus, I think it's just attacked the nerves and done damage.*
• *I think it was a result of a viral infection.*
• *I am an outdoors person and I did a lot of skiing in the cold and the wind and all of a sudden it hit me big time.*
• *I got it at an early age and I really think that it was caused by the dentist, maybe using mercury filling in my teeth as it came right after.*
• *I had a tooth extracted and during the extraction my jaw was broken and two weeks later I had pain on that side.*
• *I think stress has a major impact on weakening the immune system and then the trigeminal neuralgia comes.*
• *Radiation from a radar console whose cathode ray tubes focused on a point right on my head.*

Before we begin to discuss the causes of trigeminal neuralgia, it is important to understand how nerves work in general and how the trigeminal nerve in particular functions.

1. WHERE IS THE TRIGEMINAL NERVE?

The trigeminal nerve is one of twelve sets of cranial nerves (which are called either by a name or a number) that are particularly adapted to carrying out complex activities in the head and neck. Table 1 on the following page shows the names of the others and their roles. Some of them may be damaged during surgery for trigeminal neuralgia.

The cranial nerves are organized in pairs, one on each side. The word trigeminal comes from the Latin tres, meaning three and geminus, meaning twin, and it refers to three main sensory branches of the nerve. The trigeminal nerve is made of numerous nerve fibers that perform a wide variety of functions. The most important function is that of sensation, which includes information about light touch, temperature, pain, and proprioception (position sense), from the face and scalp. These are termed incoming fibers, since they tell the brain what is happening around the face. A smaller component of the nerve is made up of motor fibers, which are termed outgoing fibers, since the messages flow from the brain to the muscles of mastication and tell you how to move them. The smallest nerve components are the so-called visceral motor nerves ("visceral" refers to nerves innervating smooth muscle and glands such as the salivary and lacrimal glands). These fibers do not appear to be involved in trigeminal neuralgia.

Table 1

CRANIAL NERVES — THEIR NAMES AND ROLES

No.	Nerve	Function	Results from malfunctioning
I	Olfactory	Smell using several different smells	Loss of smell
II	Optic	Sight, pupil response to light	Loss of vision, poor field of vision
III	Oculomotor	Eye movements including eyelids, pupil size	Inability to lift upper eyelid, leading to closure of the eye, inability to move eye in certain directions
IV	Trochlear	Eye movements	Inability to move eye outward and downward
V	Trigeminal	Sensation of the face, muscles of mastication	Pain, lack of sensation, inability to eat
VI	Abducens	Movement of one eye muscle	Inability to turn eye inwards, squint and double vision
VII	Facial includes nervus intermedius	Movement of the face i.e. muscles of facial expression, taste	Face sags, unable to close eye, smile, frown, dribble saliva
VIII	Acoustic	Hearing, balance	Deafness, motion sickness, ringing in the ears, vertigo
IX	Glossopharyngeal	Sensation to throat, back palate and tongue, taste	Pain in the throat or ear, difficulty swallowing
X	Vagus	Complex nerve, both motor and sensory, and has effects well beyond the head.	Difficulty swallowing, hoarseness, speech difficulties, many others
XI	Accessory	Elevation of shoulder, neck rotation	Torticollis, i.e. contraction of muscles leading to abnormal position of the head
XII	Hypoglossal	Movement of the tongue	Deviation of tongue, tremor and wasting of the tongue

It is important to understand the anatomy of this nerve, since it helps to explain the surgical procedures that are done and why these procedures result in certain complications. You may want to come back to this section later. The trigeminal nerve emerges from the side of the pons (part of brain stem, near its upper border), by a small motor and a large sensory root known as the trigeminal nerve root. It is in close proximity to other cranial nerves as shown on the diagram below. This part of the brain is located in what is called the posterior fossa of the skull.

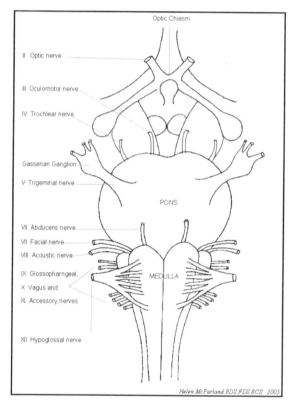

This diagram shows the ventral side view of the brain stem. The front end of the brain is at the top, and points at which each of the cranial nerves enter the brain are indicated.

The nerve then passes forward to the Meckel's cave where there is a large crescent-shaped ganglion, the Gasserian or semilunar ganglion. A ganglion is a collection of nerve cell bodies. In this ganglion lie the cell bodies of the sensory nerve fibers of the trigeminal nerve.

Meckel's cave can be identified on the skull by an impression near the apex of the **petrous** part of the temporal bone. From its convex border three large nerves form: the **ophthalmic, maxillary,** and **mandibular.** The ophthalmic and maxillary consist exclusively of sensory fibers; the mandibular is joined outside the skull by the motor root. This latter branch emerges from the skull through a hole called the foramen ovale.

The top smallest branch, known as the ophthalmic division, often annotated as V1 or VA, provides sensation to the forehead, eyes and the bridge of the nose. The middle branch, which is called the maxillary division, shortened to V2 or VB, supplies sensation to the inside of the mouth in the region of the upper jaw, upper teeth, lips, cheeks and palate, sinuses and also on the skin of the cheek and the nose. The third division, called the mandibular division, also referred to as V3 or VC, supplies sensation inside the mouth to the lower jaw, lower teeth, lower lip, the front of the tongue and outside of the skin and part of the ear. It does not supply sensation to the skin at the angle of the jaw as shown on the diagram.

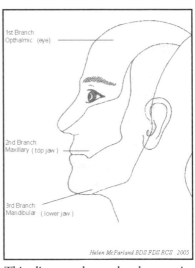

This diagram shows the three major sensory divisions of the trigeminal nerve and the area that they supply, which includes the inside of the mouth.

This diagram shows the major sensory branches of the trigeminal nerve and the Gasserian ganglion where all the sensory branches meet.

These major nerve branches are subdivided even further, and each branch is then given another name, e.g. the mandibular nerve is made up of a long buccal nerve, inferior dental nerve, lingual nerve and auriculotemporal nerve. Ultimately every tooth has its own small nerves.

The motor division of the trigeminal nerve supplies a group of muscles called the muscles of mastication. They are called the temporalis, the masseter, the medial pterygoid and the lateral pterygoid. These muscles enable us to eat and chew and open and close our jaws. It also supplies motor sensation to two small nerves to the muscles called the tensor veli palatini and tensor tympani. The word "tensor" means stretch and they stretch open the Eustachian tube.

The Eustachian tube is a small tube that helps to equalize pressure between the middle and inner ear, i.e. helps to unblock our ears when we have a cold or during flying when pressure changes occur. These two tiny nerves are occasionally damaged during surgery, which results in a feeling of fullness in the ear. The rest of the muscles of the face, so-called muscles of facial expression, are supplied by the facial nerve, also called the seventh cranial nerve. This therefore accounts for lack of a visible change in the face when suffering from trigeminal neuralgia, since the seventh nerve remains undamaged.

More details on the anatomy of the trigeminal nerve can be found both in anatomical textbooks and on Web sites, some of which are listed at the end of this chapter.

2. WHAT ARE NERVES AND HOW DO THEY WORK?

How nerves work is extremely complex and there are many unanswered questions. We still not know how nerves function in health, and we know even less about how they respond to damage. Any damage to nerves of sensation results in what is termed neuropathic pain, which may be associated with structural, neurochemical and functional changes that result in widely different presentations.

In attempting to describe the role of nerves in health and disease, we need to understand what is happening at various levels:
- molecular
- anatomical
- physiological
- psychological

I will try to explain it as best I can, beginning with excerpts from George Weigel and Ken Casey's book, **Striking Back! The Trigeminal Neuralgia and Face Pain Handbook** These writers have done a wonderful job in trying to explain these mechanisms:

"The job of nerves in general is to report contact with the world around us. They're the body's messengers that make it possible for the different parts of the body to work together as one coordinated unit. Nerves make sure the heart beats as needed. They signal your legs to move faster when you are

about to miss the bus, and they let you know when there is something crawling around on the back of your hand.

Nerves do all of this by way of billions of miniscule nerve endings or "receptors" that are stationed throughout the body. These receptors constantly monitor the environment in, on and around the body for changes. They then report this contact with the world back to the brain.

Each receptor has a specific job. Some report only when there's heat, some report on cold, some report only light touch, some monitor for pinpricks, some monitor for pressure and so on. A receptor whose sole purpose in life is to monitor heat in the left little finger, for example, only springs into action when there's a significant enough change in heat in the left little finger to alert the body.

Each of these receptors is connected to a nerve fiber – a tiny strand of tissue whose job is to carry signals from the receptor. When enough of a change in the environment occurs that a receptor activates, a chemical change occurs in the cells of the nerve fiber connected to it. This sets off a chain reaction called a "nerve impulse" that's somewhat akin to an electric current.

Instead of electricity, nerve fibers use body chemicals (sodium, potassium and chloride) to move nerve impulses. As these biochemicals move through microscopic channels across nerve-cell membranes, the impulse is handed from cell to cell down the length of the nerve fiber."

Here is another explanation by Patrick Wall, who was one of the world's leading neuroscientists, from his book, **Pain, the Science of Suffering**. This segment describes how nerve fibers move nerve impulses:

"Sensory nerve fibres detect events occurring at their ends in the tissue and signal them to the spinal cord by two methods. One method is by the production of nerve impulses, which are abrupt events in the membrane of the fiber that sweep over the fiber from its peripheral end all the way to its central end in the spinal cord. These impulses travel along the fiber-like fire in a fuse. But unlike the fuse, the surface of the fiber rebuilds itself after the fire has passed. The impulse lasts only one thousandth of a second and travels at between one and 100 meters per second, depending on the thickness of the fibers.

The second method of sensory nerve communication is much slower. The ends of nerve fibers in the tissue, particularly the thin C fibers, absorb chemicals from the tissue and slowly transport these chemicals all the way to the cell bodies in the ganglia and on to the central terminals. This transported signal takes a few hours to reach the ganglion cells if the injury is close and many days if the damage is as distant as the foot."

It is also worth remembering that the trigeminal nerve is highly represented in the brain because the face is a very complex organ and of extreme importance to our survival. If you touch the sole of your foot with a sharp pin, it will not feel nearly as sharp as that same pin applied with exactly the same pressure on the tip of the tongue.

The following is another insightful excerpt from the book by Weigel and Casey::

"A nerve fiber isn't one long, continuous strand that goes the whole way to the brain, however. Fibers are a lot like highways that sometimes come to an intersection. To continue down the right road, impulses have to jump from one fiber to another across microscopic gaps called "synapses." At each synapse, the body has a chance to modify the receptors' messages. That can mean reducing a message's pending impact on our consciousness or increasing our awareness of it."

Many drugs are targeted at these points and so they are called receptor antagonists. One receptor that is of special interest in trigeminal neuralgia is the NMDA (N-Methyl-D-aspartate) receptor, which is blocked by gabapentin. On the other hand, the sodium channels are blocked by carbamazepine. This explains why two drugs may sometimes be better than a single drug in controlling neuropathic pain.

This is actually a very clever gatekeeper system to filter out changes that aren't worth alerting the brain. The nervous system sets certain thresholds of change that need to occur in order to continue to send the impulse. If the threshold isn't met, the signal ends, and the brain isn't "bothered" by every little change. This is why you may not experience pain from a tiny scratch or feel a speck of dust that lands on your head.

Without this sort of filtering system, the brain would be overwhelmed by all of the minor sensations bombarding our bodies every second. The last stop is the brain itself, and it, too, has a built in system of "checks and balances" that grades the nerve signals and decides which are "normal" and which need some sort of response by the body.

This grading system is what allows us to decide, for example, whether that hot tub of water is just perfect, hot enough that we need to wiggle our feet around a little first, or so hot that we'd better pull our foot back out right away.

Up to a point, we can also decide to "overrule" a sensation. That's why we can tolerate heat from a heating pad. It's hot, but we're aware that it's intentional and that it's not immediately threatening. And so we put up with it and even adjust to the initially uncomfortable feeling. Introduce that same degree of heat from a sudden, unexpected source, on the other hand, and we might jump back with pain.

We're even able to temporarily snuff out quite intense pain signals for an overriding good or protective reason. For example, a person who twists an ankle and falls in the middle of a road may be able to hobble out of harm's way while suppressing the pain signals the ankle is sending out. When the emergency's over, the pain then comes through loudly and clearly.

The thresholds and grades that determine how we'll react also are able to adapt to changes in our body and the environment around us. For example, a warm shower normally feels good, but use the same temperature of water on newly sun-burned skin and suddenly you feel burning pain. Or use that heating pad on your back for *too* long and the sensation goes from comforting warmth to unbearable heat.

A sample impulse

Here's the way it's all supposed to work.

Let's say the receptors in your fingertips have picked up a sudden change in heat. An impulse is sent along the nerve fibers in that region, the "gatekeeper" cells are convinced it's definitely significant, and now the thalamus (the "central switching station" of the brain) gets the impulse.

This is where you first perceive or "feel" something hot. The thalamus then alerts the cerebral cortex, another part of the brain whose job it is to locate the source of the problem, assess any damage going on and fire off new impulses that tell your hand and arm muscles to get your fingers off the hot stove.

The cerebral cortex also will dispatch white blood cells to fight potential infection, activate nutrient reserves that are needed to start the healing process and send out "stop-pain" signals once the threat is under control. This is called the "inflammatory response." This sequence of events has been summarized in Table 2 key facts and the drawings on the following page.

Table 2: Key Facts

POSSIBLE SEQUENCE OF EVENTS WHEN SENSORY NERVE DAMAGE OCCURS

---

1. receptor stimulated
2. sends message through sensory nerve
3. other cells enhance or diminish the message, depending on whether it has caused damage and release of chemicals
4. attention mechanism selects the incoming message as worthy of entry
5. brain analyzes it and responds in a number of ways, which are also affected by psychological factors:
    a. perceives that something unpleasant has occurred
    b. informs muscles to move away from damage if possible
    c. sets up an inflammatory response to start healing process
    d. creates a memory of the event and how responded to it
6. cut nerve tries to regenerate and sends out sprouts for reconnection. This may be successful and so result in resolution of pain. But if the connection is not re-established correctly, pain will persist. Cut nerves may absorb unusual chemicals and these can then cause the nerve to send out different signals or even transport the chemicals to the ganglion and increase its sensitivity to pain.

Researchers now are beginning to explore the role of the immune system in neuropathic pain and how it leads to the amplification of pain.

It is now being appreciated that specific inflammatory substances such as cytokines, nitric oxide and reactive oxygen species may do more than just kill the harmful factors; they could also increase nerve excitability, damage myelin and alter the blood-nerve barrier. This latter effect results in the nerve being infiltrated by immune cells, antibodies and other immune molecules. For instance, there is some evidence that these substances can change the acidity of the nerve environment and so cause more pain.

It is now being proposed that these antibodies, which gain access to the nerve through the damaged blood-nerve barrier may exert an effect in two ways. They could alter the ion channel function, i.e. the sodium, potassium and chloride needed to move a nerve impulse along a nerve. The second way is much more complex and ultimately leads, among other things, to the formation of autoantibodies – i.e., antibodies directed at one's own nerves and/or the formation of new antibodies against pathogens - i.e., outside factors such as viruses that invade the nerve.

When the body is next subjected to the **pathogen,** the nerve reacts much more severely. It is also being proposed that the immune mechanism may also be involved in damaging the blood vessels that supply nerves and so indirectly affect nerve function. Most of these changes have been studied in peripheral nerves, but these changes may also be occurring more centrally in the brain.

So now back to the brain and its other reactions. Again, co-authors George Weigel and Ken Casey explain:

> "One other thing the thalamus does is alert the limbic center of the brain, which determines your emotional response to sensations such as the hot-stove incident.
>
> Depending on factors such as your mood, past pain experience and social setting, your reaction and even perception of the pain could vary greatly. At home by yourself, you may jump up and down after touching the hot stove and yell a few choice words at the profuse pain. Around dinner guests, you might say "ouch" and calmly go for some ice cubes. Around a date you're trying to impress, you might just grin and bear it.
>
> The limbic system also creates a memory of this episode and etches a link in our mind between hot stoves and pain so we learn not to touch one again.
>
> This kind of elaborate pain-sensing system is quite different from other mammals, which respond to all painful stimuli with pre-conditioned responses."

This complex mechanism for responding to a pain stimulus was first proposed by Melzack and Wall and is known as the Gate Control Theory of Pain. It has revolutionized the whole field of pain, and provided explanations for many phenomena that had previously been observed but not validated structurally or physiologically.

New functional magnetic resonance imaging technology is providing concrete evidence for this theory, since this advanced type of scanning can show which areas of the brain are activated at any one particular time. Patients who tend to magnify or exaggerate the threat value or seriousness of an event have been shown to exhibit twice the activation in the somatosensory cortex (areas of the brain known to be associated with anticipation of pain, attention to pain, emotional aspects and motor control) than patients who do not exaggerate a threat or problem.

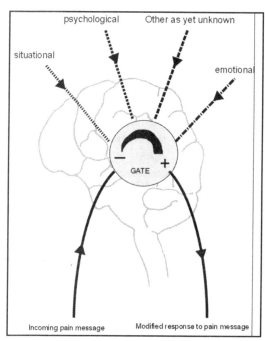

This is a very simplified diagram of the gate control theory of pain showing that any incoming signal can be modified by a number of factors, which then affect the resulting response.

It has been shown through brain imaging that individuals report less pain when asked to concentrate on visual, auditory or olfactory stimuli rather than a pain stimuli. This explains why distraction plays a crucial role in pain management and explains why the same intensity and type of pain results in so many different responses.

This concept is exemplified by this sufferer's statement: *"I feel a bit sorry for myself, but I usually try to go on with my life as though I had no problem. If I choose not to dwell on my problems, I seem to get along much better."*

Knowledge of this theory enables some sufferers to find ways to control their pain other than solely through medical and surgical management. This will be discussed further in later chapters.

George Weigel and Ken Casey again provide valuable insights in their book, **Striking Back:**

"People typically envision a nerve as a spaghetti-like strand of tissue that branches out into a few smaller tentacles. Actually, a nerve is more like a phone cable that's really a bundle made up of many smaller individual phone lines, or in this case, nerve fibers.

Each of the thousands of fibers in a typical nerve has its own specific purpose, since each is attached to one of those narrowly focused receptors.

This is what allows the same nerve to tell the difference between a feather tickling our cheek and a pin pricking it. Each trigeminal nerve, for example, has an estimated 125,000 individual fibers – some that signal heat, some that signal pain, some that signal light touch and even some that control the jaw muscles we use when chewing.

Nerves come in different sizes, depending on the number and types of fibers they contain. The more complex the nerve's duty, the more fibers it has and the bigger it is. Since the trigeminal nerve performs such a complex duty and has so many fibers, it's the biggest nerve in our head.

The fibers themselves also differ in size and number, depending on the types of message they carry and how fast those messages need to travel. Fibers that sense pain, for example, are larger than those that sense light touch. There are even different types of pain fibers – some that spring into action quickly (i.e., the so-called "A fibers" that give the brain sharp, immediate feedback when you hit your thumb with a hammer) and some that kick in for the longer term (the "C fibers" that carry that aching, throbbing pain that may last minutes or hours after you whacked your thumb)."

Table 3: Key facts

TYPES OF SENSORY NERVE FIBERS AND THEIR ROLES
A beta fibers are sensitive to gentle pressure. A delta fibers are thinner and are sensitive to heavy pressure and temperature. C fibers respond to pressure, chemicals and temperature.

The nerve impulse speed can vary, and one reason for the difference in speed of these different nerve fibers is due to the nerve structure. The fast fibers are covered by a fatty substance called myelin, which "coats" the nerve along its course. However, if the coating was continuous, then nerve transmission would not occur and so from time to time there is a break in this myelin sheath (nodes of Ranvier).

So far, we have mentioned myelin only as a universal cover for nerves. However, there are subtle differences in myelin and some of the myelin is produced by cells that are specific for the brain, and other parts of myelin are derived from what are called Schwann cells.

As the trigeminal nerve approaches the brain stem, the myelin coating changes from that produced by the Schwann cells to that produced centrally. This area has been called the route entry zone and is thought to be particularly sensitive to pressure. However, the length and exact position of this area remains debatable. It has been suggested that it is within three to five millimeters of the brain stem, but others suggest that this area could be anywhere between the brain stem and Meckel's cave.

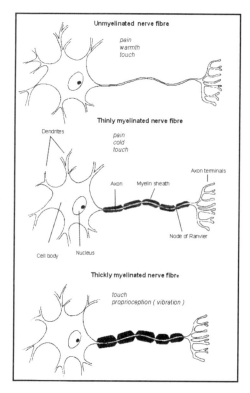

This diagram illustrates the basic differences between sensory nerve fibers.

3. WHAT IS NEUROPATHIC PAIN AND HOW DOES IT RELATE TO TRIGEMINAL NEURALGIA?

Damage to sensory peripheral nerves results in loss of sensation, with the amount being related to the extent of the nerve damage. However, in many instances not only is sensation lost, but abnormal pain is experienced. This is called neuropathic pain. It is thought to be due to dysfunction of the pain-processing neurons in both the peripheral and central nervous system. These central changes explain why so often there is nothing to demonstrate on examination of the patient. It also suggests that the pain is not necessarily resulting in further ongoing structural damage, but is more the result of a process that has gone wrong and therefore avoidance behavior is not going to make things worse.

Sufferers of trigeminal neuralgia will avoid touching the face because it causes pain, but they need to be aware that touching the face does not

result in more damage. Neuropathic pain results in severe persistent pain associated with allodynia (pain due to a stimulus, which does not normally provoke pain). In summary, the features of neuropathic pain are:
- continuous spontaneous pains, no remissions
- pain located within an area where sensation is disrupted due to a nervous system lesion
- abnormal evoked pain, i.e. allodynia
- hyperexcitability with increased response to **suprathreshold stimuli**
- a build-up of pain following repetitive stimulation
- relatively refractory to medical treatments

Table 4 below lists examples of neuropathic pains.

Trigeminal neuralgia is classified as a neuropathic pain, but it has several characteristics that do not fit with the above features, especially when considering the classical type:

- paroxysmal with refractory periods, i.e. an interval of seconds to minutes after a paroxysm during which triggering stimuli fail to launch another paroxysm
- completely pain -free intervals between paroxysm
- remissions lasting for weeks or months
- in some patients a trigger in one spot leads to pain in another area, but there is no intervening pain
- rarely have abnormal sensations
- responds well to carbamazepine

We do not as yet have an answer for this difference.

Table 4

EXAMPLES OF NEUROPATHIC PAIN
Peripheral pain syndromes
Diabetic neuropathy
Phantom limb pain
Post herpetic neuralgia
Trigeminal neuralgia
Central pain syndromes
Central poststroke pain
Multiple sclerosis pain

4. WHAT CAUSES TRIGEMINAL NEURALGIA?

Everyone is in agreement that the trigeminal nerve is no longer functioning in a normal way in patients with trigeminal neuralgia. Patrick Wall postulates two possible causes. One could be that a process as yet unknown results in the amplification of incoming signals by the peripheral nerve. The other is that the brain stem cells that receive the sensory fibers have developed an extreme hyperexcitability so that they explode in synchronized action when stimulated by normally innocuous input.

There is evidence to show that in trigeminal neuralgia, hyperex-citability of the nerve occurs and that it can be blocked by the use of anti-epileptic drugs that have been specifically developed to reduce epileptic episodes (another manifestation of hyperexcitability in the brain).

The question, therefore, is how or why does a nerve become hyper-excitable? Most would say that this is due to the loss or change in the myelin sheath of the nerve. This is borne out by epidemiological studies, which show that patients with multiple sclerosis in whom the principle cause of disease is loss of myelin, are at 20 times higher risk of develop-ing trigeminal neuralgia than any other group of people.

At the molecular level, this could be due to the inflammatory and immune response as described earlier in this chapter. On the gross anatomical level, this loss of myelin could be due to compression of the trigeminal nerve by an artery of the brain in the posterior fossa.

Electron microscope sections of the trigeminal nerve, taken from patients with trigeminal neuralgia undergoing posterior fossa surgery, have shown areas of external swelling and demyelination adjacent to the areas of arterial compression. This theory of neurovascular compression is based on three concepts:

- **Normal blood vessels compress the nerve in its course from the brain to the gearing ganglion.**
- **The nerve is compressed at an area of transition of central myelin to peripheral myelin at the route entry zone – a potentially vulnerable area.**
- **This continual mechanical pressure on the nerve results in damage and even loss of the protective covering of the nerve (myelin) and so leads to abnormal transmission of impulses from light touch transmitting nerves to pain- transmitting nerves. This so-called ephaptic transmission results in the generation of the typical paroxysms of pain. This is illustrated in the figure on the following page.**

Neurosurgeon Peter Jannetta suggests that the location of the nerve compression can be predicted from the patient's history, which empha-sizes yet again the need for care with this part of the patient manage-ment. Support for this theory comes from the fact that other cranial nerves, when compressed, also result in abnormal functioning, e.g. glos-sopharyngeal neuralgia, hemifacial spasm, twitching of the muscles of facial expression due to compression of the facial nerve. Trigeminal neu-ralgia is more commonly found in older people. It is well known that in older people blood vessels become harder and more convoluted. Blood pressure also rises in the elderly and all these factors could result in nerve damage.

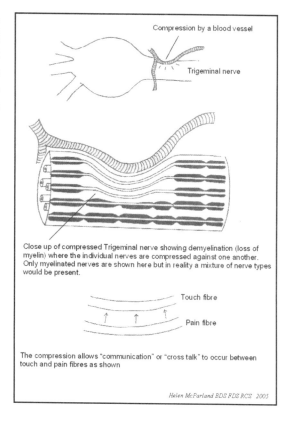

Close up of compressed Trigeminal nerve showing demyelination (loss of myelin) where the individual nerves are compressed against one another. Only myelinated nerves are shown here but in reality a mixture of nerve types would be present.

The compression allows "communication" or "cross talk" to occur between touch and pain fibres as shown

Helen McParland BDS FDS RCS 2005

This diagram shows how a blood vessel may compress a nerve and result in destruction of the myelin sheath.

Why is compression of the nerve by a blood vessel an insufficient explanation?

However, not all patients have vascular cross-compression of the trigeminal nerve. Up to 10 % of patients may have a negative exploration, i.e. no convincing compression is found. Jannetta thinks this may be due to inexperience and failure to look in less likely places. Some patients also report this after undergoing an microvascular decompression.

One post-surgical patient reported, *"The surgeon left the blood vessel, so I went for another five years thinking I was atypical and then I saw another doctor and he said no, you're classic and I had an endoscopic procedure and I am better."*

This theory does not explain adequately the approximate 25 % rate of recurrent facial pain. It has been argued that a recurrence of pain is due either to a failure to identify all the areas of compression or to the fact that recompression occurs by new vessels or even by the materials used to relieve the compression.

However, this does not explain adequately why there may be initial pain relief, nor does it explain the high recurrence rate within two years. Even if the compression has been corrected, the myelin has been damaged and needs time to regenerate. Some sufferers will always describe the same trigger points and areas of pain, but others report changing areas of pain. In our work on cryotherapy of peripheral nerves, we showed that the pain migrated in 38 % of patients. Why should this occur if the compression is already established?

Most surgeons would consider cross-compression to be significant if the artery is of sufficient size to displace and/or produce a groove in the nerve. It also often leads to discoloration of the trigeminal nerve and in some cases the nerve may become significantly thinner (atrophic). In approximately one third of those found to have this arterial cross-compression, this will be found more lateral to the route entry zone, the vulnerable area.

In other instances, surgeons find vessels such as veins and small arteries lying close to the trigeminal nerve, and it remains unclear whether these low-pressure vessels are capable of causing a change in myelin. Yet surgeons have shown that sometimes just gentle manipulation of the nerve, either in the posterior fossa or at the level of the Gasserian ganglion, results in pain relief at least for some time.

In those patients in whom no compression is found, many surgeons will cause damage to the nerve by performing what is termed a partial sensory rhizotomy. In this procedure, a section of the trigeminal nerve is divided. The pain relief period experienced by patients who have partial sensory rhizotomy is the same as those who undergo a decompression procedure.

It remains difficult to explain why damage to the nerve can also result in pain relief rather than a worsening of the symptoms. Other procedures done at the level of the Gasserian ganglion all cause damage to the nerve and yet also provide pain relief. It could be argued that the extent of damage may be crucial. Thus a neurovascular compression may play a substantial role in causing trigeminal neuralgia, but it is not the sole cause.

What is the ignition hypothesis?

Studies are also being undertaken to look more closely at how neuropathic pain is generated on the molecular level. This has led to the ignition hypothesis, which tries to incorporate our knowledge of the role of ion channels with operative and post-mortem anatomical observations.

George Weigel and Ken Casey describe the hypothesis this way:
   "In a healthy nerve, a gentle touch of the lip or a slight breeze on the cheek will create an impulse, which is sent to the brain by nerve fibers that sense light touch. But in a nerve with damaged myelin, impulses are thought to "jump" or "leap" from light-touch fibers to pain-signalling fibers, thereby sending an altered signal to the brain. Much of this fiber jumping is thought to occur either at the Gasserian ganglion or at the point of vessel compression near the nerve root where the pain light touch fibers are closest to one another.

   In other words, a sensation that starts out as an innocuous impulse on a light touch nerve fiber crosses over into a neighboring pain fiber, turning that impulse into a pain signal instead. The brain then misreads the gentle touch of the lip or slight breeze on the cheek as pain. This creates major havoc in the nervous system and brain; suddenly all sorts of intense conflicting signals are coming in from the face. The entire nerve pathway is reacting to what started out as a very minor and very focused signal. Instead of a limited or proper reaction to a minor stimulus, many wrongly recruited nerve fibers are firing by themselves.

   The pain processing parts of the brain don't know what to make of this. The logical brain responses don't work because the incoming signals aren't accurately reporting what's taking place. Confused, the brain summons other parts of its response arsenal into action.

   When a nerve is injured for whatever cause, it often becomes highly sensitive or hyper-excited. Recent research suggests this happens, at least in part, because the body tries to compensate for the injury by creating new channels for biochemicals to carry signals through the nerve. Impulses travel when sodium potassium and chloride move through those channels from one nerve cell membrane to another. It's as if the body builds several new highways to convey traffic that can no longer travel over the damaged original highway. The result is that nerve fibers tend to over-report or fire off signals at the slightest provocation. That creates a situation in which things that didn't upset the nerve before, now do.

   Nerve injuries may also interfere with the brain's ability to send standard pain signals, hindering a switching off of the pain once an attack such as trigeminal neuralgia starts. Nerve monitoring in research animals has confirmed that background nerve activity goes up when myelin is injured. This means that it might not take much of a stimulation to trigger a trigeminal neuralgia pain attack — sometimes a simulation that is not noticed at all. Once an attack is triggered, it may not stop until the nerve has worn itself out and is physically incapable of firing any more.

Rappaport and Devor believe that what finally stops attacks is that the nerve discharges all of its potassium, sodium and calcium, the elements that the body uses to create a nerve impulse in the first place. Until the supplies of those body chemicals replenish themselves, the nerve is incapable of firing again.

Both the rate at which these chemicals replenish and the levels needed to cause the nerve cells to ignite in the first place (the threshold levels discussed above) vary from person to person and time to time. Drs. Rappaport and Devor say that may explain why one person with a compressing blood vessel ends up with dreadful TN pain, while another person with a similar compression might not.

This may also explain why some patients are able to "overload" their pain. Some people say they endure one big attack when they start to eat and then get a pain-free window of 10-15 minutes to finish the meal before another attack occurs.

Depleting the nerve of nerve-firing chemicals means that there is not enough left to ignite a new chain reaction until later. The only mystery here is why a person can feel a light touch right after a pain blow-out, but that light touch no longer triggers pain. If the chemicals are depleted, in other words, how can the nerve fiber send any signals?

Another possible explanation is that the gatekeeper system in the nerve cells and brain, after being overwhelmed initially by a wave of pain signals, resets the threshold levels to quell the errant overtly sensitive nerve firings. Eventually, the threshold returns to normal levels, setting the stage for a possible new attack.

This scenario is much like putting out a fire. A fire flares and burns out of control until the fire company has time to respond and put it out. But if the cause of the original fire isn't eliminated, the blaze will rekindle after the firefighters are back at the station.

How does this theory try to explain remission periods and worsening of the condition?

We all know that sufferers with classical trigeminal neuralgia typically experience periods of pain remission. We also know that areas of skin which, during an attack of trigeminal neuralgia, were exquisitely sensitive, are no longer sensitive to light touch during these periods.

Electron microscopy studies of samples of nerves taken from trigeminal neuralgia patients show that the myelin is capable of regeneration. How quickly this occurs and how effective it is varies from patient to patient. It is postulated that when the repair is effective, the pain ceases completely, but if only partial repair is achieved, there is residual pain that may not be as severe. From the history of the disorder, it would appear that attacks of pain get progressively worse. This would be explained by the nerve's decreasing capacity to recover.

This theory of myelin regeneration has led to treatments aimed at improving repair of myelin. With this end in mind, sufferers have increased their intake of Vitamin B, and some report improvement, as indicated by these patients' comments:

- *"I found large doses of vitamin B1, 6 and 12 helped to keep the pain under control."*
- *"I began weekly B12 shots for 6 weeks and then converted to sublingual methylcobolamin."*

There have, however, not been any formal trials to test this hypothesis.

5. WHAT CAUSES ATYPICAL OR TYPE 2 TRIGEMINAL NEURALGIA?

This type of pain has many more features of neuropathic pain, and there could be two reasons for this. The mechanism for the pain may not be mechanical irritation, but some as yet unknown factor. It could also be that the initial mechanism may be the same, but the continual compression could lead to increasingly more nerve damage, resulting in not only the fast myelinated A nerves being affected, but also the thinner unmyelinated C fibres. If the thin C fibers are damaged, they result in burning continuous pain.

It could also be postulated that more frequent attacks result in more damage and less repair, thus leading to more rapid progression of the disease. Data from surgical management of trigeminal neuralgia provide some evidence that sufferers who have had trigeminal neuralgia for less than eight years have better long term pain relief after microvascular decompression than those who have had the condition longer.

There is also evidence that patients with atypical trigeminal neuralgia often do not experience complete pain relief after medical or surgical treatment. The factors causing their pain could be those described in the next section.

6. How does secondary or symptomatic trigeminal neuralgia differ?

In secondary or symptomatic trigeminal neuralgia, which is much rarer (1-2 % of all cases), it is thought that the cause of the trigeminal neuralgia is known, as shown in Table 5 below. The symptoms are often indistinguishable, but there are likely to be fewer periods of pain remission, and the severity of the symptoms increases progressively. There may also be other changes such as loss of sensation, since in these conditions, all nerve fibers are involved. This can be due to direct pressure on the nerve anywhere along its anatomical route or due to direct damage to the nerve itself by a disease process. The table below lists some of these very rare causes.

Many of these causes have not been well validated and so further research is needed to prove that they cause trigeminal neuralgia rather than being coincidental. Such studies would require large numbers of patients with and without the conditions.

Table 5

Possible causes of trigeminal neuralgia – many unproven scientifically
• Multiple sclerosis
• Tumors – acoustic neuromas, Schawnnomas, meningiomas, cholesteatomas, angiomas, epidermoids, trigeminal neurinomas, pituitary tumors
• Abnormal blood vessels- arteriovenous malformations, aneurysms
• Infective – herpes virus, tuberculosis of the brain, cavitational osteonecrosis in the jaws, and cysts – arachnoid cysts, hydrocephalus
• Bone diseases – Paget's, osteochondromas, osteoporosis, osteodysplasia
• Autoimmune conditions- scleroderma, lupus, mixed connective tissue diseases

Multiple sclerosis

One of the diseases for which there is good evidence for causation is multiple sclerosis; the evidence for this comes from epidemiological studies as discussed earlier in the chapter. The nature of this disease is still not well understood and it could be an infective cause. However, it needs to be remembered that some patients with multiple sclerosis also have compression of their trigeminal nerve and have therefore responded well to a decompression of their nerve.

Conditions in the brain:

One of the commonest major causes is a tumor, many of which are of a benign nature, i.e. not cancer. Patients may have abnormal blood vessels that can lead to deprivation of blood supply to the trigeminal nerve and hence to its malfunction. Among these are aneurysms — enlarged, bulging but thin blood vessels that transmit their pulsations to the trigeminal nerve.

In other circumstances, arteriovenous malformations may form. These are collections of abnormal blood vessels that can grow around the trigeminal nerve and compress it. In other circumstances, the arachnoid (lining of the brain) becomes thickened and scarred and can therefore act as a compressive force on the nerve. This is particularly the case if surgery has already been done in this area. These sufferers also have their theories, as expressed in these patients' comments:

- *"Twenty years ago I had a head injury and received 13 stitches in the top of my forehead at the edge of my hair line. My thoughts are that, as the years went by and gravity took over, the more pressure there was to the blood vessel on the trigeminal nerve."*
- *"Was the trigeminal neuralgia caused by the compression to the bones of my skull from diving?"*

Dental causes:

Nearly a century ago, Black showed (in cats) that removal of a root canal from inside a tooth, which contains among other things a very fine branch of the trigeminal nerve, could result in changes in the trigeminal nerve close to the brain. However, the significance of this has not been evaluated.

The trigeminal nerve is especially well adapted to coping with damage, both complete and partial, especially if the damage has occurred **distally** and not damaged the cell bodies (found in the ganglion). The cell bodies are essential for nerve regeneration. When we lose our deciduous (baby) teeth, we also lose the fine nerves that provided sensation to these teeth. Every root canal filling or tooth extracted will result in nerve damage. Drilling of teeth may also cause changes to very fine nerve fibers.

A local anesthetic can inflict further damage on the trigeminal nerve. Either the needle can damage the nerve directly or this can be damaged indirectly by reducing blood supply to the nerve. Any trauma or surgery to the face will inevitably result in nerve damage. Damage to nerves can occasionally result in only a local reaction, in that the injured nerve endings can sprout new abnormal nerve branches, which then send different messages to the brain. These are called neuromas and are often found in patients who have lost their limbs. They continue to feel as if that limb is still present. This probably also occurs in the trigeminal nerve.

Dental problems could contribute to trigeminal neuralgia in that they could aggravate a nerve that is already partially damaged. A nerve fiber may already be firing abnormally, but not quite enough to cause pain. However, the addition of a dental stimulus means the nerve then reaches the required threshold and begins to send out painful stimuli. This is a feature of many neuropathic pains in which a light touch is interpreted as painful stimuli. It also needs to be remembered that trigeminal neuralgia and dental pain can coexist, since dental problems are common.

Reading through sufferers' histories, I find many link their pain to dental causes as some of these quotes illustrate:

- *"result of an infected root canal which went undetected for a few years, resulting in damage to the infraorbital nerve."*
- *"I had a root canal a month before I had my sinus surgery and the sinus surgery is what seems to have triggered my severe pain; it started about 30 days after the sinus surgery I had."*
- *"occurred after broken zygomatic arch."*

Infective and immune causes

Inflammation around a nerve due to infection can change the way a nerve transmits and result in hyper excitability. This is particularly well exemplified in postherpetic neuralgia, which sometimes follows an attack of shingles. Postherpetic neuralgia is a neuropathic pain like trigeminal neuralgia, and results in a burning or throbbing pain and extreme sensitivity to even the most delicate touch. Many patients link their trigeminal neuralgia with viral causes, as indicated by these statements:

- *"All my life I have more than normal share of persistent fever blisters. I suspect that it is damage to the nerve track and nerve ending caused by the herpes virus."*
- *"Brought on by Bell's palsy."*

Other patients link the inflammation to the immune system. One stated, *"I think stress has a major impact on weakening the immune system and then the trigeminal neuralgia comes in."*

7. WHAT OTHER FACTORS COULD BE CONTRIBUTING TO TRIGEMINAL NEURALGIA?

Genetics, heredity and gender

Since chronic pain states only occur in some individuals, susceptibility to chronic pain could be genetically pre-determined through lowered pain thresholds or altered pain sensitivity, but only become manifest after exposure to an appropriate noxious insult, the type of pain condition being determined by the nature of the insult.

Alternatively, poor adaptive responses in the central nervous system could result in a persistent sensitized pain state in some, and recovery in others, following a noxious insult. Apart from a few very rare disorders, such as congenital insensitivity to pain and familial hemiplegic migraine, there are only a few pain syndromes that have a familial pattern of inheritance.

A search of the literature has identified 18 case reports and small series of familial trigeminal neuralgia. However, familial patterns of inheritance only become obvious when **alleles** confer a relative risk of 50 or more for the disease in question. Therefore, it could be that the inheritance of specific gene **polymorphisms** could account for such differences.

Genetic polymorphism is the occurrence together, in the same population, of two or more genetically determined phenotypes (characteristics) in such proportions that the rarest of them cannot be maintained merely by recurrent mutation. Seltzer proposes that pain syndromes are "a heritable complex trait determined by a combination of alleles of **polymorphic** genes and environmental variables."

Just as different people have varying blood groups due to certain gene types, so patients with trigeminal neuralgia could have certain genes that predispose them to trigeminal neuralgia.

Psychological factors

When patients have classical trigeminal neuralgia with a known compression of the nerve, the trigeminal neuralgia is treated in a biomedical model, i.e. through surgery to remove the offending vessel. However, in the atypical forms when there is no vessel compression, patients often are labeled as having psychological pain. There has been virtually no research assessing psychological factors in patients with all forms of trigeminal neuralgia, and yet my own reading of patients' stories has shown how many patients exhibit signs of fear, depression, anxiety and catastrophizing.

The gate control theory of pain states that descending factors from the brain are potent modifiers of pain perception. They can amplify or even change pain perception and result in other bodily symptoms. We all know that psychological factors can raise blood pressure. If the blood pressure is raised, could it increase the compression that it is causing to the trigeminal nerve?

As discussed earlier, functional magnetic resonance imaging is now demonstrating the importance of psychological factors in the perception of pain. It has been shown that the presence of another person next to a pain patient will alter the areas of brain activation and hence perception of pain. These factors therefore need to be taken into account when managing trigeminal neuralgia, both by health care workers and sufferers. As this patient expresses it:

- *"I need them (doctors) to take care of me and look into possible future treatments. Why can't they do their best research for me? If I'm a challenging case, why can't they accept the challenge with enthusiasm instead of brushing me off? I see a psychologist regularly to deal with the emotions. Without the psychologist, I would be much less emotionally healthy than I am."*

Multifactorial

Basic neurosciences have offered us many potential mechanisms for the causation of trigeminal neuralgia. It could, therefore, be postulated that trigeminal neuralgia is caused by a large number of factors and that it is not until all of them have been put together that trigeminal neuralgia can be understood.

As this patient described: *"I have concluded that the trigeminal neuralgia was caused by several concurrent conditions: 1) compression by the upper cervical misalignment, 2)toxicity caused by mercury, and 3) improper diet and nutrition."*

The causes could be central, i.e. within the brain, which explains why anti-epileptic drugs work. But there could also be peripheral causes, because we know that a local anesthetic put into the trigger point identified by a patient will result in temporary abolition of all pain. Sufferers' genetic make-up, environmental and psychological factors could further influence the presentation of trigeminal neuralgia.

Trigeminal neuralgia could be likened to a series of complex large jigsaw puzzles. Until you have put all the pieces together, you do not get the full picture and there may also be more than one picture. Just one different piece could alter the way it presents. This could explain why trigeminal neuralgia is so rare, since all the pieces have to fit before the symptoms of trigeminal neuralgia appear.

8. WHAT RESEARCH IS NEEDED?

Until we know more about the causes of the disease and the functioning of the trigeminal nerve, it will be impossible to provide effective treatments. This is one of the areas that requires a vast amount of research at all levels, but principally at the molecular level. There are still no satisfactory animal models of trigeminal neuralgia to aid research. Neuroscientists must work closely with clinicians, since both need to contribute to the generation of hypotheses that can be tested.

Questions that need answering in broad terms include:
- What is the molecular basis for neuropathic pain, and in particular, trigeminal neuralgia, including identification and functional studies of neurotransmitters, neuromodulators and intracellular messengers involved?
- Is there a genetic basis? What are the gene and protein networks implicated in the initiation and persistence of facial pain? Does the inheritance of specific gene polymorphisms predispose an individual to particular orofacial pain conditions? Is chronic orofacial pain a disease in its own right and is it possible to identify individuals more likely to develop chronic orofacial pain? Are sex differences in pain response, and susceptibility to specific pain conditions, genetically determined?
- What is the role of the immune system?
- What is the role of dental, infective and compression factors in the generation of trigeminal neuralgia?
- How do psychological factors affect pain perception?
- Would a tissue bank from sufferers with trigeminal neuralgia help to answer some of these questions?

SUMMARY

- The trigeminal nerve is the fifth cranial nerve, which supplies sensation to the face and mouth and also to the muscles of mastication. Its sensory branch is made up of three major divisions, any or all of which may be involved in trigeminal neuralgia.
- Nerves are extremely complex, both in terms of structure and function. and they have multiple roles, which has led them to be specially adapted.
- When nerves are damaged, the body initiates a set of events aimed at rectifying the damage; this process is not always successful and so results in persistent pain.
- The gate control theory of pain helps to explain how pain is perceived and modified by a multitude of factors.
- In trigeminal neuralgia the nerve no longer functions normally, and this could be due to changes in the nerve, both within the brain and along its whole length.
- The ignition hypothesis attempts to explain the mechanisms involved in trigeminal neuralgia, which assumes that loss of myelin is the underlying cause and that this, in many cases, is caused by compression of the nerve inside the brain.
- There may be many other factors involved, including the immune system and infections. Psychological factors play an important role in modifying perceptions of pain.

All of these mechanisms will have a genetic basis and probably explain why people vary in their response to pain.

FURTHER READING AND REFERENCES

Web sites

Accessed January 2005

For anatomy there are numerous sites, but I found the following useful: http://medinfo.ufl.edu/year1/trigem/home.html, created by an anatomy student, Jeremy S. Melker, MS IV.

http://www.umanitoba.ca/cranial_nerves/trigeminal_neuralgia/manuscript/anatomy.html, created by a group from Canada, including Dr. A. Kaufmann, a neurosurgeon with special interest in trigeminal neuralgia. (A tutorial on trigeminal neuralgia.)

http://education.yahoo.com/reference/gray/subjects/subject?id=200 This site will enable you to search the classical anatomy textbook, Gray's Anatomy. Enter a word or phrase to look up (e.g. norma lateralis): IX. Neurology. ... 5e. The Trigeminal Nerve.

Books

Wall P.1999) Pain, The Science of Suffering, Weidenfeld & Nicolson. ISBN 0 297 84255 2

Weigel G., Casey K. (2004) Striking Back – The Trigeminal Neuralgia and Face Pain Handbook. Trigeminal Neuralgia Association, Gainesville, Florida, ISBN 0-9672393 -2-X

References

Adams CB (1989) Microvascular Compression: an Alternative View and Hypothesis. *J Neurosurg* **70**:1-12.

Cheng TM, Cascino T L and Onofrio B M (1993) Comprehensive Study of Diagnosis and Treatment of Trigeminal Neuralgia Secondary to Tumors. *Neurology* **43**:2298-2302.

Devor M, Amir R and Rappaport Z H (2002a) Pathophysiology of Trigeminal Neuralgia: The Ignition Hypothesis. *Clin J Pain* **18**:4-13.

Devor M, Govrin-Lippmann R and Rappaport Z H (2002b) Mechanism of Trigeminal Neuralgia: an Ultrastructural Analysis of Trigeminal Root Specimens Obtained During Microvascular Decompression Surgery. *J Neurosurg* **96**:532-543.

Feinmann C and Newton-John T (2004) Psychiatric and Psychological Management Considerations Associated With Nerve Damage and Neuropathic Trigeminal Pain. *J. Orofacial Pain* **18**:360-5.

Love S and Coakham H B (2001) Trigeminal Neuralgia: Pathology and Pathogenesis. *Brain* **124**:2347-2360.

Moller AR (1999) Vascular Compression of Cranial Nerves: II: Pathophysiology. *Neurol Res* **21**: 439-43.

Nurmikko TJ and Eldridge P R (2001) Trigeminal Neuralgia— Pathophysiology, Diagnosis and Current Treatment. *Br J Anaesth* **87**:117-132.

Seltzer Z and Dorfman (2004) Identifying Genetic and Environmental Risk Factors for Chronic Orofacial Pain Syndromes: Human Models. *J Orofacial Pain* **18**: 311-317.

Villemure C and Bushnell M C (2002) Cognitive Modulation of Pain: How Do Attention and Emotion Influence Pain Processing? *Pain* **95**:195-199.

In 2004 the Journal of Orofacial Pain devoted its Volume 18 Number 4 issue to papers presented at the Vancouver symposium on nerve damage and neuropathic trigeminal pain. This edition includes many articles discussing mechanisms, investigations and management of neuropathic trigeminal pain.

CHAPTER 3

How common is trigeminal neuralgia? Epidemiology

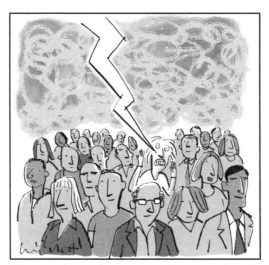

Trigeminal neuralgia is a rare disease resulting in lack of knowledge about it, both by the lay public and health care workers.

For years this has been my story
Each time I go, it is the same
Yes, that tooth. No, that tooth
They all hurt just the same.

This has been by story
for so many years...
Then one day a light appears
and these words I hear:
Trigeminal Neuralgia...
Please tell me what that means!

"*When the doctor told me, I didn't know what it was, and he told me that it happens in one in 25,000 people and I thought, why me? Why am I that one person in 25,000?*"

"*My doctor had only one patient in seven years who had it, and that was me.*"

"*I'd never heard of it before. I thought I was the only one that had it.*"

"*It's terrifying, really, because you've no experience, you don't know anybody who has had it; it's like some unknown disease. You're shaking with fear.*"

1. WHAT IS EPIDEMIOLOGY AND WHAT CAN IT CONTRIBUTE TO OUR KNOWLEDGE OF TRIGEMINAL NEURALGIA?

Epidemiology is the study of the distribution of health and disease in different groups of people and the study of the factors that influence this distribution. An epidemiological study will answer questions such as how many people get the disease, what types of people fall ill, whether the frequency of the disease varies with age, gender, social class, race, occupation, or geographic distribution. It will also provide details on how common a disease is overall, and can give us an indication of how likely we are to find a particular disease in a group of people at any one time (prevalence). These types of estimates are done through surveys, which usually involve either questionnaires or interviews with researchers.

Some of the terminology used in epidemiological studies is defined in Table 1 on the following page.

Epidemiology is closely linked with statistics, since large amounts of data need to be summarized in order to describe the findings. Data can never be collected from a total population and thus samples are taken. How these are collected is crucial to the data that is subsequently obtained. Statistical deductions are then made from the sample to indicate the extent of a characteristic in the total population.

For example, the US TNA group has collected over 11,000 survey questionnaires on the characteristics of members' pain. It is impossible at present to say whether this data is representative of all sufferers of trigeminal neuralgia, since it relied on sufferers finding details of the survey and on the motivation of these individuals to complete the questionnaire.

Using this data, we can evaluate the characteristics of these trigeminal neuralgia patients: signs, symptoms, social and demographic data. However, we cannot estimate the occurrence of disease, nor can we estimate the risk factors because we do not have a control group. A control group would be a random sample of the population whose social and demographic characteristics are similar to those of the trigeminal neuralgia sample group. But we can assess factors related to this specific sample.

Table 1: Key facts

DEFINITIONS USED IN EPIDEMIOLOGY
Incidence: Rate of onset of the disease among persons with no prior history over a given time period, often a year.

Prevalence = incidence x mean disease duration
Expressed as :
  • Point - at any given time
  • Period - during a defined period
  • Lifetime –over their lifetime

High risk groups – populations that are more likely to develop the disease
Risk factors: Risk factor is an aspect of personal behavior or lifestyle, an environmental exposure, or an inborn inherited characteristic e.g. age, gender, which on the basis of epidemiological evidence is known to be associated with heath-related condition(s) considered important to prevent. These can be modifiable factors, e.g. smoking. Can also include the determination of factors that will influence episode duration and recurrence rates.
Prognosis and natural history: what happens with time and what factors may affect progression or regression of the disease.
Prevention: what can be done to prevent the disease or minimize its effect.
Economic evaluation: what is the cost of the disease to the individual, to society.

High risk groups and risk factors

Epidemiologists have made major contributions to determining the **causes** of diseases. Indeed, epidemiological studies have often given us the answer before the biological mechanism has been known. We only need to look back into history to see examples of this. For example, John

Snow realized that a certain water pump in London was linked to outbreaks of cholera long before it was known that bacteria existed and were carried in the water.

These studies are especially useful in chronic diseases in which there are often multiple contributory factors. Epidemiologists will investigate associations between potential risk factors and the development of the disease, as well as identifying which factors are truly **causal**. Their studies have enabled us to link heart disease with lifestyle and mount large preventive health campaigns before we truly defined all the biological factors involved. Epidemiological studies to determine risk factors and high-risk groups are called observational studies.

Observational studies are those in which "nature" determines who is exposed to the factor of interest and who is not, or who among those exposed has a higher risk to develop the disease. Such a study will show whether there is an association between this factor or not. Researchers can also assess the association between a specific factor and a disease. Thus if we were to show that trigeminal neuralgia sufferers on average had lower Vitamin B12 levels than non-sufferers, we could say there was an association of Vitamin 12 with trigeminal neuralgia. But it would not prove that Vitamin B12 deficiency was the cause of trigeminal neuralgia.

Observational studies can be of three different designs and each has its role to play.

1. The *cross-sectional study* looks at all measurements at any one point in time. If we were to look at high blood pressure and trigeminal neuralgia and find an association, the design of this study would not enable us to say which came first. Put another way, if a cross-sectional study observed a significant association between high blood pressure and trigeminal neuralgia, this study could not indicate that this exposure (high blood pressure) was a cause of the trigeminal neuralgia because it is not possible to establish whether the exposure preceded the disease.

It is possible that both blood pressure and trigeminal neuralgia are the result of some other common cause we have not yet thought of. These types of studies are useful for assessing causality when the risk factor does not change (gender, race).

2. In a *case control study* of, for example, deficiency of Vitamin B12 and trigeminal neuralgia, the investigator starts with all the trigeminal neuralgia cases and with controls. The control group must be similar to the

base population from which the cases came from. We need to match for social and demographic characteristics. Such a control group is often called a matched group and the closer the match, i.e. the same number of women who are the same age as the group with the disease, the more likely that any differences found will be significant. Vitamin B12 levels are then measured in both groups.

Statistics are then used to determine whether there is a higher than expected level of low Vitamin B12 levels in trigeminal neuralgia sufferers compared to the control group. However, things are not as simple as this and matching needs to be done with great care to avoid confounding variables.

A confounding variable is one that is closely associated with both the independent variable and the outcome of interest. For example, a confounding factor in a study of coffee drinking and heart disease may be smoking. We need to be aware that some coffee drinkers are also smokers, so if researchers found a relationship between coffee drinking and heart disease, it could really mean that it is the smoking that caused the heart disease rather than the coffee. These types of studies are called retrospective studies, since the disease is already present in one of the groups.

3. A *prospective cohort or longitudinal study* is needed for stronger suggestion of causality. The investigator selects a cohort of persons who will be followed for a specific time period. During this follow-up period, factors (exposure) that we think may be causing the disease, e.g. nerve compression on **magnetic resonance imaging** (MRI) will be measured. The investigator will calculate the odds ratio, or the probability of disease among persons exposed and those not exposed.

This method is much more robust, but very difficult to do in diseases such as trigeminal neuralgia because the cases are rare and also because the disease takes decades to show itself.

The final test for proving causality would be a **clinical trial** (see **Chapter 5**) in which participants are assigned to groups on a completely random basis and all factors are kept constant except for the one being studied, and the outcomes are then compared. This could be done for Vitamin B12 if we are sure that all the other factors are controlled for.

Prognosis and natural history

Whenever we are given a diagnosis, we want to know, among other things, what is the prognosis and natural history of the disease.

Questions that can be answered through the use of epidemiological studies in relation to trigeminal neuralgia include:
- How quickly will I recover?
- Will I suffer a further attack?
- When might this occur?
- What will bring it on?
- Will future attacks get successively more severe or last longer?
- What can I do to prevent further attacks?

These are other questions a sufferer may ask, such as this one:

"It comes so suddenly, and I wish it would go so suddenly as well. I just wonder why suddenly one day it's there? I've usually had maybe five or six months without it, and when it comes back, it does come back with a vengeance."

Prevention of disease

If we knew the risk factors for trigeminal neuralgia, it might be possible to focus on primary prevention. It might not always be possible to prevent the disease from occurring, but early detection could help with interventions to reduce the subsequent progression of the disease. It would therefore be useful to know what brings on an attack of trigeminal neuralgia — that is, which factors bring about a relapse, and which contribute to a subsequent remission? If these were known, then it might be possible to prevent or delay the next attack.

Some sufferers have long remission periods, some hardly have any – what accounts for this? Research into prevention may identify factors that help to minimize the effect that an incurable disease may have on the patient, and may provide ways of adjusting to this permanent condition. It is important to identify factors that contribute to the development of disabilities and sub-groups of patients who are most susceptible to them.

Further details on the epidemiology of pain and, in particular, epidemiology of facial pain and temporomandibular disorder, can be found in the book titled **The Epidemiology of Pain**, by The International Association for the Study of Pain.

2. HOW COMMON IS TRIGEMINAL NEURALGIA?

Although to members of support groups, trigeminal neuralgia may seem to be a common disease, at the present time it is classified as rare. High quality epidemiological data is difficult to obtain, since there are very few studies that have looked specifically at trigeminal neuralgia.

Most of the data comes from surveys carried out for other purposes, since it is not economical to conduct a large population survey to look for a rare disease.

The principle characteristics of trigeminal neuralgia are still controversial, as is the question of whether there are two types and how these can best be delineated through the use of questions. Can the questions be specific and sensitive enough to diagnose trigeminal neuralgia and nothing else? Let us try it. Try answering these questions:

- Do you have pain that has been present for over three months?
- Do you have sharp, shooting electric shocklike pains?
- Do you also have a dull aching pain?
- Is the pain felt only on one side of the face/ mouth?
- Does each pain last just a few seconds?
- Do you get several of these sharp pains one after another so it becomes difficult to distinguish each individual pain?
- Do you have no pain between these attacks?
- Have you at some stage had periods of weeks or months when you have had no pain?
- Does touching parts of the face start up the pain?
- Does eating or talking make the pain worse?

Does a reply of "yes" to all the questions mean you have trigeminal neuralgia? What about the more atypical forms, would they be missed as they would not have a positive answer for each? Some forms of toothache and chronic idiopathic pain could also have the same pattern, and sufferers could answer in the affirmative for many of them.

What is the incidence of trigeminal neuralgia?

Most of the data we have on the incidence of trigeminal neuralgia comes from the Mayo Clinic in Rochester, US. All of this data was entered into a computerized diagnostic system that allows for epidemiological studies of the community. Study patients had all attended one of the hospitals in the Rochester area and had their diagnosis confirmed by a neurologist. It was assumed that all patients with trigeminal neuralgia would be seen in the secondary care sector. The diagnostic criteria were clearly set out and the patients included in the studies were residents of Rochester for one year and over. All reported their pain began between 1945 and 1984. The crude annual incidence for women and men was 5.7 and 2.5 per 100,000 per year, respectively, and incidence rates increased with age, but not with sex.

The annual incidence, when age adjusted to the 1980 USA population, was 5.9 per 100,000 women and 3.4 per 100,000 men. The average annual incidence increased with age and was highest in those over 80 years of age when the figure was 25.9 per 100,000. It was higher in females than males for nearly all age groups. However, the highest average annual incidence rate was recorded in males aged over 80 years when the figure was 45.2 per 100,000. The annual rates fluctuated somewhat from one decade to another, and the highest rate is found in those over 80.

It is therefore rare in younger patients, and this was a reason why, for example, a 23-year-old sufferer was not diagnosed. The young patient later reported, *"I went to my primary care physician and showed her the book with the information on trigeminal neuralgia and she proceeded to argue with me because of my young age."*

Table 2

AGE AND GENDER SPECIFIC AVERAGE ANNUAL INCIDENCE RATES PER 100,000 POPULATION IN ROCHESTER (1945-1984) OF FIRST EPISODE OF TRIGEMINAL NEURALGIA						
Age years	Total		Women		Men	
Groups	No.	Rate	No.	Rate	No.	Rate
0-39	3	0.2	2	0.3	1	0.2
40-49	7	3.7	6	6.0	1	1.1
50-59	14	8.9	9	10.4	5	7.1
60-69	21	17.5	16	22.8	5	10.1
70-79	20	25.6	17	33.7	3	10.8
Over 80	10	25.9	5	18.2	5	45.2
TOTAL	75	4.3	55	5.7	20	2.5
Age adjusted		4.8		5.9		3.4
Age and sex adjusted		4.7				

It would be of great value to update this data now and see if there have been changes over time. It must be remembered that any increase in incidence could just be due to improved diagnosis and increased numbers of referrals to the secondary care sector as more treatments become available.

How prevalent is trigeminal neuralgia?

There is one study, by Munoz et al, of the prevalence of trigeminal neuralgia. This was carried out in 1988 in a French village with a population of 1,144, where the researchers were trying to determine the prevalence of neurological disease in an elderly population. All patients who responded to a questionnaire indicating that they had some form of neurological disease were then examined. Out of 1,000 inhabitants, one male was diagnosed with trigeminal neuralgia, which makes the prevalence of trigeminal neuralgia that of 0.001%. They found in this survey that 2.7 % of the population suffered from some form of facial and head pain.

A British study, based on 27,658 patients in 13 primarycare practices in London, found a lifetime prevalence of 0.07/1000.

3. WHAT IS THE DISTRIBUTION OF THE DISEASE WORLD WIDE AND IS THERE ANY LINK WITH RACE OR OCCUPATION?

The geographic distribution of the disease is difficult to estimate. There is anecdotal data to suggest that trigeminal neuralgia is rarer in the Far East and yet a higher incidence of hemifacial spasm, compression of the facial nerve, is reported from China and Japan.

The importance of **race** and **ethnicity** in pain, and other areas of medical science, has been heavily influenced by the prevailing socio-political environment. Some differences have been identified in laboratory-based pain studies and epidemiological studies of pain conditions. These differences mainly relate to differences between Caucasians and African Americans. Differences in socio-economic status, access to health care, pain coping styles, and socio-cultural connotations on the emotional and behavioral response to pain, are likely to exert major influences. This would be in addition to any genetic influences on pain responses by different racial or ethnic groups.

In the Rochester study, trigeminal neuralgia sufferers were less likely to be Jewish and immigrants, in comparison with control cases. There are currently no published data on the educational and occupational details of trigeminal neuralgia sufferers.

MRS. G CASE STUDY

When Mrs. G first developed her severe pain she thought she had toothache. She went to her dentist, who suspected it might have been a decayed tooth. He did a filling. After eight weeks the pain settled and Mrs. G thought the dentist was right. When the pain returned one and a half years later in the same place, Mrs. G again went to her dentist. This time the dentist could not really account for it and said it could just be a temporary infection; he prescribed a course of antibiotics. The pain did not abate and became so severe that Mrs. G had to go back as an emergency patient. The dentist did not know what it was and decided to send her as an urgent referral to the local oral surgery department. She was given an emergency appointment. A careful history was taken and Mrs. G was told she had trigeminal neuralgia and that she needed some anticonvulsant drugs. Mrs. G was totally taken aback by the diagnosis, since she had never heard of it and did not even know how to spell the words. She was referred back to her primarycare medical practitioner for further treatment. Neither Mrs. G's. dentist nor her medical practitioner had seen a patient with trigeminal neuralgia, but both had heard of the condition.

1. Should the dentist have recognized the condition?
2. Why had Mrs. G never heard of it?
3. Should treatment have been left in the hands of the primary care physician?
4. How many patients do specialists see?

Discussion

1. As has already been discussed in Chapter 1, given the rarity of trigeminal neuralgia and the high frequency of dental care, the dentist was right to think of a dental cause first. However, on the second presentation, the dentist should have reflected on the symptoms and signs and realized that they did not fit the characteristics of any dental disease, especially since he could not detect anything. He did the right thing and referred her to a specialist.

2. Given the rarity of the condition as discussed above, it is not surprising that Mrs. G could not find another sufferer among her friends, who could have helped her diagnose herself. It is very common for sufferers to feel isolated and misunderstood because nobody else in their environment has had it or even seen someone else with the condition. Friends will not be able to offer anecdotal advice on the progression of the disease or of treatments that can be used. This is why support groups for rare disorders are so crucial; they provide an opportunity for sufferers to meet and compare experiences, and gain psychological support and understanding.

3. Initially, Mrs. G could be treated by a primarycare doctor, since there are published guidelines on management. However, it is crucial that the doctor is aware of the need for a referral to a specialist. Preferably, both the doctor and Mrs. G need to know who the specialists are, since only specialists who deal with large numbers of patients know how to manage rare diseases.

4. It has been estimated that a primarycare doctor may only see one or two trigeminal neuralgia cases in their practicing lifetime. It has been proposed that a neurosurgeon, who does more than five microvascular decompression operations a year, is experienced. A specialist such as myself, running a facial pain clinic on a weekly basis, will see 30 new cases a year.

4. Has epidemiology provided some answers to the characteristics of trigeminal neuralgia?

Studies assessing the laterality of the trigeminal neuralgia (side of the face that is affected) have found no predominance of one side of the body, although data from the US suggest a right-sided dominance. Bilateral cases are found in around 3 % of the patients with trigeminal neuralgia, and often only one side is active at any one time.

Questions frequently asked by patients about timing of the condition are:
- For how long will the remission period last ?
- For how long will the acute pain episode last ?
- Will it get more severe with time?

A natural history study, based on a survey of 75 patients, found that the median length of an episode of pain was 49 days, and the mean (average) was 116 days. Rasmussen, in his study of 109 patients, showed that only 6 % of patients would have no pain for years, whereas 36 % of sufferers had pain-free periods that lasted for several months.

Patients who had weeks with no pain, and patients who recorded only days with no pain, each amounted to 16 % of the total number. He also found sufferers more likely to report pain in the winter months. It has been estimated that 65 % of patients would experience a second episode of pain within five years and 77 % within 10 years. Rothman and Monson found that trigeminal neuralgia does not shorten life span.

Table 3

What can sufferers do to improve epidemiological research?
• Keep a careful diary of your condition as detailed under the nine headings in Chapter 1, especially things that affect onset or remission of pain. • Keep a record of all your results, e.g. MRI scans and blood tests. • If you know of any family members with facial pain, arrange for them to be assessed by a neurologist. • Answer surveys from validated researchers. • Participate in clinical trials conducted by validated researchers, especially genetic specialists.

5. DOES TRIGEMINAL NEURALGIA RUN IN FAMILIES?

There are reported cases of trigeminal neuralgia running in families, and it has been estimated at 5 %. In the material I have received, I also found accounts of familial trigeminal neuralgia. One patient reported, *"I am 73 years old and have had trigeminal neuralgia for four years. My sister, who is 82, also has trigeminal neuralgia."*

As we have learned, facial pain is common and so it would not be surprising for some relatives to report pain of this type, thinking that it was trigeminal neuralgia. This would then lead to the wrong assumption that trigeminal neuralgia ran in families. Therefore, a precise diagnosis, using well-established **diagnostic** criteria, is essential. In the studies reported above, all the patients were seen by specialists to ensure as accurate a diagnosis as possible.

To date, there are some proposals about how **genetics** may play a role, and it may be that a combination of genes are needed before the disorder becomes apparent (see Chapter 2 for details). Therefore, patients need to check whether other family members and relatives have trigeminal neuralgia and encourage them to come forward for diagnosis and possible genetic studies. This is a concern many patients raise in discussions through questions such as these:

- *"Can you pass it on to your children? I don't mind having it, but I would sure hate to pass it on to my children."*
- *"Can the grandchildren get it, can it skip a generation? My kids are okay, but will their kids be okay? Are they going to come down with it, that worries me."*

6. ARE SOME INDIVIDUALS AT GREATER RISK OF GETTING TRIGEMINAL NEURALGIA OR ARE THERE FACTORS THAT INCREASE THE LIKELIHOOD?

"Is it predictable? Can they do some sort of a test to see if you have it or are susceptible?"
These are commonly posed questions.

Cohort and case control studies have been used to answer these questions. The disease most frequently linked with trigeminal neuralgia is **multiple sclerosis**, in which the estimated relative risk is 20 times higher among those exposed to multiple sclerosis in comparison to those not exposed. This is relatively low as illustrated by the comment of this nurse with multiple sclerosis and trigeminal neuralgia: *"The MS group has no one with TN, and the TN group has no one with MS. I cannot find literature on TN progression with MS."*

The **researchers** also found that in the majority of cases, the multiple sclerosis pre-dated the onset of trigeminal neuralgia. The Rochester group analyzed a very large number of potential risk factors using their extensive database. One of the factors they looked at was a viral etiology, but it was not found to be associated, and no other relevant risk factors were clearly identified.

Neurosurgeons report that around 60 % of patients have dental treatment around the time of onset of trigeminal neuralgia and suggest that this may be a risk factor. The exact timing of the pain is crucial if an association is to be established. When did the pain really start? Sometimes it is difficult to remember which came first — the pain and then treatment or was treatment given and the pain then started? This could be a vitally important distinction in attempting to determine what factors may predispose patients to trigeminal neuralgia.

A large multinational survey of people, both with and without trigeminal neuralgia, or with other **orofacial** pains, might resolve the question regarding a dental link. —- whether dental treatment is a risk factor for trigeminal neuralgia, or whether dental treatment is an additional factor that, in a vulnerable individual, predisposes to the development of trigeminal neuralgia. This is why it is important that sufferers write down all the facts about their trigeminal neuralgia, even if they do not seem to be obviously related, since the information may help others in the future.

Prognostic features that have been looked at in the surgical cases include age, gender, duration of condition, previous surgery, preoperative sensory loss, type of pain and its distribution, number of involved nerve divisions and previous response to **anticonvulsant** therapy, as well as the ease of operation and the amount of nerve compression. But none of the data have been validated with controls using explicit diagnostic criteria, objective assessments before and after surgery and a clear definition of the measures applied.

7. CAN ANYTHING BE DONE TO STOP TRIGEMINAL NEURALGIA OR REDUCE THE CHANCE OF A RECURRENCE?

Currently there is no scope for prevention of trigeminal neuralgia, due to the lack of identified risk factors.

8. WHAT ARE THE COSTS INVOLVED IN TREATING TRIGEMINAL NEURALGIA?

One study has been done in the US, using insurance claims databases, to determine the health costs associated with painful **neuropathic** disorders (Berger et al 2004). Among the 55,686 cases studied, 1 % had a diagnosis of trigeminal neuralgia. In this group, they found that patients with neuropathic pain tended to have other health conditions and their health costs were three times higher than those of matched controls.

The economic costs of trigeminal neuralgia alone have not been estimated. They are likely to be high for trigeminal neuralgia, given the fact that many clinicians advocate CT or MRI scans prior to treatment. Microvascular decompression is a major neurosurgical procedure and, therefore, has significant cost implications. The newer **radiosurgery** is also very expensive. Patients managed medically may require a range of drugs, some of which are new on the market and hence expensive. Many patients will need regular monitoring to reduce side effects to a minimum and ensure maximum pain relief. Over time these costs could be considerable, and could be higher than for surgical treatment.

9. WHAT RESEARCH IS NEEDED?

Any epidemiological studies of trigeminal neuralgia must use very clear diagnostic criteria to ensure that the same condition is being assessed. However, population studies on trigeminal neuralgia alone would be too expensive given the rarity of the condition Thus they need to be embedded in other studies of facial pain or be assessed through large databases used for all diseases.

Revisiting the Rochester data to determine whether changes have occurred over time, and doing more focused case control studies, could be invaluable.

The following are areas in which epidemiological studies could provide help:
- further epidemiological studies to estimate the prevalence of trigeminal neuralgia and its subgroups
- cohort and case control studies to establish possible risk factors and causality risk factors currently being discussed include dental treatment, trauma to the head (including mouth), blood pressure, infections, diet, Vitamin B12, weather, radiation and even skull shape.

- longitudinal studies to determine natural history
- determine predictors for progression
- determine role of hereditary and genetics
- establish whether there is a geographical, racial distribution that may provide a clue about causality
- economic evaluations of the cost of this disease to the individual and society as a whole (desperately needed in this time of rising health budgets)

SUMMARY

- Based on old data, trigeminal neuralgia is a rare disease.
- It is a disease of middle age with a slight predominance among women.
- The only well established risk factor is multiple sclerosis.
- The disease is progressive, but does not shorten life span.
- No preventive treatments are currently possible.
- The economic costs of managing trigeminal neuralgia have not been determined.
- Up-to-date incidence and prevalence data from across the world are essential.
- Case control studies are needed to identify risk factors.

FURTHER READING AND REFERENCES

Web site

The TNA US survey can be found on the TNA US Web site: http://www.tna-support.org. Look under patient registry.

Book

Zakrzewska JM, Hamlyn PJ. (1999) **Facial Pain**. In: Crombie IKCPR, et al, eds . **Epidemiology of Pain**. Seattle: IASP:171-202. ISBN 0-931092-25-6.

References

Berger A, Dukes, EM and Oster G. (2004) Clinical characteristics and Economic Costs of Patients With Painful Neuropathic Conditions. *J Pain* **5**: 143- 149

Katusic S, Beard C M, Bergstralh E and Kurland L T (1990) Incidence and Clinical Features of Trigeminal Neuralgia, Rochester, Minnesota, 1945-1984. *Ann Neurol* **27**:89-95.

Katusic S, Williams D B, Beard C M, Bergstralh E J and Kurland L T (1991) Epidemiology and Clinical Features of Idiopathic Trigeminal Neuralgia and Glossopharyngeal Neuralgia: Similarities and Differences, Rochester, Minnesota, 1945-1984. *Neuroepidemiology* **10**:276-281.

MacDonald BK, Cockerell O C, Sander J W and Shorvon S D (2000) The Incidence and Lifetime Prevalence of Neurological Disorders in a Prospective Community-Based Study in the UK. *Brain* **123** (Pt 4): 665-676.

Munoz M, Dumas M, Boutros-Toni F, Coquelle D, Vallat J M, Jauberteau, MO, Ndzanga E, Boa F and Ndo D (1988) A Neuro-Epidemiologic Survey in a Limousin Town. *Rev Neurol (Paris)* **144**:266-271.

Rothman KJ and Beckman T M (1974) Epidemiological Evidence for Two Types of Trigeminal Neuralgia. *Lancet* **1**:7-9.

Rothman KJ and Monson R R (1973b) Epidemiology of Trigeminal Neuralgia. *J Chronic Dis* **26**:3-12.

Rothman KJ and Monson R R (1973a) Survival in Trigeminal Neuralgia. *J Chronic Dis* **26**:303-309.

Yoshimasu F, Kurland L T and Elveback L R (1972) Tic Douloureux in Rochester, Minnesota, 1945-1969. *Neurology* **22**:952-956.

CHAPTER 4

INVESTIGATIONS

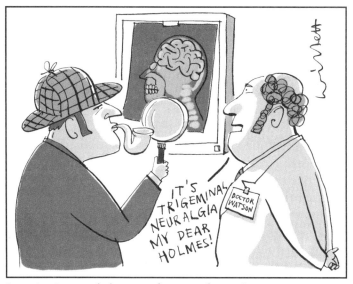

Investigation can help to confirm or refute a diagnosis.

"I had an MRI … and since they couldn't see anything on MRI – they decided I had atypical trigeminal neuralgia.

I have an MRI next week to test for multiple sclerosis because of having trigeminal neuralgia at a young age."

1. WHY DO INVESTIGATIONS AND HOW RELIABLE ARE THEY?

In reading sufferers' stories, I have noticed comments such as, *"He ordered an MRI and after seeing that, made a diagnosis of TN,"* suggesting that they believe Magnetic Resonance Imaging (MRI) can be used to prove that their pain is indeed trigeminal neuralgia.

An MRI can be used to show some of the potential causes of trigeminal neuralgia, but it cannot be called a diagnostic test for the condition. I hope this chapter will put various medical investigations into context, and you will realize that they can be erroneous and cannot be totally relied upon.

Investigation means to examine further, and in medical usage this extends to any procedure that helps to confirm a diagnosis that has been proposed based on history and examination. Investigations are therefore called diagnostic tests when they are used in order to make a diagnosis. Investigations, however, can also be used to monitor treatment or to detect side effects from treatments, or to look for some specific factor, e.g. compression of the nerve.

Before we move on to looking at individual tests that could be used in the diagnosis of trigeminal neuralgia, we need to look critically at how we judge the value of diagnostic tests. A diagnostic test needs to be reliable to identify everyone who has the disease being tested for, but it also must not diagnose someone as having the disease when they do not have it. Just as we learn to read articles on treatments critically, as explained in Chapter 5, we need to examine carefully how tests were developed and to confirm that they do what they are expected to do.

Let us look at an example of how X-ray images were found to be reliable in determining the depth of a cavity, thus helping the dentist to decide whether he needed to do a filling. This is the sequence of events that was used to determine the reliability of this test:

- The dentist found a tooth that might need to have a filling.
- He asked an independent person to take an X-ray of the tooth.
- The independent person estimated the depth of the cavity, but did not inform the dentist of the result.
- The dentist then drilled the hole without any knowledge of the X-ray finding and estimated the depth of the hole.
- The dentist then compared his estimation with the X-ray finding and asked himself how well the X-ray images predicted the depth of the cavity.

If the prediction was accurate, he can say his X-ray is reliable, especially if he does the test several times (reproducibility). Next time the dentist can rely on the X-ray and, if the cavity is small, he may decide not to do a filling. The X-ray was thus compared with the actual finding, i.e. the depth of the cavity found by the dentist, and this is called the gold standard.

Thus the three basic questions that need to be asked about the value and reliability of diagnostic tests are:

1. **"Are the results valid?"**
   - Did clinicians face diagnostic uncertainty?
   - Was there a blind comparison between the test and an independent gold standard?
   - Did the result of the test being evaluated influence the decision to perform the gold standard?
2. **"What are the results?"**
3. **"How can I apply the results to patient care?"**
   - Will the reproducibility of the test and its interpretation be satisfactory in my clinical setting?
   - Are the results applicable to the patient in my care?
   - Will the results change my management strategy?
   - Will patients be better off as a result of the test?

We will now look at this in a little more depth.

Are the results valid?

In order to be useful, a diagnostic test must be able to distinguish between conditions or disorders that might otherwise be confused. The test must perform well not only in those patients with the disease, but also those without it, and equally well in those who may have different forms of the disease.

It is important that all diagnostic tests are assessed for accuracy by comparing them to an appropriate reference standard. The reference, or gold standard, must be independent of the test being performed. The test results and the reference standard need to be assessed blindly, that is, neither party must be aware of the results. If the test is effective, there will be a close correlation between those patients who are found to have a positive test and a particular finding. For example, if all patients who complain of a set of symptoms that leads the physician to diagnose sinusitis are subsequently found to have specific changes on an X-ray image that no other groups of patients have, and all respond to a course of antibiotics, then the X-ray can be said to be an effective test.

It is also extremely important that the person assessing the diagnostic test remains blinded to the results of the gold standard. Once you know what is expected, you are much more likely to find it in the test than if you are completely unaware of the possible results. This is why the neuroradiologists in our unit do not want to know on which side the patient has the pain. The more susceptible the gold standard is to changes in interpretation, the more important is the blinding of the gold standard. For example, when scrutinizing an **MRI scan** to determine whether there is compression of the trigeminal nerve by a blood vessel, the neuroradiologist is looking for a small white dot indenting a grey/black trigeminal nerve. If you had 10 neuroradiologists looking at the same MRI scans, would they all interpret the images in the same way? The more often they all agree, the more robust is the test.

When reading original articles on the development of diagnostic tests, you also need to look at what is termed the likelihood ratios. A likelihood ratio is calculated on the basis of two questions:

1. How likely is it to obtain a given test result among people with the target disorder?
2. How likely is it to obtain the same test result among people without the target disorder?

Likelihood ratios aim to show how powerful the test is. For example, if the answer to question 1 was "very likely," and to question 2 "very unlikely," then the test would be significant in the diagnosis of the disorder. If the results were reversed, then the test would not be appropriate for diagnosis. The higher the ratio between 1 and 2, the greater the likelihood that the test will predict the disorder. This would be a positive likelihood ratio. A negative likelihood ratio may not always exclude the target disease.

Sensitivity and Specificity

You may also find the results quoted in terms of the sensitivity and specificity of the test. Sensitivity refers to the proportion of people with the target disease for whom a test result is positive. Specificity is the proportion of people without the target disease in whom a test result is positive. For example, we could say that a sharp shooting electric-like pain is always present in trigeminal neuralgia. This we may find to be true in all trigeminal neuralgia sufferers and so we could feel confident that this is diagnostic. However, if a sufferer with a particular type of dental disease, e.g. pulpitis, tells you that he gets the same sort of pain and you know he does not have trigeminal neuralgia, then you may begin to doubt the reliability of this symptom in making the diagnosis. You would then say that the test was sensitive for trigeminal neuralgia, but not specific for the disorder because it is also a symptom of a dental condition.

Below is an example taken from Drangsholt and Trueloves's paper on diagnostic criteria for trigeminal neuralgia (2001), which shows that a single question can be fairly diagnostic of trigeminal neuralgia and definitely differentiate it from common dental disease:

DO YOU HAVE ELECTRIC SHOCK - LIKE, STABBING OR SHOOTING PAINS THAT ONLY LAST SECONDS UP TO ONE MINUTE?

Compared 100 trigeminal neuralgia patients and 1000 with pulpitis (dental) pain

	TN present	TN absent	Total
Test positive	99	200	299
Test negative	1	800	801
Total subjects	100	1000	1100
Sensitivity			0.99
Specificity			0.80
Likelihood ratio of a positive finding			4.95
Likelihood of a negative finding			0.0125

False positive and negative results

There will be a proportion of patients in whom the test result will suggest a positive finding and yet they do not have the disease. Conversely, patients will get a negative result and yet in some cases will, in fact, have the disease. This is particularly important in tests to diagnose cancer. You have no doubt heard of people who were told they had cancer and did not and others who were told they did not have cancer and yet had it.

Confusion arises when these terms positive and negative results are used in a different context. A patient who has had an MRI may be told he has a positive result. He needs to ask what that positive result relates to, e.g. positive for a blood vessel compressing the nerve or for multiple sclerosis. In like manner, when told a test is negative, the patient must inquire what it is negative for, since it could still be showing other disease, e.g. positive for multiple sclerosis but negative for a compression of the nerve.

Many patients have tests performed with little thought given to their relevance, both in terms of diagnosis and monitoring. Studies with physicians have shown that when physicians are asked to categorize their tests into essential, desirable and routine, the highest yield of abnormal results is in those classified as essential. In fact, some investigators have suggested that investigations were important in making a diagnosis in only 13 % of patients.

2. WHAT BLOOD TESTS DO PATIENTS WITH TRIGEMINAL NEURALGIA REQUIRE?

There are relatively few investigations needed for patients with trigeminal neuralgia; thus patients do not need to be concerned when the doctor does not order plenty of tests. Other patients, on the other hand, will get a battery of tests as illustrated in this patient's story:

"**Results of CT, MRIs, EMGs (tests of muscle function), EEG (electrocardiograph), lumbar puncture and blood work all were unremarkable. The neurologist said, 'You don't have MS today. Maybe you could have it tomorrow, but for now you don't have MS'.... Fourteen months later, in 1996, I was diagnosed as having definite Multiple Sclerosis. The diagnosis was made strictly on clinical changes over time such as increased reflexes, paresthesias, pain, tingling, numbness, etc.**"

If the medical history suggests that a patient may be suffering from a disease that may affect the trigeminal neuralgia or its management, then tests need to be done. Some of the drugs used in the management of trigeminal neuralgia can have an effect on the blood, liver, kidneys or salt distribution. Tests need to be done so these changes are identified prior to causing symptoms as shown in the table. These may include the following:

Table 1

TESTS THAT MAY BE REQUIRED WHEN PATIENTS ARE TAKING MEDICATIONS	
Name of test	Checking
Hemoglobin and full blood count	Changes in white blood cell counts and presence of anemia
Serum levels of Vitamin B12 and folic acid	Correct levels of vitamin folic acid and B12
Urea and electrolytes	Kidney functioning well and distribution of sodium is appropriate
Liver function tests	Changes in the functioning of the liver

These tests often need to be done at the start of treatment and in the initial phases of management. In some instances, it is also useful to measure the level of drug in the blood to ensure that adequate levels are achieved.

3. WHAT TESTING OF FUNCTION OF THE TRIGEMINAL NERVE IS NEEDED?

Sensory testing

Examination of a sufferer with potential trigeminal neuralgia includes testing the trigeminal nerve for its sensory and motor functions (see Chapter 2 for further explanation). This is done in a crude way by asking the patients if they can, for instance, feel a light touch or pin prick. However, this method will not be sensitive enough to pick up a subtle dysfunction of a nerve and will not give the doctor an idea of which type of nerve fiber is not functioning.

Accurate sensory testing is complex and time consuming, and is not used in routine clinical practice. However, if medical history and physical examination suggest there are differences in sensation in different parts of the nerve, then it is important to carry out these tests. These tests, known as neurophysiological tests, are carried out by experts.

One of these is called quantitative sensory testing (QST) and is defined as an analysis of perception in response to external stimuli of controlled intensity. Detection and pain thresholds are determined by applying a stimulus to the skin in an ascending and descending order of magnitude. Specially designed equipment is used, which ensures the stimulus intensity is always the same.

QST provides some form of objective test of the functioning of the trigeminal nerve. These tests are especially useful in cases where nerve damage has occurred, since they can be helpful in establishing the extent of the damage and monitoring progress. Researchers evaluated the use of QST in 30 patients with trigeminal neuralgia who had undergone surgery, and found that even after microvascular decompression, sensory loss can occur. The tests are time consuming to perform, the equipment is expensive and they have not been fully validated because of a lack of a gold standard. The names of the tests and the fibers they are testing are shown in the table on the following page. The role of the fibers is summarized in Chapter 2

Table 2

TESTING OF THE SENSORY FUNCTIONS OF THE TRIGEMINAL NERVE			
Fibers	Sensation	Clinical test	QST test
A beta	Touch	Cotton wool	Von Frey's hairs
	Vibration	Tuning fork	Vibrameter
A delta	Pinprick sharp pain	Neurological pin	Weighted needles
	cold	Thermorollers	thermotest
C	Warming	Themorollers	thermotest
	Burning		

Testing of the nerve of hearing, eighth cranial nerve is sometimes done during posterior fossa surgery to avoid damage to the nerve of hearing.

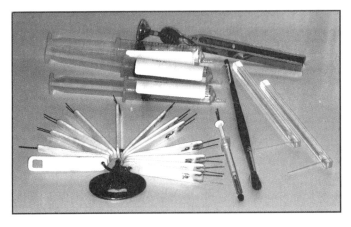

This photograph shows some of the equipment that is used to test sensation.

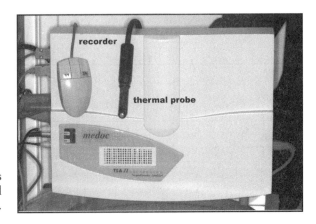

This photograph shows a computer thermal testing machine.

Reflexes

The speed at which a person blinks when the cornea is touched, or moves the jaw when the chin is tapped, is termed a reflex. The trigeminal blink reflex and jaw reflex have been found to be normal in patients with trigeminal neuralgia, but abnormal in patients with symptomatic trigeminal neuralgia, such as that caused by tumors. This may therefore be a useful test. It should be performed by a neurophysiologist.

Laser evoked potentials

These tests assess the ability of a nerve to respond to a painful stimulus. They have been proven to be useful in assessing damaged nerves, but they are currently available only in a few medical centers.

4. WHY MEASURE PAIN QUALITY AND PAIN INTENSITY?

Pain intensity and quality are subjective and therefore difficult to quantify, particularly when comparing different pain conditions. However, some attempt needs to be made to measure it. Unless pain has in some way been measured, it cannot be said to be relieved. Pain measurement is also necessary for assessing factors that affect the pain and to monitor treatment of patients who do not experience complete pain relief.

Pain can be measured in different dimensions, using questionnaires and clinical tests. These also need to be tested for validity (does the test truly measure what it purports to measure?) and reliability (are all the items in the test measuring the same idea and will the test give the same results if repeated on different occasions?).

As with other tests, the specificity and sensitivity need to be determined. That is, how accurately and exclusively does the test identify the characteristics you are interested in? This is why just making up a few questions and administering them is not a valid test, and why these questionnaires are difficult and time consuming to develop.

The use of self-complete questionnaires that have been well validated means that the doctor can have a standard against which the patient can be compared with other patients, and with themselves again when undergoing treatment. Most of the questionnaires are easy to complete, although some may be long. Scoring can be simple, although at times it is complex and special skills are required to interpret the responses. Patients would do well to bring these completed forms to their consultation as additional material to their story. The British Pain

Society Web site provides pain assessment questionnaires in a number of languages.

Pain can be measured in a number of ways:

Visual Analog Scale (VAS)

Self-reported pain measurement, using a 10 cm visual analog scale, is the most widely applied method of measuring pain intensity and has proven sensitive in detecting small changes. It can be done simply by using pen and paper or utilizing small specially designed rulers as shown in the illustration below. The Brief Pain Inventory (BPI), shown in the appendix 1, includes a VAS for pain intensity and has been validated across different cultures and languages, but has not been specifically evaluated in neuropathic pain. It has been recommended by the European Neurologists Association that both intensity and unpleasantness assessed on a VAS should be measured in all patients with **neuropathic** pain, both at baseline (start of treatment) and in assessing the outcome of treatments.

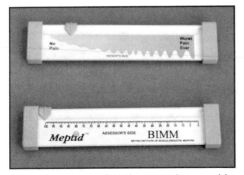

A visual analog scale. The top side is used by the patient, whereas the lower picture shows the reverse side with the scores.

Verbal Rating Scale (VRS)

This can easily be converted to a Visual Analogue Scale (VAS) if the sufferers rate the intensity of their pain on a scale of one to ten. These scales can be used for intensity, unpleasantness or even the amount of relief from pain after treatment. Scales of this type are called undimensional, since they only measure one aspect of the pain.

McGill Pain Questionnaire (MPQ)

To overcome the problem of only measuring one aspect of pain, Melzack introduced the MPQ, which provides data not just on the sensory aspect of the pain, but also the way it affects the emotions. It is one of the most frequently used ones in pain medicine. A short form of it is also used especially in clinical trials. Both these scales have been translated into various languages.

Below is shown part of the MPQ. The first ten groups of words are called "sensory" words. They describe the sensation of pain itself. The next group (10 – 15) describes what the feeling is doing to the person. Group 16 provides an overall evaluation of the pain, and the last groups are a miscellaneous group. The MPQ has been used to differentiate different types of orofacial pain (Melzack et al 1986).

MCGILL PAIN QUESTIONNAIRE

NAME: DATE:

Circle the word that describes how your pain feels right now:

Mild
Discomforting
Distressing
Horrible
Excruciating

Circle the words below that best described your current pain.
Use only <u>one word</u> in each group.
Leave out any group if the words are unsuitable.

1	2	3	4
Flickering	Jumping	Pricking	Sharp
Quivering	Flashing	Boring	Cutting
Pulsing	Shooting	Drilling	Lacerating
Throbbing		Stabbing	
Beating		Lancinating	
Pounding			

5	6	7	8
Pinching	Tugging	Hot	Tingling
Pressing	Pulling	Burning	Itchy
Gnawing	Wrenching	Scalding	Smarting
Cramping		Searing	Stinging
Crushing			

9	10	11	12
Dull	Tender	Tiring	Sickening
Sore	Taut	Exhausting	Suffocating
Hurting	Rasping		
Aching	Splitting		
Heavy			

13	14	15	16
Fearful	Punishing	Wretched	Annoying
Frightful	Grueling	Blinding	Troublesome
Terrifying	Cruel		Miserable
	Vicious		Intense
	Killing		Unbearable

17	18	19	20
Spreading	Tight	Cool	Nagging
Radiating	Numb	Cold	Nauseating
Penetrating	Drawing	Freezing	Agonizing
Piercing	Squeezing		Dreadful
	Tearing		Torturing

Brief Pain Inventory (BPI)

This is used as a standard in pain clinics throughout the UK and is shown in appendix 1. A completed one by Mrs. G can be seen in Chapter 1. It measures both pain intensity and the effect it has on the quality of life of a patient.

Leeds assessment of Neuropathic Symptoms and Signs (LANSS)

More specific scales have been developed for measurement of neuropathic pain such as the LANSS, but they have not been fully validated. Others are still working on more sensitive scales that also incorporate quality of life.

Perceptual pain matching

This is a technique where patients are asked to indicate when the intensity of pain produced by an electrically evoked experimental pain instrument is equivalent to the intensity of orofacial pain that they experience. The perceptual painmatching instrument, PainMatcher™, is a portable experimental pain stimulator that produces a constant current stimulation, controlled by a microprocessor that provides rectangular pulses with a frequency of 10 Hz and an amplitude of 10 mA. Because of the electrical stimulation, patients with a pacemaker or cochlear implant should not use this device. Patients have total control over the device and can stop the procedure at any point. The patient starts the instrument by pinching it between the left forefinger and thumb. The patient records:

  (i)   the 'sensory threshold' (the first time they feel <u>any</u> sensation from the instrument)
  (ii) the 'pain threshold' (at the very first perception of any pain)
  (iii) a 'pain matching' score (when the intensity of the experimental pain is equivalent to the intensity of orofacial pain they experience)

The readings for each point are not displayed to the patient, but are revealed to the examiner on a 0-100 scale on the liquid crystal display screen. This form of pain assessment has been validated against other methods of experimental pain assessment and has been shown to be of particular value in standardizing pain measurements in multi-center studies. It has been used in facial and neuropathic pain, but not as a routine procedure.

5. What other factors should be measured?

There is no doubt that some other measures, apart from pain measurement, are needed, as quality of life must be the final aim of any treatment and so needs to be assessed. The ability of sufferers with trigeminal neuralgia to perform physically, mentally, emotionally and socially is impaired, so some assessment of sleep, mood, functional capacity and quality of life must be measured. The current scales used can deal with a range of issues e.g. Brief Pain Inventory SF 12, SF 36 Health Survey and Nottingham Health profile or they measure specific factors such as anxiety and depression, e.g. Hospital Anxiety and Depression (HAD) scale (appendix 2), The Beck Depression Scale and Pain Anxiety Symptom Scale.

Further details can be found in Dr. Toby Newton John's chapter in the book on **The Assessment and Management of Orofacial Pain.**

Table 3: Key facts

Examples of Pain assessments in clinical use	
Pain intensity	Visual analogue scale VAS
	Verbal rating scale VRS 0-10
	Brief Pain Inventory
Pain unpleasantness	Visual analogue scale
Emotional functioning – depression, anxiety, anger	Hospital anxiety and depression scale
	Beck depression inventory
	State trait anxiety
	Pain anxiety symptom scale
Quality of life and disability	SF12 or SF 36
	Brief Pain Inventory
	Nottingham Health Profile
	Multidimensional Pain Inventory
	Oral health impact profile
	Graded chronic pain scale
Coping skills – cognitive and behavioral	Coping strategies questionnaire
Beliefs about pain – self efficacy, **catastrophizing**, future health status	Pain self-efficacy scale
Family factors	Family impact questionnaire
Treatment goals	Treatment goals questionnaire
Health care usage	Number of appointments with health-care professional, use of medication

6. ARE X-RAYS OR CT SCANS NEEDED?

To eliminate possible local dental causes of pain, **intraoral** X-rays and **ortho pontomograms** (OPG) of the upper and lower jaws are required. These should be evaluated either by a dentist or an oral radiologist. This patient recounts "*my endodontist finally agreed my pain was not in line with an infected root and the X-rays were normal.*"

Occipito-mental and **posterior anterior** views of the skull are useful for investigating sinus disease, although other structural lesions can be detected on **computer tomography** (CT) scans.

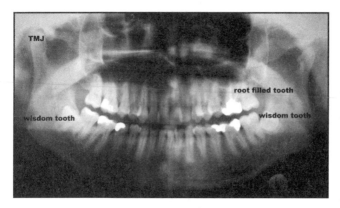

This is an orthopantomogram X-ray film. It shows unerupted lower wisdom teeth and an upper molar tooth which is root filled, all of which could cause oral pain.

What is computer tomography (CT)?

This is a sophisticated X-ray imaging procedure, which can produce pictures of a layer of the body at any depth. The detected images are then transferred to a computer. Sometimes referred to as CAT (acronym for computer axial tomography), it differs from the usual X-rays in that the images show the body in cross-sections and can reveal the internal organs.

After removal of all metal objects, the patient is asked to lie on a couch and the head is put into the machine as shown in the illustration below. The procedure can take 15- 45 minutes. In some cases the radiologists or radiography needs to inject a special dye (contrast medium)in order to provide greater detail of the internal structures. The dye is given by injection into a vein in the arm.

Anyone with a history of allergy or asthma needs to warn the staff, since they may get a reaction. The procedure results in as many as 30 images, which are then read by a **neuroradiologist** who provides a report. No one can be present in the room during the procedure because of the radiation, although the patients are monitored on closed circuit TV and there is an intercom system to aid communication.

A leaflet about this procedure can be downloaded or bought from the British Brain and Spine Foundation Web site (see the end of the chapter).

CT is useful in the diagnosis of certain tumors such as those of the nose and throat, but are often less effective for small posterior fossa **tumors** where the thick skull can make interpretation of the findings difficult. CT scans cannot differentiate between nerves and blood vessels and are not effective at picking up plaques such as are seen in patients with multiple sclerosis. CT scan relies on ionizing radiation, and this can be considerable when scanning the brain.

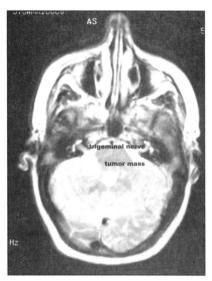

This CT scan shows a large tumor next to the trigeminal nerve.

CT scans should not be performed frequently in a patient.

7. WHAT IS MAGNETIC RESONANCE IMAGING (MRI) AND MAGNETIC TOMOGRAPHIC RESONANCE ANGIOGRAPHY (MRTA)?

These two investigations are the most frequently performed in patients with trigeminal neuralgia and they are getting increasingly more sophisticated in their ability to pick up abnormalities. MRI is a scanning procedure that uses a combination of a strong magnet, radio waves and a computer to produce detailed pictures of the inside of the body. It not only shows up the bones as do X-rays, but also details the brain, nerves, blood vessels, etc. More details on how the MRI works can be found on the Internet and at a Web site listed at the end of the chapter. Magnetic resonance tomographic angiography (MRTA) is the same as an MRI, but has been developed for use in patients with trigeminal neuralgia to image optimally the relationship of the nerve and the blood vessels in its vicinity.

In table 4 on the following page, I compare and contrast CT and MRI.

Table 4: Key facts

COMPARISON OF CT AND MRI		
	CT	MRI
Uses ionizing radiation	yes	no
Uses magnets and radio waves	no	yes
Safe and non invasive	no	yes
Repeated use is safe	no	yes
Uses computers to generate images	yes	yes
May be able to use if have any metal no implants such as hips, pacemakers	yes	
May need to use contrast medium (dye) to show up more structures	yes	yes not always
Essential to keep still for up to 45 minutes	no	yes
Excellent contrast between soft and hard tissue such as nerves and blood vessels	no	yes
dynamic	no	yes
Cost	Relatively low	High
Tolerated well by patients who are claustrophobic (fear of small places)	yes	no

An MRI is not suitable for everyone, and particular problems can arise in patients who have small metal implants or pacemakers, since these parts may move during the application of a magnetic field. Patients who are overweight need a so-called "Open Scanner." Some patients may find the procedure involved in the production of a high quality MRI scan difficult. When having an MRI scan done, a patient must keep very still, since any movement will distort the pictures.

Up to 30 % of patients may show evidence of severe anxiety that can affect the results. The anxiety can be related to factors such as claustrophobia, pain, fear of the unknown, as well as apprehension about what the test will show. Claustrophobia can be minimized by giving the patient better information about the procedure, teaching the patient relaxation techniques and using tranquilizers.

Many units will encourage patients to bring their favorite music, which can be played during the procedure. Someone else can be present in the room, provided they also have no metallic objects on their person. Some patients may be disconcerted by the loud tapping or knocking noises heard during parts of the imaging sequence.

Here is a patient's description of the process: *"My doctor arranges for an MRI the next day and the neurologist the next day. So here I am, nervous, scared of a recurrence, suffering a headache from worry and lack of sleep and they put me in the 'tube.' Nothing like a jackhammer and roller coaster chain clanking to calm you down. The MRI itself was tolerable. It was the visit next day..."*

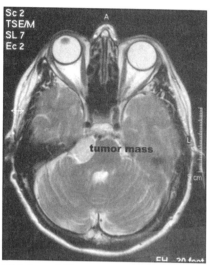

This is an MRI scan that shows a tumor mass next to the trigeminal nerve.

What are MRIs used for and how helpful are they?

MRIs are useful for the diagnosis of small tumors and for multiple sclerosis (MS). And so it is advocated that they should be routine for all patients with trigeminal neuralgia in order to detect the rare **symptomatic trigeminal neuralgia**. As this sufferer describes: *"He reviewed the two sets of MRIs I brought with me, confirmed what he saw as 'probable MS.'"*

Some centers, however, have long waiting lists for MRI scans, and their costs also limit their use. Neurosurgeons use MRI scans of patients with trigeminal neuralgia in order to look at the relationship between the trigeminal nerve and related blood vessels. MRI scans cannot be used to diagnose trigeminal neuralgia, since no comparisons have been done using patients with different types of facial pain, and with healthy controls using evaluations by neuroradiologists **blinded** to the condition and the side of the face that is in pain.

In order to achieve high quality results, neurosurgeons use special methods such as the MRTA, which are more sensitive to the flow of blood. This increases the chance of finding a true compression or dislocation of the nerve. Technology is advancing rapidly and the scans are getting more and more sensitive.

A review of the neuroradiological literature shows that there is not a single study that could be called ideal and from which a very precise sensitivity and specificity can be calculated as described above. Very few papers quote the **diagnostic** criteria that were used to assess the patients, and it may be that some patients who have negative results did not, in fact, have classical trigeminal neuralgia. Not all the studies used **controls.** Some used the other, **asymptomatic,** side of the same patient. In other studies, control patients have been drawn from those with no trigeminal symptoms, but who were being assessed for possible tumors of the **posterior fossa.**

In some studies the neuroradiologist is not blinded and is the only one making the diagnosis, as opposed to two neuroradiologists assessing the results independently. Not all patients who have an MRI decide to undergo surgical treatment, so there is no gold standard for these patients; no one has verified the findings by direct observation at surgery. Also, there is a lack of outcome data to evaluate whether these surgical findings result in relief of pain.

If no relief of pain is obtained after the operation, even though the MRI was deemed positive and a blood vessel was found, then it needs to be concluded that the compression of the nerve by the blood vessel was not the sole cause of the trigeminal neuralgia. Results from surgery do show that some patients do not get relief of pain after a **microvascular decompression.** No studies have taken into account the length of time the disease has been present, since it is expected that changes may occur over time. The severity of symptoms may also affect the MRI findings, since they could lead to a thinner nerve harder to visualize and also could result in irreversible damage to the nerve and hence a poor outcome.

Controls have not always been age matched, and if this is a vascular abnormality, this may be of relevance, since vascular compressions could be a feature of older people. Although MRI scans are occasionally ordered after surgery for patients who have failed to get pain relief, there is no study that has reported the use of MRI in all patients after surgery to see how the appearance of the MRI has altered. This is related to the cost and time involved in doing MRIs.

From the current literature, it would seem that MRI and MRTA provide vital information for the neurosurgeons. However, more carefully designed studies are essential, especially with better correlations between radiological findings, surgical findings and final outcomes.

Most studies have shown that it is highly unlikely that an MRI scan will reveal a blood vessel compressing the nerve that is not then found at operation, i.e. false positive. However, the opposite is more common — that no vessel is found compressing the nerve on MRI, but is found by the surgeon at operation, i.e. false negative. As one patient describes,

"My MRI showed no demyelenation and also showed the trigeminal nerve to be normal." Yet this patient benefited from microvascular decompression. This is why surgeons will operate on patients even when the MRI scan is negative, i.e. shows no evidence of nerve compression.

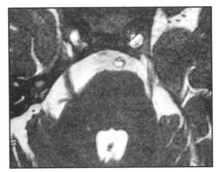

This is a special MRI scan that shows the trigeminal nerve compressed by a vessel.

What is functional magnetic resonance imaging (*f*MRI)?

Functional magnetic resonance imaging is a relatively new procedure that provides information not only about structure, as does the MRI, but also function, and there are several different forms of it. Further details of these can be found on the Internet and some Web sites are provided at the end of the chapter. This diagnostic procedure involves the same techniques as the MRI, but also maps brain activity.

When areas of the brain become active, they exhibit increased metabolic activity, evidenced by increased blood flow, among other things. It will show all the areas of the brain that are activated by different sensations or activities, including thoughts, and thus it maps not just the body but also the mind, showing how intertwined these functions are. However, these latter tests may be affected by the environment in which the tests have to be done, i.e. lying still in a large drum-like apparatus as described in the section on MRI.

The patient is put into the large opening in the machine and scanned, and then is asked, for example, to move a finger or look at a picture. The patient is then scanned again while performing this activity. A whole series of scans are performed while the activity is taking place and the first set of baseline images is subtracted from the second, and the areas that are most visible in the resulting image are presumed to have been activated by the task.

It will reveal how different parts of the brain are being activated at different times during the activity. By performing specific tasks that correspond to different functions, it is possible to locate the corresponding area of the brain that governs the function. Injuries and diseases can cause a change in function and these tests can be used to determine more accurately the causes of the disease, as well as to predict outcomes.

These techniques are now being used not just by neurologists and neurosurgeons, but also by pain physicians and psychiatrists. Experimental work has shown that in patients with chronic neuropathic pain, the thalamus on the opposite side from the pain has a decreased blood flow. But in patients with provoked neuropathic pain, such as trigeminal neuralgia triggered by touch, the blood flow to the thalamus and other parts of the brain is increased. This suggests that once an improved understanding is obtained about brain function during pain, treatments could be made more specific. The effects of drug administrations thus could be monitored to see if they are reaching those parts of the brain that are affected.

These techniques are also being used by psychologists to unravel the psychological functioning of the brain. Some experiments have shown how different parts of the brain become activated in the presence of a partner sitting next to a subject undergoing a painful stimulus. How the partner responds to the subject further influences which areas of the brain are activated.

Since these techniques are generally non-invasive, they can be performed on upgraded conventional MRI scanners, and are less expensive than the other techniques described below. Therefore, they have a greater chance of becoming available in most hospitals over the next several years. This is a rapidly expanding field and holds great promise for broadening understanding of the mechanisms involved in trigeminal neuralgia, since it could unravel the neurocircuitry and the metabolic pathways involved. Hopefully in the near future it will be possible to map which areas of the brain are activated during an attack of trigeminal neuralgia. Also it may be possible to determine whether different areas are activated in sufferers with atypical trigeminal neuralgia, what drugs have the greatest effects, what the effect of surgery is and whether future attacks of pain can be predicted.

It will also be possible to demonstrate the relationship between trigeminal neuralgia, depression and other psychological responses and how these affect response to treatment. Considerable research is needed in this area and tests, such as described at the beginning of the chapter, are needed before answers can be obtained to the questions I have raised.

8. What is Positron Emission Tomography (PET)?

Positron emission tomography (PET) is an examination that shows the chemical functioning of organs and tissues in contrast to the other techniques mentioned above, which only show the structure of organs and tissues.

PET is particularly useful for the detection of cancer, coronary artery disease and brain disease. The process involves obtaining images based on the detection of positrons. Positrons are tiny particles emitted from a radioactive substance administered to the patient. Before the examination begins, a radioactive substance is produced in a machine called a cyclotron and attached to a natural body compound, most commonly glucose. Once this substance is administered to the patient, the radioactivity localizes in the appropriate areas of the body and is detected by the PET scanner as different colored images. Tissues that use more glucose, such as cancers, will pick up more of the radioactivity and so appear brighter.

The procedure does expose patients to relatively large radiation doses and it remains very much a research tool. It is also expensive; thus as fMRI develops, it may become less useful. There are only a handful of reports on the use of it in facial pain.

9. What is thermography?

Thermography, or digital infrared thermal imaging, is a non-invasive, safe tool that does not involve ionizing radiation. It enables the examiner to visualize and quantify changes in skin surface temperature. It utilizes two pieces of equipment. One is an infrared scanning device that converts infrared radiation emitted from the skin surface into electrical impulses that are then visualized on a monitor. This color visual image is called a thermograph.

The systems measure temperatures ranging from 10° C - 55° C to an accuracy of 0.1° C., but is very sensitive to room temperature and is a time-consuming procedure. Since the images are stored on a computer, they can be statistically analyzed.

This technique has been reported in patients with a variety of neurological and vascular conditions, but there are few high quality reports evaluating its use in facial pain. Given other investigations that are now becoming available, thermography probably is of limited use in trigeminal neuralgia.

MRS. G CASE STUDY

Mrs. G's examination did not show any neurological deficit. The medical history and examination also do not suggest any evidence of multiple sclerosis or other underlying neurological condition. The attacks of pain have become more severe and difficult to control and the doses of medication have been raised significantly.

What investigations does Mrs. G need?
Differentiate which investigations would be useful for research purposes.

Discussion

1. An assessment of the pain intensity and its effects on quality of life are needed, and the results of these are shown in Chapter 1.
2. Blood tests are needed to show that the high level of drugs are not having an effect on the liver (liver function tests), the white cell count and the distribution of sodium (electrolytes).
3. Sensory testing QST and laserevoked potentials would be useful for research purposes.
4. Dental X-rays would help rule out any dental cause for the pain.
5. MRI scans of the posterior fossa, with the neuroradiologist being blinded to the side on which the trigeminal neuralgia is present. The result of the MRI scan is shown in the section on MRI. There was no evidence of a tumor or multiple sclerosis.
6. fMRI would provide some clues as to the functioning of the trigeminal nerve, but this remains a research tool at present.

10. WHAT RESEARCH IS NEEDED?

- Improved sensitive, validated scales to measure neuropathic pain and its effect on quality of life are urgently needed, since they provide the basis for all treatment evaluations.
- A simple sensitive tool to quantify pain would be extremely useful. Measurement of QST and laserevoked potentials provide details on the functioning of the trigeminal nerve, but they are still not well validated for use in trigeminal neuralgia.
- Evaluation of MRI as a diagnostic tool for trigeminal neuralgia is required and this needs to be done by comparison with other patients with other types of facial pain, healthy controls and even patients with tumors of the eighth nerve using two **blinded** radiologists.
- There is no doubt that among the investigations currently available, the future lies in *f* MRI, which provides details not only on structure but also on function. Extensive research is needed beginning with obtaining baseline data on sufferers with trigeminal neuralgia and then looking at the effects of interventions ranging from medical, surgical and psychological.

This technique has enormous potential for future trigeminal neuralgia sufferers, since it may hold clues to the cause of trigeminal neuralgia.

SUMMARY

- Pain assessment and quality of life must be recorded with the use of well validated scales such as the visual analogue scale and Brief Pain Inventory.
- Blood tests are needed to assess the effects of medication on the liver, electrolytes and blood.
- MRI scans will rule out the presence of tumors and multiple sclerosis and show the presence of a compression of the trigeminal nerve.
- CT scans can be used to detect tumors, but not evidence of compression and therefore have a limited use in trigeminal neuralgia.
- Sensory testing, thermography and PET scanning remain experimental procedures.
- Functional MRI provide details both of structure and function of the brain and open up exciting prospects for the diagnosis and management of trigeminal neuralgia.
- Research needs to concentrate on fMRI.

FURTHER READING AND REFERENCES

Web sites

Accessed April 2005

The Brain and Spine Foundation has patient information leaflets on MRI and CT scanning, which can either be ordered or downloaded from their Web site at http://www.brainandspine.org.uk/

How Stuff Works is a lay Web site that explains the mechanisms behind tests such as MRI and CAT on
http://electronics.howstuffworks.com/mri.htm
http://science.howstuffworks.com/cat-scan.htm

Radiology information resources for patients, *RadiologyInfo* is designed to answer questions related to the many radiological procedures and therapies for patients. http://www.radiologyinfo.org/content/functional_mr.htm

Many universities also have their dedicated web sites, which can be found through a search of Google, using the terminology used in the chapter.

Multilingual pain assessment questionnaires can be printed off from the British Pain Society's Web site at
http://www.britishpainsociety.org/pain_scales.html

Books

Newton-John T Measurement of Pain in Adults (2002) In **Assessment and Management of Orofacial Pain** Zakrzewska, JM & Harrison, SD (Ed) Elsevier Vol 14 in Series on Pain Research and Clinical Management London ISBN 0444509844 pp 87-104

References

Bowsher D, Miles J B, Haggett C E and Eldridge P R (1997) Trigeminal Neuralgia: a Quantitative Sensory Perception Threshold Study in Patients Who Had Not Undergone Previous Invasive Procedures. *J Neurosurg* **86**:190-192.

Cruccu G, Anand P, Attal N, Garcia-Larrea L, Haanpaa M, Jorum E, Serra J and Jensen TS. (2004) EFNS Guidelines on Neuropathic Pain Assessment. *Eur J Neurol.*11:153-62.

Drangsholt M and Truelove E. (2001) Trigeminal Neuralgia Mistaken As Temporomandibular Disorder. *J Evid Base Dent Pract* 1:41-50.

Hampf G, Bowsher D, Wells C and Miles J (1990) Sensory and Autonomic Measurements in Idiopathic Trigeminal Neuralgia Before and After Radiofrequency Thermocoagulation: Differentiation From Some Other Causes of Facial Pain [See Comments]. *Pain* 40:241-248.

Jaaskelainen SK. (2004) Clinical Neurophysiology and Quantitative Sensory Testing in the Investigation of Orofacial Pain and Sensory Function. *J Orofac Pain.* 18:85-107.

Meaney JF, Eldridge P R, Dunn L T, Nixon T E, Whitehouse G H and Miles J B (1995) Demonstration of Neurovascular Compression in Trigeminal Neuralgia With Magnetic Resonance Imaging. Comparison With Surgical Findings in 52 Consecutive Operative Cases. *J Neurosurg* 83:799-805.

Melzack R, Terrence C, Fromm G and Amsel R (1986) Trigeminal Neuralgia and Atypical Facial Pain: Use of the McGill Pain Questionnaire for Discrimination and Diagnosis. *Pain* 27:297-302.

Zakrzewska JM (2002) Diagnosis and Differential Diagnosis of Trigeminal Neuralgia. *Clin J Pain* 18:14-21.

APPENDIX 1
BRIEF PAIN INVENTORY (SHORT FORM)

FORM 3.2 **Brief Pain Inventory**

Date____ / ____ / ____   Time:_____

Name: _____ _____
                   Last   First   Middle Initial

1) Throughout our lives, most of us have had pain from time to time (such as minor headaches, sprains, and toothaches). Have you had pain other than these everyday kinds of pain today?
   1. Yes   2. No

2) on the diagram shade in the areas where you feel pain. Put an X on the area that hurts the most.

3) Please rate your pain by circling the one number that best describes your pain at its **worst** in the past 24 hours.
   0   1   2   3   4   5   6   7   8   9   10
   No   pain as bad as
   pain   you can imagine

4) Please rate your pain by circling the one number that best describes your pain at its **least** in the past 24 hours.
   0   1   2   3   4   5   6   7   8   9   10
   No   pain as bad as
   pain   you can imagine

5) Please rate your pain by circling the one number that best describes your pain on the **average**
   0   1   2   3   4   5   6   7   8   9   10
   No   pain as bad as
   pain   you can imagine

6) Please rate your pain by circling the one number that tells how much pain you have **right now**.
   0   1   2   3   4   5   6   7   8   9   10
   No   pain as bad as
   pain   you can imagine

7) What treatments or medications are you receiving for your pain?
   _____
   _____

8) In the Past 24 hours, how much **relief** have pain treatments or medications provided? Please circle the one percentage that most shows how much releif you have received
   0% 10 20 30 40 50 60 70 80 90 100%
   No   Complete
   relief   relief

9) Circle the one number that describes how, during the past 24 hours, pain has **interfered** with your:
   A. General activity

   0   1   2   3   4   5   6   7   8   9   10
   Does not   Completely
   interfere   interferes

   B. Mood

   0   1   2   3   4   5   6   7   8   9   10
   Does not   Completely
   interfere   interferes

   C. Walking ability

   0   1   2   3   4   5   6   7   8   9   10
   Does not   Completely
   interfere   interferes

   D. Normal work (includes both work outside the home and housework

   0   1   2   3   4   5   6   7   8   9   10
   Does not   Completely
   interfere   interferes

   E. Relations with other people

   0   1   2   3   4   5   6   7   8   9   10
   Does not   Completely
   interfere   interferes

   F. Sleep

   0   1   2   3   4   5   6   7   8   9   10
   Does not   Completely
   interfere   interferes

   G. Enjoyment of life

   0   1   2   3   4   5   6   7   8   9   10
   Does not   Completely
   interfere   interferes

Source: Pain Research Group, Department of Neurology, University of Wisconsin-Madison.
Used with permission. May be duplicated and used in clinical practice.

APPENDIX 2
THE HOSPITAL ANXIETY AND DEPRESSION SCALE

HAD Scale

Name: Date:

Doctors are aware that emotions play an important part in most illnesses. If your doctor knows about these feelings he will be able to help you more.
This questionnaire is designed to help your doctor to know how you feel. Read each item and place a firm tick in the box opposite the reply which comes closest to how you have been feeling in the past week.
Don't take too long over your replies: your immediate reaction to each item will probably be more accurate than a long thought-out response.

Tick only one box in each section

I feel tense or 'wound up':
Most of the time
A lot of the time
Time to time, Occasionally
Not at all

I feel as if I am slowed down:
Nearly all the time
Very often
Sometimes
Not at all

I still enjoy the things I used to enjoy:
Definitely as much
Not quite so much
Only a little
Hardly at all

I get a sort of frightened feeling like 'butterflies' in the stomach:
Not at all
Occasionally
Quite often
Very often

I get a sort of frightened feeling as if something awful is about to happen:
Very definitely and quite badly
Yes, but not too badly
A little, but it doesn't worry me
Not at all

I have lost interest in my appearance:
Definitely
I don't take so much care as I should
I may not take quite as much care
I take just as much care as ever

I can laugh and see the funny side of things:
As much as I always could
Not quite so much now
Definitely not so much now
Not at all

I feel restless as if I have to be on the move:
Very much indeed
Quite a lot
Not very much
Not at all

Worrying thoughts go through my mind:
A great deal of the time
A lot of the time
From time to time but not too often
Only occasionally

I look forward with enjoyment to things:
As much as ever I did
Rather less than I used to
Definitely less than I used to
Hardly at all

I feel cheerful:
Not at all
Not often
Sometimes
Most of the time

I get sudden feelings of panic:
Very often indeed
Quite often
Not very often
Not at all

I can sit at ease and feel relaxed:
Definitely
Usually
Not often
Not at all

I can enjoy a good book or radio or TV programme:
Often
Sometimes
Not often
Very seldom

Do not write below this line

CHAPTER 5

CREATING MORE EFFECTIVE PATIENT CARE

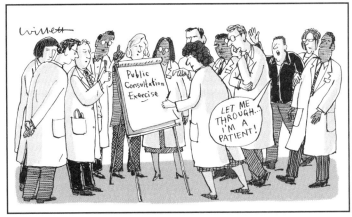

Health care workers sometimes forget that the patient should remain at the center of care.

"I am realizing that my neurologist does NOT have all the answers about every single question I might have regarding newer medicines on the market. It is MY responsibility to inform HIM of what's happening, to be articulate and as descriptive as possible, to add to his/her fountain of information, so that they have it for the next person. They will NEVER admit this, but I think they're counting on us to give them accurate feedback, as this is added to their body of knowledge. In that sense, each of us TN sufferers can teach our doctors, respectfully exchanging information and receiving it."

1. WHAT IS PATIENT-CENTERED CARE AND WHY IS IT IMPORTANT?

Health care for the 21st century must undergo transformation and the major change is in the patient's role in the process, according to Muir Gray, writing in his book, **The Resourceful Patient.**

At present it is assumed that the doctor is the responsible person and the patient is incompetent and in need of care, as described in this episode:

"I am a <u>person</u> first, after all, a person with pain, not a pain patient with an incidental personality. I told him I didn't want to take that one. That made him angry, and at that point, he got short and said, 'Then why don't you go call a surgeon?' That was probably the single most upsetting moment of my entire TN ordeal. Here was someone who should be an important team-mate and my top resource for information basically firing me for not doing exactly what he said without question. I felt abandoned."

There is growing consensus that some patients want to and should become more involved in all aspects of their health care. Patients have become experienced consumers who understand they have rights and have become less inclined to leave all the medical decisions to the doctors.

Patients' autonomy, which is what the competent informed patient wants, is more important than what the doctor thinks best for the patient. Muir Gray promotes the "concept of the resourceful patients, namely the patient who is not only aware of his rights, but is also made aware of his responsibilities and is willing to accept them, provided of course, he is given the resources to do so."

Patient involvement in care leads to better health outcomes not only in terms of reducing the severity of symptoms, but also in terms of improved life control activity and improved resourcefulness and life satisfaction. People who have life-long diseases such as diabetes know that they have to live with and manage with occasional help from a professional. In the United States, where patients have traditionally had to manage more of their care, including its payment, self-management programs have been studied and promoted for many years. The Chronic Disease Self-Management Program at Stanford University is an example of this.

In the UK, the Department of Health produced a report on these approaches to chronic disease management called "The Expert Patient," which is described in more detail in Chapter 12. Muir Gray predicts, "The expert patient with the chronic disease will not need a guide in future. Patients will find their own way to better health."

Further evidence of the importance of the patient in health care is a documented on the UK Department of Health Web site entitled, "Patient–Led Learning for the Clinical Professions: Fulfilling the Information Needs of Patients."

If patients are to manage their care they need to:
- be involved in identifying the issues or choices they need to make, e.g. drugs or surgical techniques to be used in treating trigeminal neuralgia
- know that the evidence on which to base their care is of good quality; systematic reviews and randomized control trials are the ideals, but lower quality evidence may need to be used (covered later in the chapter)
- obtain the information in a form that is accessible with minimum of bias, e.g. risks and benefits need to be highlighted
- have genuine choice, free of medical bias, as illustrated by these patients' comments:

"When I saw you, I was ready to have the operation there and then; I was ready to sign up, do you remember that? You said, go away and think about it."

"A neurologist prescribed three different medications and told me to experiment with combinations until I found the right match to control my pain."

- develop a partnership with their health care practitioner.

Patient-centered care ensures that negotiated treatment plans are decided upon; these are discussed in detail in Chapter 8 on decision making. It is therefore the patients' responsibility to reflect on what outcomes they would like from treatment so they can inform their treating health care professional. Some of these are listed in Table 1 below.

Table 1

QUESTIONS TO REFLECT UPON WHEN SEEKING TREATMENT
• What are the most important results you hope to receive from this treatment? • Are you expecting a complete cure or just relief of pain for a while? • How much reduction in suffering would be acceptable if complete reduction of pain were not possible? • Are you looking for rapid results or are you prepared to accept a slow change? • How important is your quality of life and how much can this be compromised to achieve better pain control? • How important is it to you to improve your physical and mental functioning? What help do you need to develop active coping skills?

As the table on the previous page highlights, health care for chronic diseases is not just about having one treatment and hoping that it will result in a complete cure. Many illnesses are described in physical terms and treated by physical means and yet they also have a considerable psychological impact, especially if they are chronic.

Trigeminal neuralgia is a difficult condition to classify, since it can be in some sufferers an acute condition that is treated surgically and results in lifelong relief of pain, but in others it is a truly chronic condition with, at best, some periods of no pain. Thus many trigeminal neuralgia sufferers need to change their concepts and understanding of this disease and accept that this may be a chronic long-term condition for some. They need to use treatments that deal with symptoms in a medical way, but they also need to take a more holistic view that can lead to improved pain control over a longer period of time. Many of these are described in Chapter 7.

Patients need to feel comfortable about talking to their health care provider, not just about the medical aspects of the disease but also the psychological aspects of their care and so patient-centered care begins with the patient-centered interview.

It is well recognized that patients consult for many different reasons, e.g. diagnosis and treatment of disease, relief of anxiety and validation of illness. The relationship that is built up between doctor and patient can be an ever-changing one. In his famous book, *The Doctor, the Patient and his Illness,* Balint suggests the following stages occur during consultations:
- the doctor and the patient develop an emotional relationship during the consultation;
- both doctor and patient have the power to influence the other;
- this power could be used for good or ill;
- collusion can develop between doctor and patient about which problems will be recognized and which will not;
- power flows between doctor and patient.

2. HOW TO CHOOSE THE BEST HEALTH CARE PROFESSIONAL FOR MANAGEMENT OF TRIGEMINAL NEURALGIA?

Reading through patients' stories of their disease and progression, one of the commonest emotions expressed is that of fear. This includes fear of return of pain, e.g. *"I live with the fear daily that it may return,"* fear of lack of further treatments, e.g. *"I was terrified because nothing was working. I was taking more and more and more of the pills and I* wanted to kill myself. I got to the point where I had so little quality of life," fear of the effects from treatments, e.g. *"I have taken medicine for 50 years, what is it doing to my kidneys and liver and all that? I might have liver failure by the time I'm 70 or 75." "It's not the thought of dying on the table; it's the thought of something going wrong, being paralyzed - being the worst position."*

Psychologists have shown us that fear increases pain, and I wonder how many of these sufferers actually discussed these issues with their health care providers in order to reduce their fears.

Comments such as the following, found in patients' stories sent to me about their experiences with doctors, suggest that some health care providers have not made patients feel heard and understood:

- *"You can't talk to the doctors; they haven't got time. They really aren't interested in your little problem."*
- *"The neurosurgeon just doesn't care if you are able to function at your job, let alone your quality of life."*
- *"I felt fear because none of the doctors were telling me anything and that made me frightened. I needed more information."*
- Another sufferer said, *"You need a doctor who will listen to you, work with you and is willing to learn with you."*

As Coulehan et al (2002) stress, empathy, i.e. the ability to "connect "with a patient in a deep sense, to listen and to pay attention, lies at the very heart of medical practice. This is one of the prime qualities that patients should be looking for in their doctor. This can, in part, be judged from the way the doctor takes the history at the first encounter, which is described in Chapter 1. Do they use words and statements that facilitate empathy, such as:

- Tell me a little more
- What has it been like for you?
- Hmmm … (and remaining silent and listening)
- Let me see if I have this right …
- That sounds very difficult …
- Anyone in your situation would feel like that …
- I can imagine that this might feel …

Some of the qualities patients are looking for are summarized in Table 2 on the following page.

Table 2: Key facts

WHAT QUALITIES ARE PATIENTS LOOKING FOR WHEN THEY CHOOSE THEIR HEALTH CARE PROVIDER?

Patients look for doctors who:
- want to do the best for the patient, not just for their own satisfaction
- are empathic, i.e. willing to listen and pay attention and take into account the effect the illness has on the patient and his or her community
- inspire confidence (One patient commented, *"I would much rather go to THE neurologist who does trigeminal neuralgia rather than muck around going here and there."*)
- are willing to question their own management
- have readily available sources of information about what does work
- are competent
- can be trusted

Another factor that may need to be considered when choosing a health care practitioner is personality type. Personality is a set of habits of perceiving, thinking, feeling and behaving. These can be assessed using a Myers-Briggs questionnaire and help to determine:
- How a person relates to others (either by Extraversion or Introversion)
- How a person takes in information (either by Sensing or Intuition)
- How a person makes decisions (either by Thinking or Feeling)
- How a person orders their life (either by Judging or Perceiving)

These personality types affect the way we communicate with others. If your style matches the person you are communicating with, it is likely that communication will go better than when there is more of a mismatch. Remember that not every patient wants the same style of consultation, and some doctors are willing to change their consultation styles, while others are less flexible.

Patients need to trust their doctors and feel confident in them, which is especially important when dealing with rare conditions as this sufferer expresses: *"The staff asked me to spell "trigeminal neuralgia. That didn't help my confidence level."*

The rarity of the condition means that most primary care practitioners will have limited knowledge, as indicated by this patient's comment: *"I was only my GP's (primary care doctor) second patient with TN and she wasn't absolutely sure, so I was very lucky she sent me to the hospital straight away because I don't think everyone's that lucky."*

Sufferers, therefore, inevitably need to see a specialist who has a particular interest in the condition. This is where support groups can be very helpful, since they often have lists of specialists and it can also be assumed that members of their medical advisory boards are also experts. Those who publish research papers are also highly likely to be experts. A study done in the US showed that, among surgeons, increased volume (5 or more microvascular decompression operations per year) correlated with improved results (Kalkanis et al 2003).

As mentioned above, it is essential that patients not only be given information but also the tools needed to interpret the information. They need to be able to take this information to their doctor and discuss it. No longer should the doctor be considered as a repository of knowledge, but more as a knowledge manager who can ask the right answer and then can help the patient interpret the knowledge that he has been given or has found himself.

However, providing knowledge to the patient is not sufficient, and the resourceful patient should not assume that the doctor is giving him the best knowledge. You, as a patient, need to make your own assessment of the quality and decide whether it is fit for the purpose. This next section may be fairly technical, but, if understood, will provide you with the skills to judge the available knowledge and thereby enable you to take an active role in your own management.

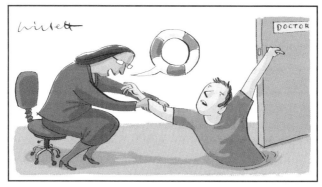

Due to the rarity of trigeminal neuralgia, it can be very difficult to find a specialist who knows how to manage the condition and when one is found, it can be a life saver.

3. HOW DO WE KNOW WHICH TREATMENTS MAY BE EFFECTIVE?

Ten years ago, going to three doctors and asking them how to manage trigeminal neuralgia would probably have yielded three very different answers, as most patients' accounts would suggest. Up until the late 1970s, only 15-20 % of medical practice was backed by scientifically and statistically sound research. Much medical practice had been based largely on intelligent guesswork and clinical experience and hence the varied answers.

According to Archie Cochrane, founder of the Cochrane Collaboration, you need to ask three key questions about a health care intervention:

- Can it work?
- Does it work in practice?
- Is it worth it?

It is impossible to interpret the results of one study in isolation; results from studies need to be critically appraised and put into context. Before the 1970s there was no systematic approach to assessing research and its effect on health care, and it was argued that patients were receiving substandard care as a result. All has changed and the Cochrane Library, published electronically, now contains systematic reviews on a very wide range of treatments. This library is open to everyone and has a special consumer section. It contains data on medical management of trigeminal neuralgia.

Despite this availability, not all doctors use these materials, so the next question to ask is whether the doctor practices evidence-based medicine and is interested in this condition?

As one sufferer pointed out, *"TN patients are not served well by doctors who are not very interested in this area of medicine. We need to 'interview' doctors and find out which ones we would be able to develop good respectful relationships with."*

Sackett defines evidence-based medicine as the "conscientious and judicious use of current best evidence from clinical care research in the management of individual patients." Evidence-based practice aims to move beyond anecdotal clinical experience by bridging the gap between research and the practice of medicine. It aims to use diagnostic tests and interventions that are as accurate, safe and efficacious as possible. The outcome measures of different clinical treatments are rigorously assessed and judged.

Evidence-based clinical decisions for the care of the patient therefore depend upon a blend of clinical expertise, research evidence and patient preferences. It places onus on practitioners to not only systematically record their clinical findings, but to make regular reference to studies, to critically examine them and, if proven of good quality, to incorporate them into practice. To help this process, a so-called hierarchy of evidence has been built up and this is illustrated in the diagram below. **We need to remember that absence of evidence is not evidence of no effect.**

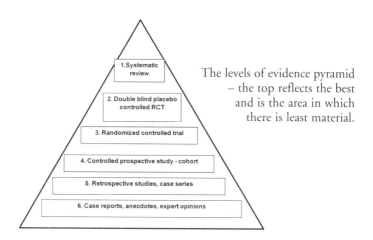

The levels of evidence pyramid – the top reflects the best and is the area in which there is least material.

The highest form of evidence is a **systematic review,** which, as its name implies, is a rigorous process of finding every single clinical study on the given topic, and then critically appraising this data and only using the high quality studies to make observations in terms of treatment. If enough high quality randomized controlled trials have been performed, then what is known as a **meta-analysis** of all the results can be performed.

This then provides an overview of the total treatment, and takes into account the fact that some trials may have had negative results and others may have shown positive results. You only then need to read this review. In the field of trigeminal neuralgia, the only meta-analysis that has been possible is on carbamazepine, since it is the only drug that has been the subject of three randomized controlled trials. Summaries of these analyses are often provided so that the whole document does not need to be read.

The next form of evidence is the high quality **randomized double-blind controlled trial** (RCT), which aims to reduce bias towards the new treatment being used by keeping both doctor and patient blinded as to which is the new treatment. Randomization means there is an equal chance in the two groups that things can be influenced by something you don't know about, as well as something you do know. For example, the results could be different if one group has HIV or you may assign more severe sufferers of trigeminal neuralgia to the new drug group rather than the **placebo** group.

More details about clinical trials are provided later in the chapter. In some cases, the doctor or patient may not have been blinded to the treatment, e.g. surgery or no surgery, and it is then called a randomized controlled trial. Currently there are several randomized controlled trials reported on drugs used in trigeminal neuralgia, and only three on peripheral surgical treatments or surgical management. Trials on surgical treatments are more difficult to design, but they are not impossible.

Controlled prospective studies or cohort studies are studies that have been planned in advance and follow patients for a longer period of time. The patients are no longer blinded to their treatment and all receive the same treatment. There are several of these types of studies reported in trigeminal neuralgia, both on the medical and surgical levels.

Retrospective studies or case series are those studies in which data is extracted from medical notes some time after they were first collected and then analyzed. The records are likely to be unreliable unless they were kept in a structured way and audited for their completeness. The investigators can also choose which records they want to use and thus can introduce considerable bias, e.g. leave out those patients who appear to have not responded well. Unfortunately, the bulk of surgical data for trigeminal neuralgia that we now have is of this type, and this makes the evidence for treatments weak.

Case reports and expert opinions are the lowest form of evidence. This is termed anecdotal evidence, in that it only reports on a small group of patients who could have been very carefully selected by the person reporting the results. A large proportion of treatments for trigeminal neuralgia belong to this category.

4. HOW TO FIND AND CRITICALLY APPRAISE
HIGH QUALITY EVIDENCE

Judging by the following comments made by patients, it is clear that they have realized the importance of obtaining healthcare information:
- *"I think it is useful to know how to use Medline, to have a tutorial on Medline and Pubmed and those sorts of things. ... we don't have access to the article, just the abstract, but it helps if we know how to navigate those."*
- *"If you have search terms and an author list. you can look up whatever you want to."*

Not only does the information need to be found, but, once found, it needs to be assessed both for quality and applicability and this is very complex even for health care professionals.

The following section is based on talks given by Dr Stephen Haines and me at the Trigeminal Neuralgia Association (TNA) Conference in San Diego in 2001, and compiled by Jillie Abbott, member of the executive committee of TNA UK. It is a short introduction to this area.

Where do you find high quality medical information?

Probably the best-known Web site for searching the medical literature is the service of the National Library of Medicine, Pub Med, which is available to everyone. It includes over 14 million citations for biomedical articles dating back to the 1950s.

PubMed includes links to many sites providing full text articles and other related resources, but not all of these are accessible to the general public. It is a searchable database that requires some experience to use. For example, typing in the words trigeminal neuralgia yields 4,500 references in August 2004, but in May 2005 the number rises to 4,658. But adding the words "and randomized controlled trial" reduces the yield to under 35 articles.

This, therefore, is not very effective. A search of the Cochrane Library, which contains systematic reviews and randomized controlled trials, may be a better source of information and will yield high quality evidence. It can also be useful to look for publications like Clinical Evidence and journals with titles that include the words "evidence based," since they often have short summarized articles many with comments by experts.

There are also sites that publish guidelines on diagnosis and management, and these are included at the end of the chapter and summarized in Table 3 below. Further information on how consumers can search the Internet for healthcare information is provided in Chapter 8.

Table 3: Key Facts

FINDING HIGH QUALITY DATA
Search: • Cochrane Library – database of systematic reviews and clinical trials   • Journals containing the word Evidence in their title, e.g. Clinical Evidence summarizes high quality data and often provide critical appraisal   • PubMed – database of millions of articles
Use articles from peer reviewed journals
Avoid promotional literature

What types of journals are you looking for?

You need to distinguish between primary and secondary sources and concentrate on primary sources. Peer reviewed journals are those whose editors ask other experts to read the articles and critically appraise them. The authors may then need to alter the articles in line with the comments made. The higher the standing of a journal, the more rigorous is this process.

The professional standing of the journal can be determined in part from what are called "impact factors," which are published yearly. The impact factor attempts to measure the way a journal's articles are used by other authors. The higher the number, the better the journal, although it must be remembered that specialty journals have lower impact factors because they have fewer issues and their articles are less frequently used.

The Lancet, New England Journal of Medicine, British Medical Journal and Journal of American Medical Association have the highest impact factors in the field of medicine. To be meaningful, one needs to look at impact factors of a group of journals containing similar articles, e.g. for articles on trigeminal neuralgia. These articles can be found in, among others, Neurosurgery, Journal of Neurosurgery, Brain, Journal of Neurology Neurosurgery and Psychiatry, Pain, Journal of Orofacial Pain and Cephalagia.

It is important not to rely on data from :
- pharmaceutical companies, since they are biased and aimed at selling drug products
- glossy medical magazines, which publish articles that are not peer reviewed and will probably have been heavily edited by the editor to make sure the content fits the image
- testimonials - they are not scientific information
- press releases and news reports – many of them jump the gun and are "selling" papers
- spurious Internet sites (These can be used to provide leads, but the information needs to be validated.)

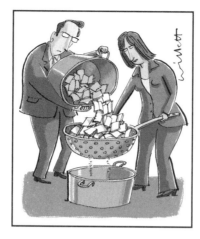

Although there is a vast amount of material to be found, only a very small percentage of it is of high quality and it needs to be carefully filtered out.

How do you screen (critically appraise) the articles you find?

The best screening device is, and will always be, your waste paper basket! There are a number of books that provide checklists for reading articles, or you can undergo a critical skills training program. Some of these are Web-based and are detailed at the end of the chapter.

Most papers should be organized along these lines, and the abstract (summary) at the start of the paper should have the same structure:
• Background (introduction)
• Aims and objective(s)
• Methods
• Results
• Discussion
• Conclusion

In Table 4 are the key features you need to ask about any medical paper:

Table 4: Key facts

WHAT TO LOOK FOR WHEN READING A MEDICAL PAPER

• Is there an abstract?
• Is the purpose of the paper clearly stated? Look for words like aims, hypothesis.
• Read the introduction - is it clear why the study is being done, what is known already?
• Have the authors chosen a good method to answer the question and described it adequately?
• Have the authors presented the results accurately?
• Have they made valid conclusions or have they over inflated the results?

Aims and objectives

The purpose of the paper should be stated as a question, e.g.,
- How is an accurate diagnosis of trigeminal neuralgia made?
- What is the prognosis of patients with anesthesia dolorosa?
- Does the Gamma knife cure trigeminal neuralgia?"

Method

When reading this section of a study, you need to determine whether the right method has been chosen to answer the question. The methods often fit under these three broad categories: diagnosis, prognosis and treatment.

Diagnosis

These studies help doctors determine whether you have a certain disease and would include tests. Some points to look for in the methods include:
- The study should include people *with* and *without* the disease.
- There should be a "gold standard" test for comparison.
- There should be tests of agreement among different observers, and among the same observers at different times.
- Measures called "sensitivity" and "specificity" should be calculated and included if tests are being discussed.
- Look for diagrams that look like this:

	Disease + (disease present)	Disease - (disease not present)
Test +		
Test -		

Prognosis

These articles discuss approaches to determining what happens to patients over a period of time, following patients for a longer time.
Check that the following have been addressed:
- The patients should be reliably diagnosed using validated diagnostic criteria.
- The investigation should start at a clearly defined point in their disease, ideally early.
- Measurements – the outcome should be measured frequently, objectively and accurately in order to make sense.

- Patients must all be followed long enough to understand their fate.
- Every patient must be accounted for.
- Patients could have had treatment and the study is then looking at factors in the disease that predict outcome (so-called prognostic factors).

Treatment

When looking at treatments, ideally we need to only assess systematic reviews and well conducted randomized controlled trials. There are high and poor quality trials, and there are methods described to grade their quality using some agreed-upon criteria. More details on clinical trials are given later in the chapter. In Table 5 are listed the basic questions that need to be answered when reading these studies.

Table 5: Key facts

QUESTIONS TO ASK WHEN READING A STUDY OF A CLINICAL TRIAL

- Were the patients allocated to the treatment groups in a completely random way?
- Were details of the randomization kept concealed?
- Were patients and clinicians blind to the treatment?
- Were the patients analyzed in the groups to which they were assigned?
- Was the follow-up long enough, and were all the patients accounted for?
- Were the groups of patients similar at the start of the study?
- Were all the groups treated equally except for the experimental treatment?
- Were the measured outcomes appropriate and of importance?
- Were all the side effects and adverse events reported?
- Were the patients similar to my patient in their characteristics and condition?
- Who funded the study?

If the answer to all these questions is yes, the study is likely to be a high quality, double-blind, randomized controlled trial and hence significant.

It is important to ascertain who funded the study, since there could have been a conflict of interest, e.g. a pharmaceutical company paid for the research and the company expects to get a good result; this is often stated at the end the paper.

Evaluation of treatments would be easier if there was a standardized way of doing this. This has been appreciated for some time and led to the following statements:

"The CONSORT statement is an important research tool that takes an evidence-based approach to improve the quality of reports of randomized trials. The statement is available in several languages and has been endorsed by prominent medical journals such as The Lancet, Annals of Internal Medicine, and the Journal of the American Medical Association. Its critical value to researchers, healthcare providers, peer reviewers, journal editors, and health policy makers is the guarantee of integrity in the reported results of research.

CONSORT comprises a checklist and flow diagram to help improve the quality of reports of randomized controlled trials. It offers a standard way for researchers to report trials. The checklist includes items, based on evidence, that need to be addressed in the report; the flow diagram provides readers with a clear picture of the progress of all participants in the trial, from the time they are randomized until the end of their involvement. The intent is to make the experimental process clear, flawed or not, so that users of the data can more appropriately evaluate its validity for their purposes."

The diagram below is an example of a flow diagram.

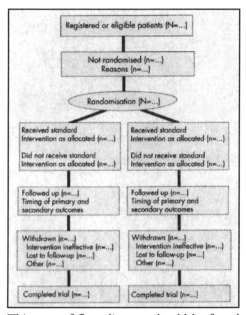

This type of flow diagram should be found in all publications describing randomized control trials it is reproduced from the British Dental Journal.

Otherwise you need to look for tables such as these:

	New Treatment	Standard Treatment
Success	A	B
Failure	C	D

We have provided some guidelines on how to assess the quality of surgical papers, which are discussed in chapter 8 (Zakrzewska and Lopez 2002).

How are judgements on health care made?

Once the knowledge has been found, it needs to be put into a format that will aid decision making, just as a tailor can get his material together, but then needs to decide how to put it together for his individual client. This gathered evidence needs to be assessed for applicability to the individual. The way this is done has now changed as shown below.

The Old Way	The New Way
Expert opinion (reviews) (1)	Critical analysis (3)
Consensus statement (2)	Systematic review (4)
	Evidence-based guidelines (5)

1. Review article – the reviewer may be biased, choosing only articles that support the argument
2. Consensus statement – all the same experts who do not look at problems objectively
3. Critical analysis – focused question predetermined
4. Systematic review – covers a broader topic and includes all articles with a very clear statement as to why articles included and excluded
5. Enables evidence-based guidelines to be developed, which give some indication on the level of evidence and recommendations

5. WHAT ARE GUIDELINES?

A guideline is a statement or rule that serves to guide conduct in accordance with policy. It is not practical for individual clinicians to make high quality clinical decisions unaided; therefore, clinicians and patients commonly use clinical practice guidelines as a source of support to help decide on treatment. They are not a rigid constraint on clinical practice, since they are only used if they apply to the patient. Some uses of guidelines are shown in Table 6 on the following page:

Table 6

WHY ARE GUIDELINES USED?
• improve health outcomes for patients
• enable clinicians to stay abreast of clinical research findings
• provide medico-legal protection
• prevent errors
• reduce practice variation
• influence hospital policy
• promote efficient use of resources
• identify research priorities based on lack of evidence

Guidelines for management of trigeminal neuralgia in the primary care sector have been developed, but those for specialists are currently being developed by an international panel of neurologists. Users need to be confident that the guidelines they are using have been systematically developed by panels of people with access to the available evidence who have an understanding of the clinical problem. Guidelines are developed in the following stages:
  • Establishing the need for a guideline
  • Developing the clinical question
  • Searching the literature
  • Grading quality of evidence and strength of recommendations
  • Making the recommendation
  • Implementing and keeping up to date
There are methods available for screening guidelines called "Appraisal of Guidelines Research and Evaluation," which are available on the Internet.

The better the evidence the more confidence can be put into guidelines, and the best evidence is from several high quality trials. In order, however, for these types of evidence to be available, clinical trials are urgently needed.

6. WHAT ARE CLINICAL TRIALS AND WHY DO WE NEED THEM?

When a new treatment becomes available, everyone is naturally enthusiastic, hoping the new treatment will be an advance. This enthusiasm for a new treatment has just been seen with the introduction of the gamma knife for trigeminal neuralgia. However, some diseases and conditions tend to get better anyway. We know that this is the case in trigeminal neuralgia, and it would be easy to assume that the new treatment brought about the good result, whereas it was in fact the natural history of the condition.

Furthermore, trigeminal neuralgia varies in severity, and making a judgment about whether a given treatment has made any difference is extremely difficult. There is therefore a need for an independent, unbiased view of a large enough number of patients to determine whether the difference is really due to the new treatment. Many trials will also assess the patients' quality of life as a result of the new treatment.

New treatments can be compared with standard treatments, i.e. with controls or with placebos when there are no standard treatments. A placebo is a treatment that has no effect, positive or negative, on the patient or illness. Mechanisms of how placebos work still remain poorly understood, but it is recognized that chemicals such as endorphins are released as a result of placebo use and this may result in treatment improvements when they are not expected.

It also needs to be remembered that the doctor himself may act as a placebo, especially if charismatic. Without a control it is impossible to measure how much of the improvement in the patients is due to the new treatment and how much would have happened by chance or with standard treatment.

It is interesting to find that a significant number of patients not only report improvement in symptoms when on placebo, but also develop side effects such as headaches, vomiting, rashes etc. Just the anticipation of having treatment is sufficient in some people to produce an effect. This reinforces the importance of being able to discriminate between the true effect of the proposed treatment and the placebo effect or even the psychological effects.

How many patients are needed for trials?

In most trials done in patients with chronic pain, an improvement of 50 % is thought by patients to be significant and will be considered useful. If it is thought that a 100 % improvement is needed in order to classify the new treatment as successful, then it is likely that the new treatment will need to be used in a larger number of patients.

In most trials the expected difference between an old and new treatment is not as large and thus even larger numbers are needed. If a difference of 10 % between treatments is expected, a valid study would require 1,000 patients to be recruited. If, on the other hand, a difference of only 5 % between treatments is expected, then it requires 4,000 patients to be recruited. In drugs used for trigeminal neuralgia, we often expect much higher improvements.

This means that for a rare condition like trigeminal neuralgia, several centers may need to be collaborating in order to have enough patients. The length of time the trial lasts will also affect the size of the sample needed.

What types of trials are there and what are they?

Open controlled trials are trials conducted without a control group and should only be used to assess the safety and effectiveness of a new drug. They are very biased, since both doctor and patient know that a new treatment is being tried.

Cross-over trials are designed to allow a patient to be given both the new and old treatment or placebo, so that a direct comparison can be made. For example, in one trial some patients were given lamotrigine in addition to their carbamazepine, while others were given only a placebo in what is called the first arm of the trial. After a few weeks, in the second arm of the trial, those who got the placebo were given the lamotrigine and those who had lamotrigine were given the placebo. The treatments were thus crossed over.

This method overcomes the problem that treatments could be affected by factors such as age, gender, disease severity, ethnicity, dietary and smoking habits. However, bias can creep in because when patients are taking different treatments, their disease severity can change. The other problem can be that the effects of treatment can carry over to the other part of the treatment even if you leave a period of time between treatments —- the washout period.

In the above study on the use of lamotrigine, just this effect was seen. Those patients who received lamotrigine in the first arm did better on placebo in the second arm than those who got placebo first.

Double-blind or single-blind trials refer to whether the patient or investigator knows the actual treatment being carried out. In double-blind trials, both investigator and patient are unaware of which treatment is being given. In single blind trials, either the patient or investigator knows which treatment is being carried out. In double-blind trials, only the trial organizers know who is getting which medication.

Blinding of surgical procedures is much harder, but one way of getting around this is to have a third researcher evaluate the treatment but not to be told what was done.

The use of "blinding" reduces bias, since it may be that if the patients knew they were receiving the new treatment, they would feel more positive or negative about it, and thereby influence what they report to the researcher. Similarly, if researchers know the patients are taking a new treatment for which they had high hopes, this may affect the way they judge the patients' responses to it.

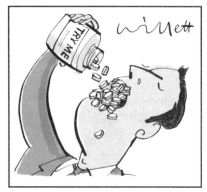

All treatments need to be carefully evaluated to see if they are really effective and to do this, clinical trials provide the only unbiased way of making this evaluation. A single patient does not provide sufficient evidence of effectiveness.

In randomized double-blind controlled trials, the allocation of patients to the treatments is totally random, often done by a computer to ensure an equal similar mix of patients in both arms of the treatment. At the end of the trial researchers will look at how effectively this was done. In good quality trials the two groups should represent a good match.

Who does trials and how are they organized?

The idea for a trial usually comes from a leading expert in the field who realizes that a question needs answering, e.g. which surgical treatment for trigeminal neuralgia gives the best long-term results or which is associated with the fewest side effects? The idea is then discussed with a range of people, which should include the consumers. If a new drug is being used, help will also be given by the pharmaceutical industry.

A protocol, i.e. the design of the study, is prepared. This provides details of the whole trial, including the size of the study. It is especially important to provide an estimate of the expected effects and specify clear end points, which can include:
- complete response – 100 % relief of pain
- partial response – 50 % relief of pain
- time to recurrence
- improvement in quality of life
- cost effectiveness of treatment

The protocol will also include a patient information sheet, free of medical jargon, so the patient understands everything about the trial.

This protocol is then submitted to an ethics committee. The ethics committee is made up of an independent group of people, including medical and nursing staff, lawyers and members of the public, all of whom have received training.

The ethics committee checks that:
- the researchers are qualified to carry out the trial
- protocol is suitable for the needs of the trial
- the probable benefits of new treatment outweigh the side effects
- there is enough information for the participants
- the consent form is valid
- the way in which people will be recruited is correct
- there is provision for compensation to participants if something goes wrong
- the local health facilities can support the trial

Designing and running clinical trials is difficult, since the medical researchers need to ensure that patients' health is not put at risk and everything must be very carefully documented in special case record files. This makes the trials costly and time consuming, especially with increasing new legislation. All trials in the UK are now covered by strict regulations and many are externally audited. Any personnel undertaking trials must have completed training in "good clinical practice." Considerable enthusiasm and commitment is needed from the team.

The advantages and disadvantages for patients taking part in clinical trials are shown in Table 7.

Table 7

WHAT ARE THE ADVANTAGES FOR PATIENTS OF TAKING PART IN CLINICAL TRIALS?	
advantages	disadvantages
• patients are managed by experts • extra attention is given to any changes in health as continual monitoring is carried out • some patients may get the very best new treatment, but all will get the best of current treatments • patients are given high quality information about the whole trial • patients help influence future treatments	• may not get the very best treatment, but will get the current best treatment • may need to make extra visits to see the realists • may not be able to get the treatment after the trial has ended • may undergo extra tests

Why are there so few high quality trials in the field of trigeminal neuralgia?

Due to the rarity of the condition and the difficulty of designing trials that take into account the natural pain remission periods, there are few high quality randomized controlled trials focused on trigeminal neuralgia . There are also difficulties in funding research into rare disorders. A number of factors can affect the results of trials, including those listed below.

- Choice of patients – it is essential that patients who enter the trial fulfilled the diagnostic criteria that have been suggested by organizations like the International Headache Society. If other types of patients have been used, this needs to be clearly stated. It may be important to assess specific symptoms, e.g. shooting pain or dull ache and severity.

- Age of the patients may influence the outcome of treatments.

- Duration of the condition may affect results. It is known that pain-relief periods are longer initially and that with time the pain free intervals decrease. We have shown that oxcarbazepine became less effective with time, not because it was not achieving the same serum concentrations, but because the disease itself had become more severe as shown on the outcome measures we used.

- Standardized outcome measures have not been agreed upon, although several clinical trials researchers have attempted to measure several parameters in order to improve evaluations. Quality of life is as essential to measure as pain relief and side effects.

- Not all patients who entered the trials are analyzed, i.e. an intention-to-treat analysis has not been done.

- Placebos are difficult to justify due to the severity of the pain, which has resulted in the use of either cross-over trials or trials in which the new drug or placebo is added to the current sub optimal therapy. Placebos that reproduce the side effects of the drug being tested have also been used to try and reduce bias.

- Carbamazepine is used in most trials as the cross-over drug, and this poses problems, since the effect of carbamazepine can take 3 weeks to disappear. It also interacts with many drugs.

- Size of trials - randomized controlled trials have been done with various sizes. The largest involved 77 patients and the smallest had only three patients. Few centers have enough patients to enter into trials of sufficient size to show a significant treatment effect. In other areas of medicine, trials involve thousands of patients.

Trials in surgery are more difficult, but not impossible, and McCulloch et al describe some solutions in their article in the British Medical Journal. In research in the area of trigeminal neuralgia, only have a handful of trials have been done in more than one center.

There is an urgent need for more centers to work together, not only nationally, but also internationally. As one patient pointed out, *"I kind of wish all the medical people associated with trigeminal neuralgia would get together, including the neurosurgeons and the neurologists and the dental people."*

We need solid databases and agreed-upon criteria to achieve what has been done in areas such as migraines and cluster headaches. Only then will we begin to lose some of this uncertainty and help to fulfil the goal defined by the TNA: "Together we will end the pain."

**What can consumers do to improve the number of
high quality trials being done?**

- MUST demand that ALL new treatments, surgical or medical, are subject to randomized controlled trials (RCT)
- must be represented in the group designing the protocol
- need to agree to take part in RCTs
- pressure grant giving organizations to fund RCTs

Only randomized controlled trial will enable us to significantly improve treatments for trigeminal neuralgia.

7. WHAT DO WE DO IN THE ABSENCE OF GOOD QUALITY DATA FOR TREATMENTS?

We need strategies for dealing with uncertainty, and pressure is needed to ensure that high quality trials are carried out. In the UK one way of dealing with uncertainty has been the setting up of the National Institute for Clinical Excellence (NICE). As stated on their Internet site, "The National Institute for Clinical Excellence works on behalf of the National Health Service in the UK and the people who use it. It is the independent organization responsible for providing national guidance on treatments and care for people using the NHS in England and Wales. Our guidance is intended for health care professionals, patients and their caregivers to help them make decisions about treatment and health care."

It is important to identify these uncertainties, which are reflected in dramatic variations in clinical practice as observed in any group of trigeminal neuralgia sufferers. The uncertainties also suggest the need for increased knowledge. Some may reflect ignorance of existing evidence, while others will be due to lack of appropriate evidence. These uncertainties need to be more publicly acknowledged.

Admission of uncertainty can sometimes undermine patients' confidence and even reduce the therapeutic effect, but it is important that patients also accept this uncertainty as this patient would have done:

"I'd have appreciated it if they were at least honest".….

Ian Chalmers (BMJ 2004) argues that an alliance of clinicians, patients, researchers and managers to discuss how to deal with them is essential.

Gamma knife surgery for trigeminal neuralgia is a good example of this uncertainty. There has only been one randomized controlled trial in this area, in which researchers tried to determine the best dose to use. Yet there is still no objective high quality evidence for its efficacy in terms of both pain relief and quality of life. In view of this, NICE has issued a range of documentation on this topic. A booklet designed to help patients understand this uncertainty is available on their Internet site or by postal mail.

8. Why do doctors use treatments that do not work?

Voltaire once said, "The art of medicine consists in amusing the patient while nature cures the disease."

The British Medical Journal, in February 2004, devoted an entire issue to the topic "If it doesn't work, stop it." One of the articles discusses the question posed above and puts forward the following reasons for using ineffective or harmful treatment:
- clinical experience
- over reliance on indirect outcomes
- natural history of the illness
- ritual and mystique
- a need to do something
- no one asks questions
- patients' expectations (real or assumed)

Only 30-50 % of patients get better due to drugs. In many cases, patients get better or worse on their own, no matter what the doctors do. Clinical experience has been shown to be a poor judge of what works or what does not, hence the need for adequate randomized controlled trials.

In other instances, the wrong outcome measures are looked at or we may ignore the severe side effects of a drug. Pimozide was shown to be effective in trigeminal neuralgia, but it is now well known that its side effects do not warrant its use for this condition.

Doctors continue to order tests as part of a ritual, but they rarely change outcomes or even management. This is particularly common in pre-operative assessments. Doctors want to relieve suffering and find it difficult to stand back and do nothing. They also do not want to feel as if they are missing some treatment. But it can be argued that missing a rare diagnosis may cause less harm than over testing vast numbers of patients.

Although we would like to think of medicine as a science, but it remains a human activity and we need to remember it is not the disease that needs treatment, but the patient!

MRS. G. CASE STUDY

Mrs. G has now had three episodes of trigeminal neuralgia and the time interval between the attacks has become shorter and the attacks themselves longer lasting. She is now on her fourth drug. She has heard there are new drugs on the market and she would like to try them. She finds out that one center is doing a clinical trial on leviteracetam, whereas in the other center, her fellow trigeminal neuralgia sufferers tell her that gabapentin is being used routinely.

To which center should Mrs. G go for treatment?

Discussion

A search of the literature needs to be done to ascertain the evidence on the use of these two drugs. This shows that there are some case reports on the use of gabapentin in trigeminal neuralgia, but that there is nothing about the use of leviteracetam in trigeminal neuralgia. If she goes to the center where gabapentin is being used routinely, she may find the drug helpful, but, on the other hand, it could be of no value. The results are unlikely, however, to be recorded in any high quality journal, since the results would classify as low level – just a case series.

If she goes to the other center, she will be given full information about the trial of leviteracetam and if she is eligible, she would be asked to enrol. Mrs. G will again have an equal chance of the new drug working as in the other center. However, this time the results will be analyzed careful and the randomized controlled trial will be published in a high quality journal. It will therefore help to establish the efficacy of this new drug and thus help other patients in the future.

---

9. WHAT RESEARCH IS NEEDED?

- Randomized controlled trials of medical, surgical and psychological treatments, with comparisons between them, are crucial.
- What outcomes for treatment are needed? This study should be done in discussion with patients, health care workers and other stakeholders.

- Guidelines for specialists on management of trigeminal neuralgia and related facial pain.
- What effect does provision of information and sharing of experiences with other sufferers and health care professionals have on treatment expectations and outcomes?

SUMMARY

- The patient of the 21st century will be at the center of health care and will work in partnership with his doctor.
- The choice of health care practitioner for a trigeminal neuralgia sufferer depends not just on expertise, but also on ability to be empathic.
- To make decisions about their care, patients need high quality evidence, which is found in systematic reviews and randomized controlled trials.
- Doctors and patients need to know how to critically appraise the literature they read.
- Randomized controlled trials are essential for high quality evidence; physicians must perform them and patients must agree to take part in them.
- Managing trigeminal neuralgia in the absence of good quality evidence and guidelines is difficult and results in wide variations of treatments.
- Funding is essential if randomized controlled trials are to be carried out.

FURTHER READING AND REFERENCES

Web sites
Checked May 2005

BMJ series, "How to Read a Paper" 1996-7,a series of papers that appeared over a period of time and can be downloaded from the British Medical Journal web site www.bmj.com

Centre for Evidence Based Medicine NHS Research and Development, an excellent site from which to start to learn how to read a paper critically. http://www.cebm.net/index.asp

Clinical Evidence – short articles updated every 8 months (will *only* accept randomized trials) www.clinicalevidence.com

The Cochrane Library www.update-software.com/cochrane

Bandolier easytoread short articles on evidence based medicine http://www.jr2.ox.ac.uk/bandolier/

National Institute for Clinical Excellence NICE provides guidelines on treatments, and provides an extensive section on gamma knife http://www.nice.org.uk/

Netting the Evidence is intended to facilitate evidence-based health care by providing support and access to helpful organizations and useful learning resources, such as an evidence-based virtual library, software and journals. http://www.shef.ac.uk/scharr/ir/netting/

Evidence based tool kit provides checklists for use when reading the literature. Adapted from the Users' Guides series prepared by the Evidence Based Medicine Working Group and originally published in JAMA. http://www.med.ualberta.ca/ebm/ebm.htm

Sites on guidelines that have been peer reviewed and deemed useful, such as www.guidelines.gov

Guidelines given to UK GPs on management of trigeminal neuralgia
http://www.prodigy.nhs.uk/

AGREE stands for "Appraisal of Guidelines Research and Evaluation."
It originates from an international collaboration of researchers and
policy makers who work together to improve the quality and effectiveness of clinical practice guidelines by establishing a shared framework
for their development, reporting and assessment. The site address is:
http://www.agreecollaboration.org/

Patient-Led Learning for the Clinical Professions
http://www.nhsia.nhs.uk/informatics/pages/resource_informatics/

J.A. Muir Gray, The Resourceful Patient,
http://www.resourcefulpatient.org/

Books

Sackett DL, Straus SE, Scott Richardson W, Rosenberg W, Haynes RJ
(2000) **Evidence -Based Medicine. How to Practice and Teach EBM** .
Edinburgh, Churchill Livingstone, ISBN 0-443 06240-4. This small
book is in its second edition and includes a CD Rom and further
updates on the Web at http://www.cebm.utoronto.ca/

Crombie IK. (1996) **The Pocket Guide to Critical Appraisal**. London,
BMJ Publishing Group, ISBN 0-7279-1099- X. Enables the reader to
judge papers based on preset criteria.

Greenhalgh T (2000) **How to Read a Paper: the Basics of Evidence
Based Medicine. Second edition** BMJ ISBN 0727915789. This is
based on the series of articles that appeared in the BMJ, and is very
useful.

Evidenced Based Medicine Working Group. (2001) Edited Guyatt,
Rennie **Users' guides to the medical literature.** JAMA press.
ISBN 1-57947-191-9

Muir Gray JA. (2002) **The Resourceful Patient**. Alden Group ISBN 1-
904202-00-

Balint M (1964) **The Doctor, His Patient and the Illness.** London: Churchill Livingstone, (May be out of print)

References

Journal of American Medical Association (JAMA) series, 1993 onwards, Users' Guides to the Medical Literature. These articles appear regularly on a very wide range of topics and are illustrated with case studies.

Doust J and Del Mar C (2004) Why Do Doctors Use Treatments That Do Not Work? *BMJ* **328**:474-475 Can be read on Internet, issue 28 February 2004, at www.bmj.com

Coulehan JL, Platt FW, Egene B, Frankel R, Lin CH, Lown B and Salazar WH. (2001) Let me see if I have this right... words that help build empathy. *Ann Intern Med.* **135**:221- 227

Kalkanis SN, Eskandar E N, Carter B S and Barker F G (2003) Microvascular Decompression Surgery in the United States, 1996 to 2000: Mortality Rates, Morbidity Rates, and the Effects of Hospital and Surgeon Volumes. *Neurosurgery* **52**:1251-1261.

Kitt CA, Gruber K, Davis M, Woolf C J and Levine J D (2000) Trigeminal Neuralgia: Opportunities for Research and Treatment. *Pain* **85**:3-7.

McCulloch P, Taylor I, Sasako M, Lovett B and Griffin D (2002) Randomised Trials in Surgery: Problems and Possible Solutions. *BMJ* **324**:1448-1451.

Rabinowitz I, Luzzat RI, Tamir A and Reis S (2004) Length of Patient's Monologue, Rate of Completion, and Relation to Other Components of the Clinical Encounter: Observational Intervention Study in Primary Care. *BMJ* **328**:501-502

Zakrzewska JM and Lopez B C (2003) Quality of Reporting in Evaluations of Surgical Treatment of Trigeminal Neuralgia: Recommendations for Future Reports. *Neurosurgery* **53**:110-120.

CHAPTER 6

MEDICAL MANAGEMENT

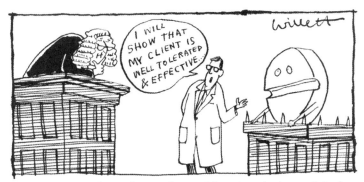

There are many drugs that can be used for trigeminal neuralgia, but they need to be rigorously tested.

There is a medicine you can take
But it's not the cure
It may make you drowsy
It may make you sick
Now he was not kidding
For this it quickly did
There are more pills to take
And there's no miracle fix
Well days have come and gone
The nausea is still the same
I feel I'm fighting a battle
With little coasting along the way.
Betty Price
West Columbia, SC

1. HOW TO MAXIMIZE TREATMENTS?

It is well known that some treatments fail because patients do not take the treatment (non-compliance, non-adherence) and this could be for a wide range of reasons even as simple as this patient describes, *"I hate taking medication but I can't live without it."*

Previously it was considered that compliance was entirely the patient's responsibility, but it is now appreciated that this is a two-way process, and that the doctor also has a part to play in the process.

Maximizing compliance involves identifying barriers to patient understanding, identifying barriers to compliance, and helping the patients to develop their own treatment plans. Educating the patient is one of the prime roles of the doctor and is something that was understood in the ancient world. The word "doctor" derives from the Latin *docere,* meaning to teach. Patient education is not just about knowledge but about a change in behavior.

Improved compliance is seen when patients:
- **are given more information**
- **report satisfaction with doctor**
- **establish trust with a caring doctor**
- **consult a doctor with good communication skills**
- **are warned of likely side effects of medication**
- **are given clear explanation of the purpose of treatment**
- **feel part of treatment planning**

Thus some poor compliance is due to poor communication between doctor and patient, as suggested in this quote: *"It is difficult to explain to someone medical sitting at a desk opposite you, who is saying in a matter of fact way 'well this is what you need to take and this is what you need to do', and you're sitting there thinking I am terrified and I can't explain that to this person because I don't think he'll be able to understand."*

Other reasons for non-compliance are technical factors, e.g. cannot open a bottle because of arthritis of the hands. A lack of symptoms leads to forgetfulness in taking regular medication. There is also good evidence that taking drugs twice a day improves compliance, as compared to taking medication four times a day. Patients prefer a once-a-day regimen as expressed by this patient, *"I would cut down on my medication just to have the one tablet a day, because I don't like living on tablets."* However, patients need to realize that sometimes a once-daily regime is not always possible due to the drugs' properties.

Drugs are handled by the body in a wide variety of ways, which accounts for the reason why they are differently prescribed and why some may react with other drugs that are being taken. Some drugs pass through the body very quickly and therefore need to be given on a frequent basis, whereas others take a long time to be broken down and removed from the body. This is expressed as a half-life of a drug, and the shorter it is, the more frequently it needs to be given. This may need to be explained to patients in order to optimize their use of the drug. The following is a patient's account of her discovery of this phenomenon:

"It gradually got worse until I was taking 1200 milligrams a day, and it still wasn't controlled. It was about a year ago I saw your registrar who said, how do you take them? No not all at once but two, two, two, ...absolutely fantastic, cut down by half and no pain at all."

Most simple painkillers work within 30 minutes, but their effect has totally worn off after 6-8 hours, whereas drugs such as antidepressants drugs may take up to three weeks to reach their peak. Drugs used in trigeminal neuralgia need to be slowly built up so that the body adapts to them. Equally importantly, they need to be withdrawn slowly to prevent effects such as this patient reported:

"My doctor said, 'just stop taking them,' and it's the worst thing that he did because he didn't realize that it had to be done gradually, and I didn't know any better, so I did stop and was ill for about three weeks. I couldn't move. I've gone back to it now and there is no problem because I've done it gradually."

Over a three-week period drugs such as carbamazepine alter the way the liver enzymes work and so can result in the drug being less effective and the patient needing a larger dose. These effects on the liver enzymes are not permanent and revert to normal after about three weeks.

Some newer drugs have been specially formulated so that they are released slowly (the word retard is added after the names of these drugs), and a more even level of the drug is achieved in the body. Care must be taken when using retard versions together with normal formulations as an overdose can be taken. Others have been formulated as liquids, as well as tablets, to enable them to be taken more easily when the pain is severe. Some capsules can be opened and sprinkled onto food but this could affect their effectiveness.

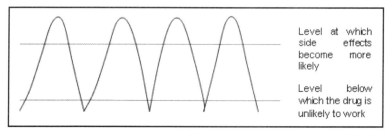

This graph shows the blood concentrations of a standard type drug when taken four times a day. There are peaks following each dose, and these correspond to the time when the drug is most likely to cause side effects. The troughs are times when the drug is likely to be least effective.

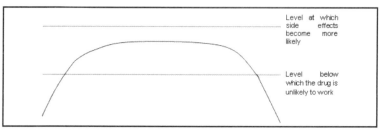

This graph shows how the blood concentrations of a slow release drug (retard) when taken once a day. It does not peak as sharply, but gradually increases before gradually decreasing. This may result in fewer side effects, but could also mean less pain relief.

To maximize treatment, it is essential that physicians have ensured that they have a full history from their patients, including their medication history. The patient then needs to be given accurate information about the medication and how to take it. This is summarized in the Table 1 on the following page.

Table 1: Key facts

WHAT THE PATIENT NEEDS TO DO BEFORE TAKING TRIGEMINAL NEURALGIA MEDICATION

Before beginning treatment with drugs ensure that

- The doctor is fully aware of your medical history including the possibility that you may be pregnant or are breast feeding
- The doctor knows of all treatments you are currently taking, including those bought over the counter, herbal preparations, homeopathic preparations
- The doctor knows of drugs you have taken in the past for trigeminal neuralgia
- The doctor knows of any drugs that you have particularly reacted against
- You have discussed with the doctor the different forms of the drug, e.g. slow-release drugs, liquid or capsule (Some forms can be more effective than others)
- You understand how the medication you have been given is going to work
- You know how to take it, how frequently and whether it is taken before or after meals
- You understand why the drugs need to be slowly increased over a number of days
- You know what side effects to expect and how to deal with them
- Make sure you know how you react to the drug before driving, using machines or doing anything else that can be dangerous, since it can affect your alertness and coordination
- You are given some way of recording your response to the drug
- You have given consent for the treatment
- You are going to be regularly reviewed, since you may need to have blood tests taken
- You know how to stop the drugs, preferably slowly, although you may need to stop them quickly if you develop a severe side effect
- Appreciate that these types of drugs can take a couple of weeks to really give maximum benefit

---

To improve outcomes from medication, the patient needs to be aware that just taking the medication does not necessarily give the best results. Table 2 on the following page provides practical hints for the patients on how they can maximize their treatment. With trigeminal neuralgia, the pain can get worse but can also disappear. During periods of pain remission, drugs do not need to be taken, since the ones currently being used are not curative, but merely diminish **ectopic** impulses.

Table 2: Key facts

HOW CAN YOU IMPROVE THE TAKING OF YOUR MEDICATION?

- Ensure that you understand how your pain is generated and why it may persist despite taking medication
- Gain a better understanding of how the treatment you are going to be taking leads to pain relief
- Ensure the doctor understands your life-style and how treatment may need to be modified as a result
- Take control of your medication by learning to understand how you respond to it
- Learn to understand factors that might influence the effect of the drug
- Involve close members of your family in your treatment
- Determine from the doctor exactly how long the treatment will work and how good a response the doctor expects you to gain
- Take notes during the consultation
- Keep a pain diary and take it to your doctor so that he can give you feedback on how you take your drug
- Be sure you go to regular follow-up appointments with the doctor
- Tell the doctor if you experience side effects from the treatment (immediately if severe) or if the treatment itself is not effective
- Record details of any effects the medication may have on you with details of how long it lasted and what drug and what dosage of the drug you were taking at the time and also whether you were taking any other drug
- Remember to check with your doctor if you start taking any other medications, even those you buy over the counter, in case they interact with the current drug you are taking
- Do not be afraid to ask questions and to clarify issues you do not understand
- If you miss your medication and remember within an hour or so, then take the medication as soon as possible. However, if it you do not remember until just before taking the next dose, then skip the dose and go back to the usual schedule. Do not double the dose
- Ensure you store the medication correctly and discard outdated medication

---

What are pain diaries?

No one can remember their pain experience over a long period of time; one tends to remember the best and the worst times and forget about the intervals in-between. It is therefore useful to keep a regular diary of painful events to aid the following:

• monitor response to treatment
• record potential side-effects
• establish what factors other than drugs might be affecting the pain
• determine whether the pain is still active or has gone into remission

Pain diaries also provide evidence that pain is present, as explained by this patient:

"Sometimes people see you and think, well you look fine, you have nothing to show them, but if you have pages of pain charts which I have done, then it's different, it's oh gosh, there is something here."

The use of diaries has shown us that patients with trigeminal neuralgia need to take their medication 30 to 60 minutes before eating or engaging in activity that will involve touching their face in order to gain maximum benefit from the drugs. However, this can increase the chances of nausea or vomiting. By using a pain diary, the patient can work out the optimum dosage schedule, remembering that this may be different for different drugs.

Diaries can be very simple recordings of day-to-day events. In a conventional diary, however, a sheet that is more structured can be more useful, since it is quicker to "read." An example of one is shown in the appendix. This also provides space for the physician to provide guidance on how to take the drugs, which is especially useful when first using a new drug or changing drugs. The patient can record the severity of the pain in a variety of different ways. Activities that were limited by the pain, and an emotional component showing how the patient is coping with the pain, can also be shown.

With the use of electronic data, it is now possible to record pain in electronic format, especially through the use of personal data assistants (PDA's). Some of these can be programmed to load into a spreadsheet, which makes it easier for analysis.

We have remarkably little data on the temporal characteristics of trigeminal neuralgia, and these new methodologies may yield further insight into this condition and how drugs work best. They may also give us an idea of how the pain changes over time, how frequently it gets worse, and how long are the pain-relief periods.

2. WHAT MEDICATIONS (DRUGS) ARE USED FOR TRIGEMINAL NEURALGIA?

In the appendix is a list of the trade (brand) names given to the drugs described in this chapter.

It is well known that conventional, over-the-counter analgesics such as aspirin, paracetamol (acetaminophen), ibuprofen, and even the potent narcotics, have little effect on trigeminal neuralgia, as explained well by this patient: *"I was given so many different types of tablets to try at first, and nothing worked and it was getting worse and worse, and I was getting pain every ten minutes and in the end I went to the hospital and I begged them for carbamazepine because I had it before, and I knew that was the only thing. I took one tablet and within a matter of a few minutes the pain had completely gone."*

This is because trigeminal neuralgia is a **neuropathic** pain (pain originating in nerves), and we now know that anticonvulsant drugs or antineuralgic drugs are the most effective. How we came to use these drugs is explained in Table 3 on the following page. It is important to remember that none of these drugs are curative; they simply stop transmission of the pain. These drugs are particularly effective at stopping sharp shooting pain, but appear to be less effective for dull aching types of pain. Not every patient will have a 100 % response.

It is estimated from randomized controlled trials that 70 % of patients will respond to carbamazepine. Doctors have often said that response to this drug can serve as a diagnostic test as indicated in the above patient's story. Sometimes the intensity of the pain attacks will be reduced, while in other instances the frequency with which the attacks occur is reduced. We still do not know why this varied response occurs, but it could be due to genetic factors in the way different patients handle drugs. Until we know the cause of trigeminal neuralgia and exactly how the drugs act, it will remain difficult to treat trigeminal neuralgia with medications.

The gold standard drug remains carbamazepine and this should be used for firstline treatment. The following statements from patients provide evidence for this effectiveness of carbamazepine (Tegretol):

- *"He gave me Tegretol and that immediately started making a difference."*
- *"Within minutes of chewing that first Tegretol 100 mg. tab, I got IMMEDIATE relief."*
- *"I started on Tegretol and immediately realized this was a very powerful and sedating drug. I got up to 800 mg a day and never really did get total relief. Also, the sedating symptoms never really improved much. I felt like a zombie all of the time. I had about two or three points where the pain went into remission and I was able to reduce and get off of Tegretol for a few weeks."*

It is crucial when using any drug to keep a diary of its effect. I have read in the accounts patients have given me that far too many patients are taking drugs that neither the doctor nor the patient know the efficacy of. Some patients may be taking six or seven drugs and experiencing severe side effects, still not knowing if the drugs have a beneficial effect. If the drugs do not provide any pain relief when used in the correct way, it is important to consider discontinuing them.

Table 3

How did we come to use anti-epileptic (anticonvulsant drugs)?
In the mid 1880s, a French physician, Trousseau, suggested that trigeminal neuralgia, because of its intermittent activity, was similar to epilepsy. The disease was therefore renamed neuralgia epileptiform. A very wide range of drugs then came to be used for trigeminal neuralgia, including poisons such as hemlock and venom of bee and cobra, metals, purgatives, quinine, ferrous carbonate, galvanic therapy and even radiation and X-ray therapy.
In 1876 the anti-epileptic drug potassium bromide was first used. However, it was not until 1942 that Bergouignan proposed the use of a new anti-epileptic drug called phenytoin. However, this drug was not as effective as the next one (carbamazepine) reported in 1962 by Bloom. Carbamazepine has become the gold standard against which all other drugs are compared. Since then, most of the anti-epileptic drugs have been tried for management of trigeminal neuralgia. Drugs used to treat spasticity, such as baclofen, were first used in 1972, but these have not been shown to be as effective as the anticonvulsant drugs.

Medications should be used in sequence as illustrated by this patient's comment: *"The first couple of years I took Neurontin and was totally pain free. Then they put me on Tegretol, which I couldn't take and then they tried Dilantin and the same thing. Oxcarbazepine it is the only thing that works. I have been on that now for two and a half years. I am basically pain free as long as I take it. As soon as I stop, I get the pain back."*

When patients are on medication, it is essential for the physician to regularly review them and ascertain:
- how much of the drug is being taken, and how often. This is most effectively done by discussing the pain diary with the patient
- the effectiveness of the drug, in terms of both pain relief and side effects
- that pain is still present; then determine its intensity, character and effect on daily activities
- that the drug is not causing any side effects, either as reported by the patient or as ascertained through blood tests

- the need for further use of the same drug at the same, higher or lower dosage, adding on of other drugs, or changing the drug
- whether the gradual withdrawal of the drug should be considered if pain control has been achieved and a period of remission has occurred
- whether referral for a neurosurgeon's opinion, include performing an MRI scan, is indicated because of continuation of pain
- whether the signs and symptoms have changed in any way, e.g. the patient developed multiple sclerosis or tumor
- whether the diagnosis continues to be correct or a different diagnosis should be considered, e.g. idiopathic facial pain, dental problems, or cluster headache
- that the patient's wishes in respect to treatment have been taken into consideration
- that the patient feels in control

Drugs that have been evaluated in randomized controlled trials for trigeminal neuralgia are shown in Table 1. Other drugs, which are mentioned in the next table, are those that are based on reports of the lowest level of evidence, i.e. case reports. Although all these drugs have undergone formal testing and are available in most countries, some of the drugs have not been specifically licensed for use in trigeminal neuralgia. Doctors may therefore be reluctant to prescribe drugs that are "off-licensed use" or "off label."

Specialists may have to provide general practice doctors (GPs) or primary-care doctors (PCs) with written instructions about the drug and how to optimize treatment. On the other hand, some pharmaceutical companies do such good marketing on their products that doctors are convinced that they are effective. A recent study in Germany showed that 94 % of advertising material sent by drug companies to GPs (PCs) contained statements that were not scientifically supported by identifiable literature.

Gabapentin (Neurontin), for example, has never been tested in a randomized controlled trial in trigeminal neuralgia and the only evidence for its use in trigeminal neuralgia is based on a few case reports as shown in Table 8. Yet surveys done by the TNA US show that it is very widely used.

Is there a benefit in taking more than one drug to control trigeminal neuralgia?

In the treatment of epilepsy, it is common practice to use more than one drug, and this same principle has been used in the management of trigeminal neuralgia, especially when one drug has not worked. Baclofen (Lioresal) and lamotrigine (Lamictal) have been evaluated as add-on medications to carbamazepine and shown to be effective. There is no evidence for other drug combinations.

Sometimes the drugs provide relief for the severe, sharp, rapid pain, but do not help with the other so-called background pain. This type of pain is much more difficult to manage. It is often treated, as other chronic pains are, with antidepressant drugs, especially the tricyclic drugs, as can been seen from this patient's statement, *"I take gabapentin 2400 mg daily, baclofen 40 mg, amitriptyline 10 mg and propoxyphene 100 mg. When I combined this with oxcarbazepine 1200 mg, it gave me no extra pain relief, but pain in the back of the head."*

There is currently no evidence to show whether this is effective, but their addition no doubt increases the risk of side effects.

Why do patients get so many side effects with drugs?

Anticonvulsant drugs decrease the excitability of nerves and so help to stop the pain fibers of trigeminal nerve from firing. Unfortunately, since these drugs affect the nervous system, they also result in a reduction of side effects such as drowsiness, dizziness, unsteadiness on the feet and double vision. Other drugs that act on the nervous system can make the effects of these drugs even more severe. These also include things such as alcohol as described by this patient:

"The other thing is, with tablets you shouldn't be drinking too much. I've never drunk excessively, but I do like a drink and there again, with the nature of the business, I often used to have a drink socializing with people."

Side effects from drugs are often related to the level of the drug in the blood and so can sometimes be reduced by decreasing the dose. They can also decrease as the body gets used to the new drug. Some side effects are common, whereas others are less common or even rare. The drug information that is included with drugs will list all of them. Development of side effects may also affect the way that drugs are taken.

A survey I conducted at Trigeminal Neuralgia support group meetings in America and in England, showed that all patients suffered from side effects while using these drugs and they complained of an average of three side effects. These are some of the comments they make about side effects:

- *"It is a double-edged sword; if you do not take your medication, you are in pain and you do not function. If you take the medication you cannot have a coherent conversation, so it is horrible."*

• *"I have been very, very tired trying to hold down a job where every-thing was critical – dates, times, etc. where I had to be 100 percent all day."*
• *"Medications gave me such side effects as double vision, walking into walls, dizziness, muscle pain, swelling of extremities, shaking."*
• *"Mind-dulling, robot-inducing side-effects."*

Experts, on the other hand, have estimated that only 70 % of patients would have side effects.

Some patients will develop a true allergy to a drug, which means they must never use the drug again. An allergy to a drug most frequent-ly shows itself as an itchy body rash. This can come on slowly over a few days or it can be sudden. The more quickly the reaction occurs, the more serious it is likely to be. In the more severe cases, it can also result in ulceration of the mouth and, in very rare cases; it can cause a life-threatening reaction called an anaphylactic shock.

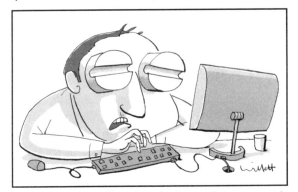

Many drugs used for trigeminal neuralgia cause side effects and can interfere with the quality of life.

The drugs have a high potential to interfere with other drugs the patient is taking and lead to:
• more side effects
• reduced effect of the anti-neuralgia drug or the other drug
• increased effect of the anti-neuralgia drug or other drug

Drugs need to be developed that will be much more specific in their mode of action and, as a consequence, will decrease side effects and improve quality of life.

Which drugs have been well tested in randomized controlled trials?

This next section should be read in combination with Table 4. The drugs are listed in alphabetic order. All drugs have at least two names, a generic one and a trade name. Drug names that use the name of the pharmaceutical product are called generic and are written in lower case, whereas the ones marketed by companies, i.e. trade (brand) names, of which there may be more than one, are capitalized. While a drug is under patent, only the pharmaceutical company that produced it can market it and it enables them to recoup some of the money used in its development. Once the drug is no longer covered by a patent, then any company can produce it and thus several versions become available.

The use of the generic name enables one to recognize which drugs are actually the same. The same drug may also have different trade names in different countries. I will use the generic names, but will provide in brackets some of the trade names used principally in the US and UK. The data provided below is not exhaustive, and more data can be obtained either from the pharmaceutical companies or from pharmacists who have access to detailed texts as cited in the reference section at the end of the chapter. Most drugs are now dispensed with further detailed information written in jargon-free language that highlights major and minor side effects.

The photograph below shows just some of the drugs now available for trigeminal neuralgia.

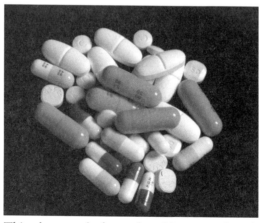

This photograph shows the wide range of medications now available for trigeminal neuralgia sufferers.

Table 4

DRUGS USED IN RANDOMIZED CONTROLLED		
Type of trial (no treated)	drug daily dosage	Number improved NNT
2 Controlled trials, cross-over (10)	Baclofen (Lioresal) 50 – 80 mg	7/10 active, 1/10 placebo NNT 1.4
1 Controlled trial, cross over (15)	L-Baclofen 6-12mg	9/15 L baclofen, 6/15 baclofen 2 (1-4)
3 Randomized controlled trials, cross over (178)	Carbamazepine (Tegretol) 400mg – 2.4gm	178/315 active, 41/224 placebo (same patients entered several times during sequential trial) NNT 2.6
1 Randomized controlled trial, cross over (3)	Dextromethorphan 120-920mg	0/2 more pain on active drug, but wide fluctuations
1 Randomized controlled trial, cross over (14)	Lamotrigine (Lamictal) 200 – 400 mg	10/13 active, 8/14 placebo NNT 2.1
1 Randomized controlled trial, cross over (48)	Pimozide (Orap) (4-12mg)	48/48 pimozide, 28/48 carbamazepine NNT 3
1 Randomized controlled trial, parallel. (47)	Proparcaine hydrochloride 2 drops of 0.5% solution	6/25 active, 5/22 placebo NS
1 Randomized controlled trial, parallel (12)	Tizanidine 6 –18 mg	1/6 tizanidine, 4/6 carbamazepine NS
1 Randomized controlled trial, cross over (12)	Tocainide Tonocar 60mg/kg	8/12 tocainide carbamazepine 9/12 NS
1 Randomized controlled trial, cross over (3)	Topiramate 75-600mg	0/3 NS

NNT is number need to treat – the lower it is, the better, e.g. NNT of 2.6 for carbamazepine means that every third patient will get a good result or 70 % will report a 50 % reduction in pain.

TRIAL — BEST FORM OF EVIDENCE

Side effects/withdrawals/ number of side effects in reports	Comments
unsteadiness, fatigue, nausea, vomiting 1/10	In some cases baclofen used as an add-on. Slow withdrawal, since may cause seizures and hallucinations
Dizziness, confusion, lethargy 6/15 on baclofen, 1/15 L-baclofen	L-baclofen not available commercially
side effects: unsteadiness, dizziness, double vision, tiredness 71/150 NNH=3.4 withdrawal 6/114 NNH= 24	Reduced white cell count, low salt levels higher doses, folate deficiency in prolonged use
1 withdrew due to poor pain control 2 non-trigeminal neuralgia patients withdrew 1 sedation, 1 rash on placebo. All had mild side effects altered concentration, dizziness and unsteadiness	Very small trial
dizziness, drowsiness, constipation, unsteadiness, double vision, irritability 7/14 active and placebo withdrawal 1 due to poor pain control	Rapid dose rise increases incidence of rashes. All patients were on some other anticonvulsant
tremor, rigidity, memory loss 40/48 pimozide, 22/48 carbamazepine NNH 3	Side effects too severe to recommend routine use including sudden death
None reported	Eye problems in long- term use
2 withdrew due to poor pain control	Effect is short lasting
Nausea, numbness 2/12. Withdrawal rash 1/12	Severe damage to red blood cells resulting in death, precludes its routine use
Irritability, memory gastrointestinal, fatigue 3/3	May provide some reduction in pain but trial was very small

NNH is the number needed to harm – same idea, this is not always available.
NS not stated. The side effects only refer to those reported in these trials; there may be others.

BACLOFEN
(Lioresal) available as a tablet

Baclofen is one of the few drugs that is not an anticonvulsant; it was first introduced for use in trigeminal neuralgia by a neurologist named Fromm in 1972.

How does the drug work?

Baclofen is easily absorbed when taken by mouth, and reaches its highest concentrations between 3 and 8 hours after its taking. It is, however, very quickly removed from the body in an unchanged form, through the kidneys. The half-life of the drug is 3 to 4 hours, which means it needs to be taken on a fairly frequent basis, such as three or four times a day.

What side effects does it cause?

The most common ones include tiredness, unsteadiness, unusual weakness, nausea and vomiting. Great care needs to be taken when stopping this drug, since rapid withdrawal can result in hallucinations (seeing or hearing things that are not there), as well as fits and anxiety.

What drugs does it react with?

Since the drug remains unchanged in the body, it is rare for it to react with other drugs and so is safe to use in patients who are taking other drugs or can even be added to other anticonvulsant drugs.

Does it work in trigeminal neuralgia?

In clinical trials the drug has been shown to be highly effective, but Fromm suggests that it works best when taken in combination with carbamazepine. Table 5 provides a possible dosage schedule.

It is important to stop at a point at which good control of pain is gained and few side effects are experienced. Normally this is around 50-60 mgs daily. When using higher dosages, it is better if the drug is spread out in four- times-a-day schedule. The drug needs to be withdrawn slowly over 3 to 4 weeks to reduce it.

Table 5

SUGGESTED DOSAGE SCHEDULE FOR BACLOFEN				
Daily Dosage	Day	Morning	Mid-day	Night
15mg	1-3	5mg	5mg	5mg
25mg	4-6	10mg	5mg	10mg
30mg	7-9	10mg	10mg	10mg
40mg	10-12	20mg	10mg	10mg
50mg	13-15	20mg	10mg	20mg
60mg	16-18	20mg	20mg	20mg
70mg	19-21	30mg	20mg	20mg
80mg	22-24	30mg	20mg	30mg
You do not need to go up the full scale and you can change more slowly. The amount of drug you need is related to your body weight and age, so you may start at a different point in the scale as instructed by your doctor.				

CARBAMAZEPINE

(Also called Tegretol, Tegretol Retard, Teril Retard, Timonil Retard, Atretol, Carbatrol, Epitol). It is available as suspension, tablet, chewable tablets or capsules.

The short report in the Lancet in 1962 on the use of carbamazepine in patients with trigeminal neuralgia has proven to be a landmark publication that has revolutionized the management of trigeminal neuralgia.

How does the drug work?

Carbamazepine works slowly, but is nearly completely absorbed within 2-8 hours. Its absorption, however, is very erratic and accounts for why patients show wide variations in response to it. The drug has a powerful effect on liver enzymes, causing them to act differently and resulting in a more rapid breakdown. This accounts for why 3-5 weeks after beginning treatment with carbamazepine, the drug may appear to have lost its effectiveness. This effect of the drug on the liver enzymes also results in side effects, since these enzymes are normally used for routine bodily functions.

Other drugs also use this liver enzyme and so they enter into competition with carbamazepine if given together. This means that drug activity can be enhanced or reduced in different situations. The drug is fairly quickly eliminated and therefore should be given on a frequent basis to prevent loss of efficacy. It is for this reason that a slow-release form of carbamazepine has been developed. Recent works suggests that the slow-release medication is more reliable in achieving fairly constant drug levels in the blood.

What side effects does it cause?

Carbamazepine results in a multitude of side effects, which are listed on the sheets included with the medication. The most common adverse effects are drowsiness, unsteadiness, double vision, lightheadedness, nausea and vomiting. The elderly appear to be more sensitive and experience more side effects. Most of the side effects are minor and reversible, but a few are potentially serious. Especially in early use, carbamazepine may reduce the level of white cells, which results in a decreased ability to protect the body against infections. It may also induce deficiency of folic acid, a vitamin that is used to make red blood cells.

Carbamazepine can also result in water retention and hence swelling of the legs. This is more likely to be seen in patients with heart problems, those who are elderly, and those who are on higher doses.

Up to 10 % of patients may develop an allergy to the drug. The allergy may be mild, limited to an itchy rash, but it can be very severe, causing widespread itchy rash, ulceration and sores on the lips and inside the mouth. Some patients may show increased sensitivity to sunlight, as indicated by a rash, itchiness or redness. Sunblock products should therefore be used.

Patients are more likely to develop serious side effects early on in the use of the drug rather than through prolonged use. It is for this reason that regular blood tests are essential when taking this drug, especially in the first year of use.

The drug can interfere with other diseases such as diabetes and should be avoided during pregnancy and by mothers who are breastfeeding their infants.

What drugs does it react with?

Carbamazepine reacts with many drugs, so it is essential for the doctor to know all the drugs the patient is taking. This is particularly important in the case of anticoagulants (blood thinners). Patients who are on these types of drugs need to have their blood tested very regularly, especially if they attempt to change the dose of carbamazepine, since this can result in excessive bleeding. It also interferes with oral contraceptives (birth control) and additional birth control precautions may be needed.

It has been suggested that any grapefruit product — including dietary supplements that contain grapefruit bioflavonoids, or even tangelos (a hybrid grapefruit) can interact with carbamazepine. Chemicals in grapefruit interfere with certain enzymes that break down carbamazepine in the gut and liver. This can result in higher-than-desired blood levels of the drug and an increased risk of serious side effects.

Does it work in trigeminal neuralgia?

There is high quality evidence that this drug is highly effective in patients with the sharp, shooting pain of trigeminal neuralgia. It is likely that 70 % of patients will respond to this drug when it is first used. The drug may prove to be less effective with time, and this is less likely to be due to tolerance than to the fact that the pain is beginning to be more severe.

Table 6 provides a suggested schedule for how it should be taken.

Table 6

SUGGESTED DOSAGE SCHEDULE FOR CARBAMAZEPINE					
Daily dosage	Day	Morning	Lunchtime	Afternoon	Night
200mg	1- 3	100mg			100mg
300mg	4-6	100mg	100mg		100mg
400mg	7- 9	100mg	100mg	100mg	100mg
500mg	10-12	200mg	100mg	100mg	100mg
600mg	13-15	200mg	100mg	100mg	200mg
700mg	16-18	200mg	200mg	100mg	200mg
800mg	19-21	200mg	200mg	200mg	200mg
The dose in the blood is dependent on body weight, so a higher schedule will be needed by a person who weighs more.					

Carbamazepine retard

A retard form of this drug, which releases the drug more slowly, may be given. This is especially good for use in the evening, since it ensures a beneficial level of drug in the blood throughout the night. It can be used during the day to cut down on the number of times patients need to take the drug, especially if the pain has stabilized. It is then only taken twice daily.

DEXTROMETHORPHAN

This drug was first evaluated for trigeminal neuralgia in 2000.

How does the drug work?

The drug is rapidly absorbed and processed through the liver and then excreted in the urine.

What side effects does it cause?

These are few, mainly related to drowsiness and stomach disturbances.

What drugs does it react with?

Drug interactions occur mainly with antidepressant drugs.

Does it work in trigeminal neuralgia?

The drug has only been reported in the use of three patients with trigeminal neuralgia, although it was a randomized controlled trial. None of the patients had good outcomes. The drug therefore needs further evaluation before being considered for general use.

LAMOTRIGINE
(Lamictal) available as tablets, and chewable tablets

This drug first became available in 1991 and the first drug trial of its use in trigeminal neuralgia was reported in 1997.

How does the drug work?

Lamotrigine is quickly and well absorbed, and peak blood concentrations are reached within three hours. In approximately 24 hours, half the dose will remain in the body. For this reason, its dosing can be on a twice-daily basis.

What side effects does it cause?

As with most other anticonvulsant drugs, it is very important with this drug to increase the dosage very slowly, since a rapid increase can lead to a rash, which is not thought to be an allergic type response. This skin reaction can be very severe. It causes the same side effects as the other anticonvulsant drugs. It has otherwise few effects on the blood and thus appears safe for long-term use.

What drugs does it react with?

It rarely interferes with other drugs and can be used with carbamazepine.

Does it work in trigeminal neuralgia?

The one small, randomized controlled trial showed that it was effective when used in combination with another anticonvulsant drug. There have as yet been no reported studies of its use as a single stand-alone drug.

Table 7

SUGGESTED DOSAGE SCHEDULE FOR LAMOTRIGINE			
Total daily dose	Week	Morning	Evening
25 mg	1	25mg	0
50 mg	2	25mg	25mg
75 mg	3	50mg	25mg
100mg	4	50mg	50mg
125mg	5	50mg	75mg
150mg	6	75mg	75mg
175mg	7	75mg	100mg
200mg	8	100mg	100mg

- After 4 weeks the dose can be increased faster, e.g. 50 mg a week.
- Most patients use a range between 100 and 200 mg daily.
- If you are taking it with carbamazepine, you will need to use doses of 200-400 mg daily.

PIMOZIDE
(Orap) available as a tablet

This drug was first reported for use in trigeminal neuralgia in 1989.

How does the drug work?

Only about half the drug is absorbed after swallowing it, and peak concentrations are reached any time between 4 and 12 hours later. It is broken down in the liver and then removed through the body both in the feces and urine. It has a very long half-life.

What side effects does it cause?

It can cause a wide range of side effects, including rigidity, muscle twitching, blurred vision, hand tremors and decreased memory. It can have severe side effects affecting the heart rate, and some of the side effects do not always disappear after withdrawal of the drug.

What drugs does it react with?

It cannot be used with any drugs used to treat cardiac conditions or psychiatric disorders.

Does it work in trigeminal neuralgia?

Although in a randomized control trial it was shown to be effective, its side effects make it unacceptable for routine use in trigeminal neuralgia.

PROPARCAINE HYDROCHLORIDE EYE DROPS

Topical analgesic eye drops were discovered by chance to have brought about relief of trigeminal neuralgia when used for an ophthalmic examination in a patient with trigeminal neuralgia in 1991.

How does the drug work?

This is a local anaesthetic with short duration of action. The speed of onset and duration of action depends on the site of administration.

What side effects does it cause?

Repeated use can lead to damage to the front of the eye.

What drugs does it react with?

None have been reported when used in this form.

Does it work in trigeminal neuralgia?

The initial case reports, including 60 patients, seemed to suggest that this could be an effective treatment for patients with trigeminal neuralgia in the first nerve division. However, when subjected to a randomized controlled trial, the eye drops were found to be no more effective than a placebo. It may have some use in the short-term control of an acute attack.

TIZANIDINE
(Zanaflex) available as a tablet

This drug has muscle relaxant properties and was first reported in the use of trigeminal neuralgia in 1986.

How does the drug work?

Tizanidine is absorbed from the gastrointestinal tract and peak concentrations are reached within 1-2 hours. It goes through the liver and is excreted via the urine as an inactive metabolite. It is eliminated within 2-4 hours.

What side effects does it cause?

It can cause drowsiness, fatigue, dizziness, dry mouth, stomach problems, and low blood pressure. Altered liver enzymes and acute hepatitis have been reported and so regular monitoring tests are important. The side effects are dose related.

What drugs does it react with?

It interacts with a wide range of drugs, including blood pressure drugs and phenytoin.

Does it work in trigeminal neuralgia?

When used in a randomized controlled trial comparing it to carbamazepine, tizanidine proved to be less effective than carbamazepine in pain control.

TOCAINIDE

This drug was evaluated in a randomized controlled trial, but because of its very toxic effect, it has been virtually withdrawn and there are no indications for its use in trigeminal neuralgia.

TOPIRAMATE
(Topamax) available as tablet, capsule)

Topiramate is a relatively new anticonvulsant, whose use in trigeminal neuralgia was first reported in 2000.

How does it work?

It is easily absorbed from the gastrointestinal tract and reaches peak concentrations within 2 hours. About 50 % of it is broken down in the liver and the rest is removed unchanged through the urine. Its half-life time is 21 hours, so it can be used twice daily and a steady state will not normally be achieved for 10-15 days.

What side effects does it cause?

The usual side effects occur, unsteadiness, impaired concentration, confusion, and dizziness. It needs to be used with care in patients with liver or kidney problems.

Does it react with other drugs?

There are complex interactions with other anticonvulsant drugs, which can be unpredictable. It also has an effect on some types of heart drugs and oral contraceptives.

Does it work in trigeminal neuralgia?

The first report in 6 patients with multiple sclerosis, who also had trigeminal neuralgia, showed it to be effective. It was subsequently used in a very small, randomized controlled trial that failed to show any benefit.

Which other drugs can be used?

This next section should be read in conjunction with Table 8 on the following page.

BOTULINUM TOXIN TYPE A INJECTIONS
(Botox)

This purified version of the botulinum toxin has been approved for use in cosmetic treatments and to treat facial spasm. There are two papers reporting a handful of patients with trigeminal neuralgia. It resulted in pain relief for 5 to 12 weeks. Since this drug works principally on muscles, it results in mild muscle spasm of the face. It could possibly be useful as a temporary measure, but needs to be evaluated in well-controlled clinical trials.

CAPSACIAN CREAM
(Axasin, Zacin) available as cream

This is a derivative of red pepper. It has been suggested that it may be effective in neuropathic pain, since it aims to deplete neurochemicals needed to transmit pain. The capsaicin cream is applied topically over the painful area three times a day for several days. It can cause transient burning, and care needs to be taken not to get it in the eye. Hands should be washed thoroughly after using it and contact lenses should not be handled until the hands have been washed. It can be useful while waiting for other drugs to start working.

Table 8

Drugs not evaluated in randomized controlled trial, but used in trigeminal neuralgia				
No. of reports (no. pts)	Drug daily dosage	Outcome reported in each study	Side effects/ withdrawals (no of side effects in reports)	Comments
2 reports (12)	Botox 25- 75 units	8/11 had 50% reduction maximum time 12 weeks 1/1 reduced pain by 50%	Temporary muscle weakness of the face	Needs careful evaluation
2 reports (17)	Capsaicin (Zostrix) 3 gm for 21-28 days	6/12 complete, 4/12 partial, 4/12 relapses, 1/5 partial, 4/5 nil or little	Burning sensation, (NS)	Rub on the skin, temporary relief in majority, avoid contact with the eye
4 reports (63)	Clonazepam (Rivotril, klonopin) 2 – 8 mg	5/7 good result, 13/19 excellent or good, 10/25 excellent, 6/25 good, 64% complete/partial	Lethargy, fatigue, dizziness, personality change (31/46)	Drowsiness is very severe and dose relat- ed. Affects blood
3 reports (20)	Gabapentin (Neurontin) 1200 – 3600 mg	2/2, 6/7 excellent, 1/7 partial, 10/11 excellent	unsteady, dizziness, drowsiness, sickness, headache, swelling of the feet (nil reported in these reports)	Some patients had multiple sclerosis. Was also used with lowdose carbamazepine or lamotrigine
3 reports (49)	Oxcarbazepine (Trileptal) 300 – 1200 mg	13/13 excellent or good, 16/21 excellent or good, 15/15 excellent short term	Unsteady, dizziness, double vision, lethargy that may be related to change in salt balance (24/49)	Side effects less severe than with carbamazepine, lowers salt levels and is dose dependent
2 reports (49)	Phenytoin (Epanutin) 200 – 300 mg	4/4 excellent, 8/20 excellent, 6/20 partial, 4/5 excellent, 1/5 partial	Unsteady, lethargy, sickness, headache, behavioral changes (NS)	Folate deficiency in prolonged use, enlargement of gums, can be used intra- venously for immediate effect
2 reports (30)	Valproic acid (Epilim, depakote) 600 – 2000 mg	9/20 excellent /good, 4/20 good if used with other drugs, 3/20 no response, 4/10 excellent/ good, 6/10 poor but if used as add on 10/10 good	Irritability, restlessness, tremor, confusion, sickness (only one study provided data 1/20)	Rash and, with prolonged use, hair loss. Also weight gain

The side effects listed in this table are those reported in the trials, but other adverse effects may occur.

CLONAZEPAM
(Klonopin, Rivotril) available as tablets

It was first used in 1975. In addition to being an anticonvulsant, it also is a tranquiller (tranquilizer). Maximum blood levels are achieved rapidly and it has a half-life of 1-2 days. Four case reports have reported excellent or good results in more than 60 % of patients. Drowsiness, which is dose related, is a major problem. This can be reduced if the dosage schedule is made more frequent.

GABAPENTIN
(Neurontin) available as tablets, capsules

This drug was recently introduced after successful trials in post-herpetic neuralgia. It causes the same side effects as other anticonvulsants, but less frequently and has a better safety profile. There are small, poor-quality case reports of its use in trigeminal neuralgia, yet it is widely used in clinical practice. A trial is being conducted currently on its use in patients with intractable pain. The drug has not been studied in pregnant women and it is not known if it passes into breast milk.

Table 9 provides a suggested dosage schedule.

Table 9

SUGGESTED DOSAGE SCHEDULE FOR GABAPENTIN				
Daily Dose	Day	Capsules / tablets to be taken		
		Morning	Midday	Evening
300mg	1	0	0	300mg
600mg	2	300mg	0	300mg
900mg	3	300mg	300mg	300mg
1200mg	4	300mg	300mg	600mg
1500mg	5	600mg	300mg	600mg
1800mg	6	600mg	600mg	600mg
2000mg	7-14	600mg	600mg	800mg
2200mg	15-21	800mg	600mg	800mg
2400mg	22-28	800mg	800mg	800mg
Most patients use a range between 1200 – 1800 mg daily.				

OXCARBAZEPINE
(Trileptal) available as tablets, suspension

Oxcarbazepine, a daughter drug of carbamazepine, was introduced in some countries many years ago, but it has only recently become available in the UK and US. Although not subject to a randomized controlled trial, it has been evaluated in a prospective cohort study over 15 years; thus there is better evidence for its use than other drugs in this section.

How does the drug work?

It is well absorbed and peak levels are reached within 2 hours. It is rapidly broken down and then excreted through the kidneys. It has a half-life of 8-11 hours and therefore should be used three or four times a day. It does not affect the liver enzymes.

What side effects does it cause?

Oxcarbazepine is related to carbamazepine. Cross-sensitivity needs to be considered if using it in patients allergic to carbamazepine. It has a side effects profile similar to that of other anticonvulsant drugs, but less severe effects than those associated with carbamazepine. It does alter salt distribution in the body when used in higher doses.

What drugs does it react with?

Relatively few.

Does it work in trigeminal neuralgia?

In case reports, it appears to be effective at controlling the pain of trigeminal neuralgia. We have recently reported a long follow-up study on its use, and shown that it was initially very effective, but lost its effect, not because of the development of tolerance but because of progression of disease. A 300 mg dose of oxcarbazepine is equal to 200 mg of carbamazepine.

Since oxcarbazepine is not licensed for use in trigeminal neuralgia in many countries, both patient and primary-care doctor need to be aware of this, and it is useful for patients to be given written information about it.

A leaflet given to my patients is reproduced in Table 10 on the following pages.

Table 10

EXAMPLE OF A PATIENT INFORMATION SHEET ON OXCARBAZEPINE

Oxcarbazepine or Trileptal is an anticonvulsant drug. Although it has been on the market in some countries for many years, it has only recently been available in the US and UK. Its chemical composition is similar to carbamazepine (Tegretol). Since it is a "daughter product," it shares many characteristics with carbamazepine. The drug is ultimately broken down in the body into the same products as carbamazepine. However, this is not done in the same way, so the same liver enzymes are not used by oxcarbazepine.

How much and how often should I take oxcarbazepine?

Oxcarbazepine should be taken in the same way as carbamazepine, using it regularly and at regular intervals throughout the day with the largest doses being taken at night. A dose of 300 mg of oxcarbazepine is equivalent to 200 mg of carbamazepine. It is important to raise and lower the daily dose slowly to avoid side effects. I suggest one dose change every three days.

The average dose required is 300 mg four times a day, but there is wide variation in the amount people need. Although it is normally recommended that drugs be taken after meals, for patients with trigeminal neuralgia the time of worse pain is, in fact, at mealtimes. I suggest that you take the drug at least 30 minutes before meal times and at times when you touch your face, e.g. washing, shaving.

Can I take carbamazepine and oxcarbazepine together?

If you are changing over from carbamazepine, it is possible to take both drugs together, gradually replacing each dose of oxcarbazepine with carbamazepine. It is not recommended that you take both drugs, since there is no benefit in this. You can take oxcarbazepine with other anticonvulsant drugs.

What are the side effects of oxcarbazepine?

The side effects of oxcarbazepine are similar to those of carbamazepine, but milder with less drowsiness, tiredness and feeling of being "a zombie." If you had an allergy to carbamazepine, you may still be able to take oxcarbazepine. Some patients can, however, be allergic to oxcarbazepine. The major side effect of oxcarbazepine is that at higher dosages it causes changes in the distribution of salt in the blood. This can lead to effects such as drowsiness, tiredness, swelling of the ankles and weight gain. If these side effects persist, your doctor can easily do a blood test to check this out. Dose reduction will quickly resolve the problem. People at highest risk of having problems with their salt balance are those on diuretics (water tablets) for blood pressure.

In my use of the drug in 18 patients over periods as long as 8 years, I have not observed any severe side effects — no effects on the white blood cells, red cells or liver.

Can I take other drugs with oxcarbazepine including warfarin?

Oxcarbazepine does not interfere with as many drugs as carbamazepine, and therefore is safer to use when you are on other medication. It is safe to use with warfarin (an anticoagulant).

Continued...

...Continued

Can I develop tolerance to oxcarbazepine if I take it for long periods?
In my experience, drug tolerance does not develop, but the condition itself gradually becomes more severe and surgery is indicated. In my group of patients, all but 3 patients eventually had surgery. No drugs cure the condition; they just prevent the nerve transmissions from occurring.

Is it safe to take oxcarbazepine long term or should I come off it as soon as possible?
Oxcarbazepine has been designed for long-term use. However, if your pain goes into remission, it is a good idea to stop taking the drug. If the pain returns, you can restart it again slowly.

How will I know that I have gone into remission?
The only way you will know that you have gone into remission will be if you slowly reduce the drug and find that the pain does not recur. It is therefore a good idea to keep a daily pain diary as shown below. This will give you an idea of how the pain changes over days. It is useful to take to your doctor so he/she can also see how your pain responds to the drug.
Date: Pain severity score 0-10; pain relief 0-10; number tablets; side effects

How do I know that this drug is effective in trigeminal neuralgia?
Unfortunately, no well conducted randomized controlled trials have been done with oxcarbazepine in patients with trigeminal neuralgia. The only evidence we have to support its use in patients with trigeminal neuralgia is that its use has been reported in three reports with a total of 45 patients. It is assumed that since oxcarbazepine is similar to carbamazepine, it will have similar properties. This is not always the case. It is therefore used on the basis of "let's try it and see."

Dr. Joanna M. Zakrzewska
Copyright Barts and the London NHS Trust November 2000

Oxcarbazepine can be taken four times a day as shown in Table 11 below.

Table 11

SUGGESTED DOSAGE SCHEDULE FOR OXCARBAZEPINE					
Daily dosage	Day	Morning	Lunchtime	Afternoon	Nightime
600mg	1- 3	300mg			300mg
900mg	4-14	300mg	300mg		300mg
1200mg	15-21	300mg	300mg	300mg	300mg
1500mg	22 - 28	300mg	300mg	300mg	600mg
If you are replacing your carbamazepine with oxcarbazepine, substitute one dose of 200 mg carbamazepine for 300 mg oxcarbazepine every three days until the changeover is complete.					

Table 12: Key facts

ADVANTAGES AND DISADVANTAGES OF DRUGS CURRENTLY BEING USED FOR TRIGEMINAL NEURALGIA – EVIDENCE IN TABLE 5 AND TABLE 8		
Drug	Advantages	Disadvantages
Baclofen (Lioresal)	Wide dosage range possible Few side effects No major drug interactions Can be used if patient allergic to other anticonvulsant drugs Can use as add-on therapy	Needs to be started and reduced slowly Needs to be taken on a three or four times a day schedule Monitor kidney function in long- term use
Carbamazepine (Tegretol)	Highly effective, rapid pain control Wide dosage range, which enables a range of dosage schemes Variety of formulations	All patients will have side effects Interferes with function of other drugs Causes changes in liver enzymes Allergy develops in 7 % Regular blood tests needed
Lamotrigine (Lamictal)	Can be used in the elderly Does not interact with common drugs Effective if used twice daily Tolerable side effects	Its use as standalone therapy has not been assessed Rapid dose rises lead to rashes, so not suitable for acute pain control Side effects noted in most patients
Clonazepam (Rivotril, klonopin)	May be effective	Not evaluated in a randomized controlled trial Side effects very common with drowsiness being a major problem and enhanced by alcohol Regular blood tests especially liver function Must not be withdrawn rapidly
Gabapentin (Neurontin)	May be effective as shown in other neuropathic pains Fewer side effects than other anticonvulsants, so well tolerated Does not interfere with other drugs	Not evaluated in randomized controlled trial Needs to be started and reduced slowly Expensive
Phenytoin (Dilantin, Epanutin)	May be effective Long history of use Appears to work well with carbamazepine	Little variation in dosage range Regular blood tests needed Interacts with drugs, especially diabetic ones Need to consider folic acid replacement if used long term
Oxcarbazepine (Trileptal)	Effective for short-term use as shown in long- term cohort studies Fewer side effects than carbamazepine Rarely reacts with other drugs	Not evaluated in random- ized controlled trial Dose-related salt imbalance Patients allergic to carbamazepine may exhibit cross sensitivity
Valproic acid (Epilim, depakote)	May be effective Numerous side effects	Not evaluated in random- ized controlled clinical trial Can cause liver failure, so regular monitoring required

PHENYTOIN
(Dilantin, Epanutin) available as tablets, chewable tablets, suspension

This drug works in a complex way with very variable effects on individuals, and its effectiveness is dependent on the form in which it is used. Due to the way it works in doses over 300 mg daily, a small increase in dosage can result in a disproportionately large increase in blood levels and hence unexpected side effects. It reduces levels of folic acid, thus it is important to check folic acid levels when used long term. Phenytoin interacts with many drugs. It is often used when patients develop an allergy to carbamazepine. It can be used together with carbamazepine. It is not recommended currently for use in trigeminal neuralgia because of all these problems. An injectable form of it, fosphenytoin, has been shown to be useful in controlling an acute attack.

VALPROIC ACID, SODIUM VALPORATE
(Depakene, Depakote, Epilim, Convulex) available as tablets, capsules, liquid

This drug was first used in trigeminal neuralgia in 1980. Although it is suggested that its two forms, one as an acid and the other as a salt, are interchangeable, care needs to be taken. It is rapidly absorbed, reaching peak levels within 2 hours and its half-life is relatively short, 6-17 hours. Its main side effects are tremor, weight gain and hair loss, all of which are reversible on cessation. It should not be used during pregnancy. It has few drug interactions, but it does interact with carbamazepine and phenytoin. It tends to be used by neurologists, since they prescribe it for epilepsy. The small case reports suggest that it is an effective drug, and it was used in one poor-quality randomized controlled trial.

NEW DRUGS

Drugs that are being evaluated, but on which there are as yet no publication regarding their use in trigeminal neuralgia, include leviteracetam (Keppra), tiagabine (Gabitril) pregablin (Lyrica) and zonisamide (Zonegran), cannabinoids and harkoseride.

What are the advantages and the disadvantages of the various drugs currently available?

Table 12 on the previous page provides some guidance on the use of these drugs. It is important to remember that not all these drugs need to be tried before referral for surgical management. In Chapter 8 you will find guidance on how decisions on further management can be made. Chapter 7 also provides additional information on how improved pain control can be achieved. You may also wish to look at other details in George Weigel and Ken Casey's book, **Striking Back! The Trigeminal Neuralgia and Face Pain Handbook.**

MRS. G – CASE STUDY

After her diagnosis Mrs. G was put on carbamazepine, 100 mg three times a day, and phenytoin, 100 mg daily. This controlled the pain and after two months she was able to withdraw it completely with no recurrence of pain. Nine months later the pain returned and she restarted slowly the same medication, but this time it gave her no relief. She went back to her primary-care doctor, who changed her treatment to gabapentin 600 mg three times a day and co-dydramol 1gm four times a day. This provided relief for two months and the pain returned very severely. Her primary-care doctor then stopped the gabapentin and restarted phenytoin 200 mg four times a day. This failed to control the pain and Mrs. G was now confused, unsteady, unable to concentrate, and felt her quality of life was very poor. She asked for a referral to a specialty center. In her medical history, Mrs. G had suffered three deep-vein thromboses and was now taking warfarin, an anticoagulant. She was also being investigated for a possible stomach ulcer. She came to the specialty clinic in severe pain, unable to talk due to the pain.

Mrs. G had classical trigeminal neuralgia as described in the chapter on diagnosis. The primary-care doctor therefore thought he could manage her pain. He put her on two drugs. What justification was there for this?

What should he have done?

Mrs. G decided she wanted to stay on medication, so how should she be managed now?

Discussion

Carbamazepine and phenytoin are the two oldest drugs used in the management of trigeminal neuralgia. There is no evidence that both should be used and there are now more drugs to choose from. Given the rarity of the disease, it would not be expected that the primary-care doctor would know the latest guidelines on treatment. Therefore, the doctor should look for guidance, and in the UK, this is provided by the NHS by PRODIGY (see the end of chapter for details).Consulting this Internet site would have helped the primary-care doctor confirm the diagnostic criteria and would have provided guidelines on treatment – carbamazepine on its own and a pain diary. It would also have recommended referral to a specialist at the second episode, when the drugs were no longer effective. There was no justification for using gabapentin at this stage, and it is known that analgesic drugs such as co-dydramol do not help. From the Web site, he could have printed out a patient information leaflet to give to the patient and provided information regarding a patient support group that the patient could have contacted.

When Mrs. G visited the specialist, in severe pain, it was necessary to first give her a long-acting local anaesthetic to give her temporary relief of pain, so she could provide a pain history and could concentrate on what the specialist was telling her.

Continued...

...Continued

Further management

Mrs. G. had responded well to carbamazepine initially, but she was now on warfarin (an anticoagulant), a drug known to interact seriously with carbamazepine, so she needed a different drug. According to the levels of evidence, the next drugs of choice would be baclofen or lamotrigine. Both are known to work better with carbamazepine, but lamotrigine doses cannot be raised rapidly. Mrs. G was in severe pain and needed to increase her drug levels quickly. The next drug of choice, based on the hierarchy of evidence, is oxcarbazepine, which has been evaluated in a long-term cohort study. Since it is a daughter drug to carbamazepine, it could therefore be assumed that this drug would give adequate pain relief. Mrs. G was started on oxcarbazepine, given a pain diary and patient information. Some routine baseline investigations were also done.

---

3. What drugs can be used to control the burning aching pain?

In some patients the sharp shooting pain comes under control with trigeminal neuralgia drugs, but there remains a dull, aching, burning, and nearly continuous type of pain. Management of this pain is difficult, since there have been no clinical trials to guide us. There remains controversy about whether this is really a type of trigeminal neuralgia (atypical trigeminal neuralgia), another form of neuropathic pain, or a chronic idiopathic facial pain (atypical facial pain).

A systematic review of management of neuropathic pain and trials in chronic idiopathic facial pain has been done. Antidepressant drugs, especially the tricyclic antidepressant type amitriptyline, and second-generation ones known as the serotonin re-uptake inhibitors (SSRIs), in particular fluoxetine (Prozac), used in smaller doses than for depression, have been shown to be effective. Treatments need to be used for a long time, a minimum of 12 weeks and up to two years. Cognitive behavior therapy is also useful and is discussed in the next chapter.

4. What research is needed?

Basic science

Basic scientists working in the area of pharmacology need to look at mechanisms of a drug's potential to target specific sites of action in order to reduce side effects. This then needs to be rapidly translated into drugs that can be used in patients. More basic pharmacologists need to work closely with clinicians.

Pharmacogenetics

Research in this area would help to identify why there are individual variations in patients' responses to drugs.

Randomized controlled trials

Any new drugs being considered for use in trigeminal neuralgia should first be evaluated in a small open-label trial and, if found to have promise, should be the subject of a randomized controlled trial. These may need to be carried out in several centers to ensure that the number of patients recruited is large enough to show a difference. It would be useful to have a template for the conduct of such clinical trials that has been approved by an international group of experts, since it would be easier to compare drugs.

Combination therapy

Trials need to be done to assess not only the combination of anti-neuralgic drugs, but also whether additions of antidepressants would optimize treatments.

SUMMARY

- Strategies are proposed on how to maximize the use of medication, which include providing patients with adequate information, giving clear instruction on the use of the medication(s), and asking patients to keep a pain diary.
- When taking medication for trigeminal neuralgia, it is important to provide regular reviews for monitoring response in terms of both pain relief and side effects.
- The main group of drugs to be used for trigeminal neuralgia is anticonvulsant drugs.
- Guidelines on the treatment of trigeminal neuralgia in primary care can be accessed from a UK primary care doctors Internet site. High quality evidence can also be found in the Cochrane Library and Clinical Evidence.
- If carbamazepine is no longer effective, there are a variety of other drugs that can be used, or referral to a neurosurgeon can be initiated.
- Future research needs to ensure that all new drugs of potential benefit in trigeminal neuralgia are tested in randomized controlled trials.

FURTHER READING AND REFERENCES

Web sites
Checked May 2005

The **Cochrane Library** consists of a regularly updated collection of evidence-based medicine databases, including The Cochrane Database of Systematic Reviews, which provides high quality information to people providing and receiving care and those responsible for research, teaching, funding and administration at all levels.
http://www.update-software.com/cochrane

The **Centre for Reviews and Dissemination** (CRD) was established in January 1994, and aims to provide research-based information about the effects of interventions used in health and social care.
http://www.york.ac.uk/inst/crd/

Clinical Evidence, from the **BMJ Publishing Group**, is the international source of the best available evidence for effective health care. This group promotes informed decision-making by summarizing what's known — and not known — about the treatment and prevention of nearly 200 medical conditions. http://www.clinicalevidence.org

Current Controlled Trials Ltd. is part of the Current Science Group of biomedical publishing companies. In response to the growing body of opinion in favor of prospective registration of controlled trials, Current Controlled Trials Ltd. launched the Current Controlled Trials Web site in late 1998, aiming to increase the availability, and promote the exchange, of information about ongoing randomized controlled trials worldwide. http://controlled-trials.com/

PRODIGY : a source of clinical knowledge, based on the best available evidence, about the common conditions and symptoms managed by primary healthcare professionals. Patient Information Leaflets (PILs) form an integral part of PRODIGY and are intended to empower patients by increasing their understanding of their health problem. There is a section on trigeminal neuralgia. http://www.prodigy.nhs.uk/

Physicians' Desk Reference (PDR) for the latest, most accurate drug information. The drug information on PDR*health* is written in lay terms and is based on the FDA-approved drug information found in the PDR. It gives consumers clear explanations for the safe and effective use of prescription and nonprescription drugs—explanations that are consistent with the information professionals are referencing in the PDR. http://www.pdrhealth.com/

Electronic, International Drug Reference from the Pharmaceutical Press, London, UK. Accessible only with a subscription. Not for the public, but for health care professionals. http://www.micromedex.com/products/martindale/

The BNF provides UK health care professionals with authoritative and practical information on the selection and clinical use of medicines in a clear, concise and accessible manner. http://bnf.org/bnf/

Books / booklets

Weigel G., Casey K. (2004), **Striking Back! The Trigeminal Neuralgia and Face Pain Handbook.** Trigeminal Neuralgia Association, Gainesville, Florida ISBN 0-9672393 -2-X

Zakrzewska JM (2002) Trigeminal neuralgia in **Assessment and Management of Orofacial Pain.** Edited Zakrzewska JM and Harrison SD Volume 14 in series, **Pain Research and Clinical Management.** Elsevier ISBN 0-444-50984-4 chapter pages 267-370.

"The Use of Medicines Beyond l\Licence – Information for Patients" This document is an information booklet prepared on behalf of The Association for Palliative Medicine and The British Pain Society. It is intended to help patients better understand drug-licensing regulations in relation to pain management. Can be downloaded from http://www.britishpainsociety.org/gen_pubs_reading.html, or obtained from their offices at The Secretariat, The British Pain Society, 21 Portland Place, London W1B 1PY, United Kingdom.

References

Blom S (1962) Trigeminal Neuralgia. Its Treatment With a New Anticonvulsant Drug (G32883). *Lancet* **i**:839-840.

Campbell FG, Graham J G and Zilkha K J (1966) Clinical Trial of Carbamazepine (Tegretol) in Trigeminal Neuralgia. *J Neurol Neurosurg Psychiatry* **29**:265-267.

Fromm GH and Terrence C F (1987) Comparison of L-Baclofen and Racemic Baclofen in Trigeminal Neuralgia. *Neurology* **37**:1725-1728.

Fromm GH, Terrence C F and Chattha A S (1984) Baclofen in the Treatment of Trigeminal Neuralgia: Double-Blind Study and Long-Term Follow-Up. *Ann Neurol* **15**:240-244.

Gilron I, Booher S L, Rowan M S, Smoller M S and Max M B (2000) A Randomized, Controlled Trial of High-Dose Dextromethorphan in Facial Neuralgias. *Neurology* **55**:964-971.

Killian JM and Fromm G H (1968) Carbamazepine in the Treatment of Neuralgia. *Arch Neurol* **19**:129-136.

Kitt CA, Gruber K, Davis M, Woolf C J and Levine J D (2000) Trigeminal Neuralgia: Opportunities for Research and Treatment. *Pain* **85**:3-7.

Kondziolka D, Lemley T, Kestle J R, Lunsford L D, Fromm G H, Jannetta and PJ. (1994) The Effect of Single-Application Topical Ophthalmic Anesthesia in Patients With Trigeminal Neuralgia. A Randomized Double-Blind Placebo-Controlled Trial. *J Neurosurg* **80**:993-997.

Lechin, F, van der Dijs, B, Lechin M.E., Amat, J, Lechin, A. E., Cabrera A, Gomez, F, Acosta, E., Arocha, L, Villa, S., and Jienez, V. (1989). Pimozide therapy for trigeminal neuralgia. *Arch.Neurol.* **46**: 960-963.

Lindstrom, P and Lindblom V. (1987) The analgesic effect of tocainide in trigeminal neuralgia. *Pain* **28**: 45-50.

McQuay H, Carroll D, Jadad A R, Wiffen P and Moore A (1995) Anticonvulsant Drugs for Management of Pain: a Systematic Review. *BMJ* **311**:1047-1052.

McQuay HJ, Tramer M, Nye B A, Carroll D, Wiffen P J and Moore R A (1996) A Systematic Review of Antidepressants in Neuropathic Pain. *Pain* **68**:217-227.

Nicol CF (1969) A Four Year Double-Blind Study of Tegretol in Facial Pain. *Headache* **9**:54-57.

Rockliff BW and Davis E H (1966) Controlled Sequential Trials of Carbamazepine in Trigeminal Neuralgia. *Arch Neurol* **15**:129-136.

Sindrup SH and Jensen T S (1999) Efficacy of Pharmacological Treatments of Neuropathic Pain: an Update and Effect Related to Mechanism of Drug Action. *Pain* **83**:389-400.

Taylor JC, Brauer S and Espir M L E (1981) Long-Term Treatment of Trigeminal Neuralgia. *Postgraduate Medical J* **57**:16-18.

Vilming ST, Lyberg T and Latase X (1986) Tizanidine in the Management of Trigeminal Neuralgia. *Cephalalgia* **6**:181-182.

Wiffen P, McQuay H, Carroll D, Jadad A and Moore A (2005) Anticonvulsant Drugs for Acute and Chronic Pain. *Cochrane Database Syst Rev*CD001133. updated regularly

Zakrzewska JM (2001) Consumer Views on Management of Trigeminal Neuralgia. *Headache 2001* **41**:369-376.

Zakrzewska JM and Lopez B C (2005) Trigeminal Neuralgia. *Clinical Evidence* updated every year also on *Internet www.clinicalevidence.com.uk*

Zakrzewska JM and Patsalos P N (2002) Long-Term Cohort Study Comparing Medical (Oxcarbazepine) and Surgical Management of Intractable Trigeminal Neuralgia. *Pain* **95**:259-266.

APPENDIX

DRUG NAMES THAT ARE OR MAY BE USED IN MANAGEMENT OF TRIGEMINAL NEURALGIA AND RELATED PAINS

Generic name	Trade name/s used US /UK	Type of drug
Amitryptyline ✗	Elavil, Tripafen	AD
Baclofen	Lioresal	Muscle relaxant
Capsaicin	Axsain, Dolorac, Capzasin-P, Zacin	Analgesic, topical
Carbamazepine	Tegretol, Tegretol retard, Teril retard, Timonil retard, Atretol, Carbatrol, Epitol	AED
Clonazepam	Rivotril, klonopin	Tranquilizer
Codeine phosphate	Codeine	Opioid
Dosulepin	Prothiaden	AD
Fentanyl ✗	Actiq, Duragesic ✗	Opioid
Fluoxetine	Prozac	AD
Gabapentin ✗	Neurontin ✗	AED
Imipramine	Norfranil, tofranil	AD
Lamotrigine	Lamictal	AED
Leviteracetam	Keppra	AED
Morphine	Oramorph, Seredol, Morcap, Morphagesic, MST Continus, MXL, Zomorph	Opioid
Nortriptyline	Allegron, Pamelor	AD
Oxcarbazepine	Trileptal	AED
Oxycodone	OxyNorm, OxyContin	Opioid
Phenytoin	Dilantin, Epanutin	AED
Pimozide	Orap	Antipsychotic
Tiagabine	Gabitril	AED
Tizanidine	Zanaflex	Muscle relaxant
Topiramte	Topamax	AED
Valproic acid	Depakene, Depakote, Epilim, Convulex	AED
Venlafaxine	Effexor	AD
Zonisamide	Zonergan	AED

AED – anti-epileptic drug (anticonvulsant), AD – antidepressant drug trade names are subject to change. Before prescribing any of these, the details must be checked in a current drug formulary. Some of the major opioid analgesics have been listed, but the non-pioid analgesics have not been listed, since there is an enormous range of these.

PAIN DIARY

Patient's name:_____Date of visit:_____

At the end of each day, please record your pain severity and ability to do activities according to the definitions below:

a) How intense (severe) is the pain ?
   On a scale of 0-10, where 0=no pain, 10=worse pain ever
b) How much has the pain interfered with your daily activities?
   On a scale of 0-10, where 0=No interference, 10=Unable to carry out activities
c.) How severe are the side effects of the drugs? You may wish to specify what they are
   On a scale of 0-10, where 0=no side effects, 10=severe side effects that stop all activities
d) Please enter number of tablets per day and which ones, by initial.

Carbamazepine (Tegretol)	100 mg (T1)	Lamotrogine (Lamictal)	25 mg (L)
Carbamazepine (Tegretol)	200 mg (T2)	Gabapentin (Neurontin)	300mg/600mg (G3/6)
Carbamazepine retard	400mg (TR)	Nortriptyline (Allegron)	10/20/30/40mg (N)
Oxcarbazepine (Trileptal)	300mg (OXC)	Fluoxetine (Prozac)	(P)
Baclofen (Lioresal)	10 mg (B)	Other	

PROPOSED DOSAGE SCHEDULES (completed with physician)
The times are just a guideline

Days	7.00 a.m.	12 MD	5.00 p.m.	11.00 p.m.

Patient to complete daily

Date	Pain	Activity	No. Tabs	Side Effects

CHAPTER 7

Additional Ways of Managing Trigeminal Neuralgia

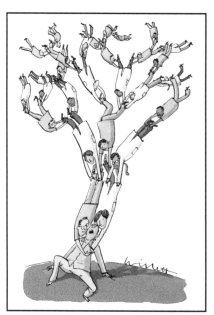

Patients with trigeminal neuralgia need support from health care workers, family, friends and support groups.

"I feel I am in control of the pain instead of the other way around, like it was years before. I have bad days and sometimes bad weeks or even months, but thoughts of death are no longer a part of my daily routine."

1. How is chronic pain treated?

The **biomedical model** of patient care is one that is adopted by many doctors and relies on finding a cause for a disease and then treating it either medically (with drugs) or surgically. This means the patients are controlled by health care workers, who take responsibility for the patients' health. The value of this model is expressed by this patient's comment:

"We need to find a medical doctor who is interested in TN as a specialty, for they have the power to prescribe medications, and to perform procedures and surgeries."

The patient can therefore be a passive recipient of care.

In the **biopsychosocial model of care,** the patients' social and psychological needs are taken into account. In this form of treatment, the patients are no longer passive recipients of care, but are encouraged to take responsibility for their health and to take control. This model takes into account the fact that all illness has a cause (unknown or unknown) — that it can in some instances be treated medically, but that it has an effect on the sufferer both emotionally and socially and that this can affect the outcome. There is good evidence to show that this approach to health care results in increased patient satisfaction, increased compliance with treatment and decreased use of health care services.

Trigeminal neuralgia has for a long time been managed along the biomedical model. In the medical literature there is virtually nothing related to a more psychological approach to the management of trigeminal neuralgia. It is assumed, particularly in patients with classical trigeminal neuralgia, that using drugs and then surgical management will deal effectively with this severe, suicidal pain. Yet my own experience over 20 years and my reading through the hundred or so e-mail messages that patients have contributed to this book, show that the emotional impact of this pain is enormous and their response to it is crucial on the road to effective management. I have alluded to these in Chapter 1.

2. What are the effects of chronic pain?

Pain is something we have all experienced and we know it is one of the most powerful senses we have. Most of us think of it negatively as something we do not want and yet if we had no pain, we would be unable to survive, as we need pain to:
- warn us about impending or actual damage
- motivate us to escape and take preventive action
- warn others around of potential threat and danger
- instigate empathy and care in others

It is when pain loses these functions that it becomes useless and a burden, and this is what is meant by chronic or persistent pain – pain that has outlived its usefulness. It is no longer warning us that further damage is occurring, so the system is malfunctioning. It is important to remember these positive aspects of pain when learning to live with pain.

Chronic pain results in a range of physical, emotional and social changes that add to the burden of the original pain and are summarized in Table 1 below.

Table 1: Key facts

POTENTIAL EFFECTS OF CHRONIC PAIN
Physical
• Immobility and consequent wasting of muscles, joints, tense stiff muscles • Depression of the immune system and increased susceptibility to disease • Alteration of the patterns of steroid production • Disturbed sleep • Poor appetite and nutrition • Increased fatigue • Lack of concentration • Dependence on medication and inappropriate use of professional health care systems
Emotional
• Anxiety, fear • Loneliness • Bitterness, anger • Frustration, depression, suicide • Helplessness • Isolation from society and family, becoming introvertive • Transfer of these emotions to caregivers
Social
• Over-dependence on family and other caregivers • Costs of healthcare services and medication • Job absenteeism and disruption in the workplace • Loss of income • Non-productivity in the workplace and in the home • Financial burden on family, friends and employers • Worker compensation costs and welfare payments

All these factors then lead to unhelpful thoughts such as **catastrophizing** and beliefs that further compound the problem. The continuous rounds of consultations, the battery of tests and the range of treatments given, become an ever-increasing spiral leading to **depression** and even

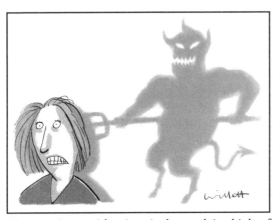

Many patients with trigeminal neuralgia think of their pain as a devil that can strike at any time.

suicide. This journey to despair has been undertaken by many, as described here by this sufferer:

"My whole life was falling apart; everything was falling apart. My husband was losing a lot of weight, New Year I spent in bed, everything was falling apart in our house, my job, everything. And there was nothing I could do about the pain. The doctor told me there is nothing else we can do for you and I thought I can just end it now because the pain is too bad and all I do is sit here in this bed holding onto the rails waiting for the pain to come and I can't take it any more."

3. HOW CAN SUFFERERS HELP THEMSELVES?

Some sufferers have found a way out of this voyage of despair, as this patient reports:

"I wanted to keep that positive approach all the time, but I could see how it could drag you down, and you go down and down and down."

How have they achieved this positive outlook?

For some trigeminal neuralgia sufferers, a "miracle cure" (drug or surgical treatment) has been found. But those sufferers with the less typical types or with other causes for their facial pain have not found any doctor to help them and they have turned from persons to patients who no longer have control over their lives. These sufferers need to realize that to get out of this downward spiral, they have to help themselves, as expressed by this patient: *"Doctors overall have been helpful, but they have their limits."*

Medicine has as yet not found a cure and, although difficult, the sufferer must learn to live with the pain, but they can reduce the impact it has on their lives. Pain patients need to learn to become a person again, and it can take time first to realize the need to do this oneself and then to achieve it. This is exactly what Ruthi Purchase has realized. She has prepared handouts for her support group and I am taking the liberty of showing you some of her work on the following page:

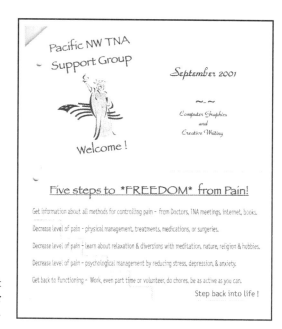

Pacific NW TNA
Support Group

September 2001

~ ~
*Computer Graphics
and
Creative Writing*

Welcome!

Five steps to *FREEDOM* from Pain!

Get information about all methods for controlling pain – from Doctors, TNA meetings, internet, books.

Decrease level of pain - physical management, treatments, medications, or surgeries.

Decrease level of pain – learn about relaxation & diversions with meditation, nature, religion & hobbies.

Decrease level of pain – psychological management by reducing stress, depression, & anxiety.

Get back to functioning – Work, even part time or volunteer, do chores, be as active as you can.

Step back into life!

This is an illustration that Ruthi Purchase prepared for her support group.

This has led organizations like The American Chronic Pain Association and the Scottish Pain Association to publish little leaflets on ten steps to move from patient to person. In Table 2 below I have listed the steps they suggest.

Table 2 :

THE TEN STEPS FOR MOVING FROM PATIENT TO PERSON, BASED ON LEAFLETS BY THE SCOTTISH PAIN ASSOCIATION AND THE AMERICAN PAIN ASSOCIATION

1. Accept pain - be realistic
2. Get involved – take an active role, educate yourself
3. Set priorities – ask yourself what matters
4. Set realistic goals – break up tasks, pace yourself
5. Recognize thoughts and feelings as they affect physical functioning
6. Learn relaxation and the value of distraction
7. Exercise and modify diet if difficult to eat
8. Know your basic rights – be treated with respect
9. Communicate – learn to get your needs met, find support
10. Rediscover hope – gain control, focus on abilities, lessen suffering

The first step to recovery, therefore, is the realization that the sufferers have to learn to manage their pain themselves. One trigeminal neuralgia patient said the following in her e-mail note to me:

"I have accepted that this will be my lifelong problem and I take responsibility for caring for myself."

Ruthi Purchase, in one of her handouts, takes it even further with her short piece called "Shifting our perspective of suffering," shown in Table 3 below.

Table 3

"SHIFTING OUR PERSPECTIVE OF SUFFERING," FROM R. PURCHASE'S HANDOUT FOR THE PACIFIC NW TNA SUPPORT GROUP

We know that at times suffering can serve to toughen us and to strengthen us. Did you know at other times it can have value by functioning in the opposite manner? It can soften us, make us more sensitive and gentle. The vulnerability we experience in the midst of our suffering can open us and deepen our connections with others.

"A deep distress hath humanized my soul" – William Wordsworth

Many sufferers, when told that they have to manage their pain, insist that they are already doing so and that it still has not worked. Like everything in life, new things need to be learned and knowledge needs to be deepened. You may have mastered a foreign language, and even passed an examination in it at school, but when you go to live in the country you will realize that your knowledge of the language is insufficient. Extra effort has to be put into learning it so that you can live and work in that country in an integrated way.

In the same way, pain management is a skill you can learn either through self-help manuals or by taking part in pain management courses. Leaflets such as *"Chronic Pain: Managing Your Emotions,"* available through the Mayo Clinic Web site, may be a useful starting point.

These types of courses are referred to as cognitive behavioral therapy (CBT). Dr. Daniel, writing in The Neuropathy Trust of the UK booklet, *"Neuropathic pain – Quality of life under the spotlight,"* describes CBT as "a non-medical intervention in chronic pain. It does not cure pain, but people can learn and develop self-management techniques to help them cope with it and improve their quality of life. Cognitive relates to knowing or perceiving, behavior refers to what people do and can include what they do to cope. By addressing thinking and behavior, cognitive behavioral pain management tries to reduce both the emotional and the physical consequences of pain. Self-management means that people learn ways to manage their pain themselves. They develop more confidence in doing this and eventually will not need as much help from the medical profession." It is essential to remember that CBT does not cure the underlying cause of the chronic pain.

4. DO WE KNOW WHETHER COGNITIVE BEHAVIORAL TREATMENT (CBT) HELPS PATIENTS WITH CHRONIC FACIAL PAIN?

Morley et al, in 1999 performed a systematic review of the literature (as described in Chapter 5) and showed that CBT is effective in the management of chronic pain. When one looks for evidence of its effectiveness in chronic orofacial pain, a number of trials have been carried out to assess its use in patients with temporomandibular (TMD) pain, and one trial involved patients with idiopathic facial pain and burning mouth syndrome. There have been no studies reporting the use of CBT in trigeminal neuralgia.

CBT is often used after all other types of interventions have failed. Amanda Williams (2003), a clinical psychologist with extensive experience in running pain management programs, argues that this may not be the correct approach. CBT aims to change the individual's relationship with pain. By offering it earlier, when it is less likely that patients will have developed pain-related behavioral problems, it will provide maximum freedom from the negative impact of pain. Keefe (2000) from the US has also proposed that pain clinicians should focus on early interventions. That is, on integrating CBT protocols into medical treatments, and developing tailored interventions, in order to prevent pain from becoming chronic and to improve the quality of life of patients suffering persistent pain. This needs to be explored further in trigeminal neuralgia sufferers.

What are the aims of CBT and what do these programs include?

The aims of CBT are shown in Table 4 on the following page.

Morley's (1999) systematic review highlights a range of problems that are encountered when reviewing the use of CBT in chronic pain. There are over 40 different types of CBT programs in which a wide variety of outcomes have been used, including variable treatment groups and variable therapists. The program used in chronic facial pain patients by Harrison and others included education about gate control theory, pain coping strategies, relaxation, assertiveness, communication training, maintenance of gains and coping with acute exacerbations (worsening) of pain.

<u>Table 4: Key Facts</u>

AIMS OF CBT

- Increase range and level of activity
- Reduce distress caused by pain
- Reduce depression
- Lessen fear
- Reduce frustration
- Increase control
- Increase independence from health care
- Decrease dependence on family, friends, society
- May reduce pain intensity

Dr. Michael Nicholas and his team in Australia have developed and assessed the effectiveness of their program, ADAPT. Full details are provided in their book, **Manage Your Pain.** Below is a modified overview version of it.

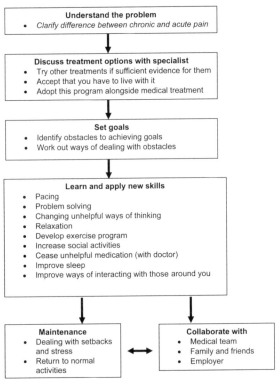

Understand the problem
- *Clarify difference between chronic and acute pain*

Discuss treatment options with specialist
- Try other treatments if sufficient evidence for them
- Accept that you have to live with it
- Adopt this program alongside medical treatment

Set goals
- Identify obstacles to achieving goals
- Work out ways of dealing with obstacles

Learn and apply new skills
- Pacing
- Problem solving
- Changing unhelpful ways of thinking
- Relaxation
- Develop exercise program
- Increase social activities
- Cease unhelpful medication (with doctor)
- Improve sleep
- Improve ways of interacting with those around you

Maintenance
- Dealing with setbacks and stress
- Return to normal activities

Collaborate with
- Medical team
- Family and friends
- Employer

There are many texts that can serve as a self-help manual. Table 5 below is based on a booklet called "*A Guide for Patients in Chronic Pain,*" produced by two nurses (Helen Henderson and Janette Barrie) and published by Napp Pharmaceuticals, which contains elements often used in CBT.

Table 5

PRACTICAL HINTS ON METHODS USED IN CHRONIC PAIN MANAGEMENT
Relaxation
• Needs practice • Keep a relaxation diary – which types are best, when and where • Practice diaphragmatic breathing • Relax all groups of muscles • Calm your thoughts using music or creating images in your mind • Spend 5 minutes a day relaxing physically and mentally • Try Yoga or tai chi
Pacing
• A technique that you can use to gradually increase your level of activity • Work out your baseline time for a given activity, divide by two, then pace up • NEVER do more than you planned • Pacing keeps you motivated by continually achieving a series of small goals
Goal setting
• Goal must be realistic • It must be something you can measure • It must be YOUR goal • Do not be too ambitious, but it needs to be important • Review progress regularly • Small steps are as important as big leaps • Enjoy your success
Managing stress
• Learn to relax • Have someone to confide in • Find a practical solution rather then worry about it • Use pacing techniques and breathing exercises

Continued ...

...Continued

Assertiveness and communication
• Be firm • Keep calm • Try not to complain, plead or be apologetic • Make your messages clear; be precise • Explain to people why you are asking them to do something • Ask for help – say I want, not "I need or cannot"
Improving sleep habits
• Do not take naps during the day • Avoid caffeine, alcohol, smoking for at least 4 hours before going to bed • Go to bed when tired, but try and go at the same time each night • Deal with your worries before bedtime • Keep the bedroom as a bedroom and do not watch TV, eat or read in it • Use breathing and relaxation techniques before going to bed • If you cannot sleep, get up and do something relaxing • Get up at the same time, regardless of whether you slept well

It is very important for other people to be involved and for the sufferers to communicate how best they can be helped. One patient expressed her need this way:

"When I need someone to help me with a procedure or trip to the doctor or something else, it feels extraordinarily lonely to have to ask friends and family to step in."

People without pain may find it difficult to understand the effects of pain and often do not know how best to help and so get frustrated. It is helpful for sufferers to agree with their family and friends exactly how and when they can help. Here are some stories from sufferers with trigeminal neuralgia who have achieved this ability to ask for help:

- *"I had to learn to get comfortable asking or telling my best friend what I needed. I still remember finally getting comfortable with lying down on her couch when I was just too tired to drive home. Once I was able to rest, we ended up having a wonderful second half of the day together. I remember her telling me days later how happy she was that I was comfortable enough to rest at her house. People want to help, but accepting the help is sometimes harder than it seems."*

- *"He takes care of our children and me when I am unable to do it myself. He has loved me through it all. We are a wonderful team. He speaks for me when I cannot and he always knows just what to say. He has been a constant support in my life."*

Table 6: Key facts

PSYCHOLOGICAL THERAPIES THAT MAY BE HELPFUL IN CHRONIC PAIN
• Relaxation techniques • Distraction • Imagery • Hypnosis • Biofeedback • Positive thinking • Reduce **catastrophizing** behavior, and developing coping strategies • Cognitive behavioral therapy - this often involves many of the above

5. WHAT IS DISTRACTION THERAPY?

This is a very simple procedure in which patients are encouraged to focus attention on a stimulus other than pain. Often another sensory modality is used, e.g. touch or olfaction. This can be as simple as reading, listening to music, talking about pleasant events or breathing rhythmically. It can be used effectively while waiting for drugs to take their effect. A number of studies have shown distraction can reduce pain.

Here are examples of sufferers using these techniques:
- *"If I choose not to dwell on my problems, I seem to get along much better. I lead a very busy life."*
- *"I'm a pretty optimistic person, and on most days I can distract myself enough to get through the day with the help of medication."*

6. WHAT IS MEANT BY IMAGERY?

This differs from distraction in that it is not dependent on an external stimulus, but is dependent on the mind evoking visual or other sensory images. It can be used as part of distraction. People can be taught the technique and they can use it for periods of 10 to 20 minutes. The pain sufferer needs to be alert and to concentrate on creating a pleasant image where pain no longer exists. If the pain is too severe, it can be incorporated into the picture such that the pain can be made to flow away or be transformed into another sensation, e.g. numbness.

Color can also be used to create images, and pain can be converted from a harsh red color to more peaceful greens and blues. If this results in a change in mood and emotional state, then the perception of pain can be altered. There is no evidence for its effectiveness in chronic facial pain.

7. HOW COULD IMAGES AND PAINTINGS BE USED IN PAIN MANAGEMENT?

The American philosopher Khatchadourian postulates that art brings order to the human world and can bring people together –"we may become more sensitive to ourselves and others and so perhaps better equipped to exist on deeper human levels." A picture can help engage patients in deep and revealing conversations, as shown by Wikstrom in her work with elderly people in nursing homes.

Wikstrom writes, "Reading a painting is a complex procedure that allows the onlooker to perceive far more than is represented. One aspect of the complexity of a painting is the reality of times, places and people interacting with the onlooker. Another aspect of complexity is the diversity of languages expressed in a painting. It could be an imitation of nature, a self-expression of the artist or it can speak for itself. Consequently, a painting can be a challenge for the onlooker to search for the language described by the artist."

Deborah Padfield, a photographic artist, took this further and worked with patients to create photographic images of their pain. She has published her work in a book called **Perceptions of Pain.** By adding a visual dimension to the language of chronic pain, Deborah found that interactions between the patient and health care provider were improved and in some instances proved to be the only way to determine the intensity of the pain.

Art has been known to have healing powers, yet it is only recently being used for these purposes in health care settings. The Massachusetts General Hospital Cancer Center has recently reported on its use of art, which has been summed up by one of their artists and cancer survivors, Brian:

"Art that distracts and engages a patient's mind with cheerful and calming colors, forms, and images can spontaneously and effectively reduce the levels of anxiety that are often present in hospital waiting rooms.... When patients are relaxed and receptive, they place themselves in the best possible state of mind and spirit for medicine to do its work."

What is meant by metaphor?

Another way of communicating about pain and managing pain is to use metaphors, and its meaning will become clear after reading this section. This section and the exercises were given to me by Kate Maguire, a psychotherapist who uses these techniques with victims of torture.

Metaphors are a symbolic and a profound means of communicating complex information, observations, reflections and feelings in simple ways.

Metaphor, among other things, enables people to speak of the unspeakable, is open but safe, is deeply effective, integrates the cognitive and the emotions, creates a safe place and provides a means by which patients can help themselves. You can find metaphors in phrases, poetry, images, dreams, stories and objects. In the box below are exercises for health care workers and patients to try. See the pictures below.

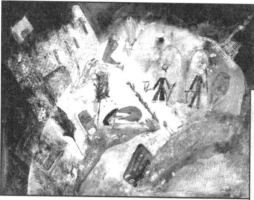

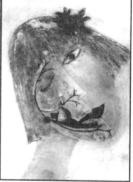

These pictures, *"A day in my life"* (above) and *"Candle"* (right), were painted by Rosa Sepple, an artist who suffers from trigeminal neuralgia. Although reproduced in black and white, try using them for the exercise described in Table 7.

Table 7

PRACTICAL WORK ON METAPHORS
For health care workers
On a table, put out a selection of pictures, postcards or objects and then ask everyone to pick out one to which they were drawn. Then go away with it individually and reflect on it. • What has drawn you to the particular image/object? • What connected you to it? • What does it make you feel? • What does it make you think of / feel in relation to yourself, to something you have experienced? • Or perhaps you are afraid to look forward to or wish for? • Think of a patient you feel overwhelmed by, you feel you cannot help, you have no connection with and imagine that they gave you this image to

Continued...

...Continued

describe their pain or something important about themselves they want you to know, but could not explain it. Can you "see" what it is?

For pain patients

Draw your pain or choose a picture that expresses your pain and then choose another one of where you would like to be or which expresses your emotions before you had pain.

Think about the following:
- How would you like to change this image?
- If you could change or color it, what would it be?
- Who or what are you in the image?

For the second image ask yourself :
- Why do you want to be here?
- So how do you get from the one picture to the other?
- What is the bridge?

What about taking your pictures to your health care worker to help them understand what you are going through?

During these types of exercises, the metaphor often shifts and changes over time, which in itself is a metaphor of progress. If it does not change, this in itself is a metaphor for the entrenchment or paralyzing features of the patient's experience and so the patient will need more help.

A dental student, Tina Chrysostomou, used the above exercises with some patients with chronic pain, including some with trigeminal neuralgia and found that a whole new dialogue was created and that patients found the process helpful ... *"with words you have to think about it, but this just expresses it straight away as opposed to writing and ticking boxes."*

A patient who felt suicidal was able to express this because she found a black and white face (The Prophet, by E. Nolde) represented her *"monster pain,"* which she said *"I would have overdosed to get rid of."* The emptiness, loneliness, fear, dread, panic, anger, and uncertainty of pain were found by many to be present in Munch's painting of "The Scream."

For patients who are able to engage in this visual way, having images at home can help them track feelings on a daily basis. This can be achieved by changing the images on the refrigerator, in the bathroom, or in a diary, depending on how the pain is that day. The physical act of changing the picture is an engagement of power. This also assists the patients in measuring for themselves the progression or other changes of the pain, and the coping factors that affect it at home. They can then use this to convey to the clinician - *I had three Munch days this month and one day of Flowers, etc.* It can be a rewarding and creative attempt to engage patients in their own therapy.

The images created by patients, whom Deborah Padfield coordinated, have been shown to aid some consultation processes. Sufferers can make use of visual and written metaphors on their own.

9. WHAT IS HYPNOSIS AND HOW CAN IT BE APPLIED TO PAIN MANAGEMENT?

Toby Newton–John discusses the use of hypnosis in our book, **Assessment and Management of Orofacial Pain.** Part of the broader family of relaxation approaches is that of hypnosis. There is an ongoing debate about the true nature of hypnotic induction – does it produce an altered state of consciousness or trance, or does it represent the manipulation of social influence between a charismatic practitioner and a receptive patient?

There is considerable overlap between the relaxation training and the use of hypnosis for chronic pain. Both involve attempts to decrease sensory and proprioceptive input, to decrease arousal, and to increase feelings of calm and well-being. However, hypnosis involves a specific induction (telling the patients that they will or are likely to experience certain things) and the narrowing of attention.

Most of the research examining the use of hypnotic inductions with facial pain has been in the context of non-chronic disorders, such as treating dental phobia or tooth extraction. One uncontrolled trial has been done in patients with TMD pain and has shown encouraging results.

Closely linked to hypnosis is meditation, an ancient technique that can decrease anxiety.

10. WHAT IS BIOFEEDBACK?

This is a technique whereby patients get feedback on the physiological effect that actions produce, e.g. they can see their heart rate on a monitor or look at the tension in muscles on **electromyography** (EMG). Increases in muscle tension due to worry or stress will result in increased pain. EMG biofeedback has been used in patients with chronic temporomandibular pain, who often have tense muscles, and it has been shown to be effective. Silver chloride electrodes are taped to a couple of the involved muscles, which detect and "feed back" the electrical activity within the muscles to the patient. The feedback is usually in the form of an audible signal, where increases in tension cause the pitch to rise.

Using relaxation or other techniques that have been discussed above, the patient learns to reduce muscle tension by lowering the pitch of the audio signal. The feedback is instantaneous, and the sensitivity can be altered to indicate very minor changes in muscle tension levels.

11. WHY ARE POSITIVE THOUGHTS IMPORTANT IN PAIN MANAGEMENT?

Negative thoughts about pain are important causes for maintenance of pain and pain behavior. These are just some that I found in the material sufferers sent to me:
- *"I am very scared."*
- *"I consider I have a curse handed out to me."*
- *"Absolutely nothing takes the pain away."*
- *"I have stockpiled the Neurontin and feel I will never be without it."*
- *"There is no fix for this."*
- *"Trigeminal neuralgia was not only attacking my face; it was attacking my family."*
- *"You take away my power, pleasure, purpose. You are my constant thorn, my ghastly, ghostly tic doloroux."*

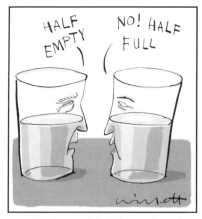

How do you label these glasses?

Effective therapy will depend on:
- identifying these thoughts
- questioning their accuracy
- looking for evidence to support or refute them
- challenging them to change them by taking a more objective view of the problem

Thinking statements that express confidence, optimism and competence are crucial. It is important to think of pain not as a problem, but as a challenge. People need to re-learn hope, remember that there are things worth striving for, even if life seems to be restricted. Here are some examples of sufferers with positive thoughts:
- *"I think that you should collect pictures of face wear to help us all laugh. Laughter gives back a feeling of control."*
- *"The days I'm feeling better are more special because I don't always know if the next day or days I will be feeling well enough to do those*

things with them. It makes me value the time God has given me and try and spend it as wisely as I can."

- *"I manage my own health rather than depend on the advice of any one medical provider. I truly believe that only a team of medical professionals could have effectively helped me, but no such teams exist. Every TN patient must become proactive. They must become the leader of the medical team. They must seek a broad spectrum of input and then they must form their own treatment plan."*
- *"You will have days when you feel crummy, but take it from one who knows ... keep fighting and just do not give up."*
- *"I thank the Good Lord for days when I do not hurt."*
- *"I just have to believe that God will not put on us more than we can handle."*

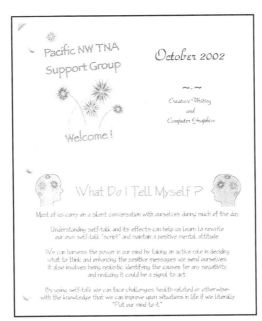

Here is another of Ruthi Purchase's handouts for her support group.

12. How can catastrophizing be diminished?

Feeling in control and having good **coping strategies** can reduce the disability caused by pain. The main methods are shown in the table below and discussed in the other sections.

Table 8: Key facts

Main coping strategies
• Increasing tolerance to pain – learning to minimize the disability by techniques described in this chapter   • Increasing role of patient in treatment and changing of beliefs – improving control and self management   • Controlling mood –feelings of anger, frustration and anxiety need to be altered   • Encouraging positive thinking, reducing catastrophizing

Ruthi Purchase, of the Pacific Northwest TNA support group, says in her preface to her monthly handouts, "They were designed so our members would have something positive and tangible to take away." But in the process of developing the materials, she says, " I found a way to impart my own thoughts and motivations about the effects of this terrible pain. By giving something back to the group, I've re-discovered some latent talents of my own."

She also goes on to say, *"I have learned the past is something to learn from – it is not something to dwell upon."*

13. How to cope with a flare-up of pain?

Trigeminal neuralgia sufferers have periods without pain, but often live in constant fear of its return and how they will cope with it. It is crucial to have a plan of action, since attacks often come quickly with no warning. It helps to think of flare-ups as challenges, not disasters. Anxiety, frustration and distress will inevitably increase the pain, whereas calmness and rational thought may stop it from getting worse. It is important to recognize what is happening and put a plan in place. Medications need to be restarted and hints on that can be found in Chapter 10. If the flare-up does not settle, it is important to seek medical help.

In Table 9 on the following page are listed some coping strategies that can be used:

Table 9

PRACTICAL HINTS ON COPING WITH A FLARE-UP
• Analyze it • Do not panic • Accept that it is rarely possible to shut it down rapidly • You can't stop it, but you can stay on your feet and flow along with it until it eventually subsides • Take or restart your medication slowly • Think positively • Be kind to yourself • Take control
Prioritize
What can you: • Leave until later • Ask someone else to do • Cancel completely • Let those close to you know what is happening to reduce fear and isolation
Relaxation
• 5-10 minutes of deep, controlled breathing can make you feel reasonably calm. • Relaxation is not the same as doing nothing; you do have to concentrate • Being in pain is about the least "relaxing" state you can be in • When the pain intrudes on your thoughts, just gently bring your mind back to your controlled, regular breathing • Keep as calm as possible, rather than go to sleep
Light activity
• Even though you are in pain, attempt 10-15 minutes of non-vigorous activity • The activities must be physically and mentally undemanding
Rest and distraction
• Give yourself complete time out —- up to 20 minutes • Give your body a chance to recoup some energy • If you "do nothing" for too long, the pain will begin to dominate your thinking *Gentle stretching* • Pain can often result in increased muscle tension • Try simple, gentle stretching of the neck, upper back, shoulders, arms and lower back for 10-15 minutes • Go for a slow, gentle walk *Distraction* • Divert your mind away from the pain for 5-10 minutes • Distraction requires concentration, so think of an activity that you get really absorbed in
Reflection
• Did the pain last as long as it usually does? • Did you feel more in control of the pain? • Were you still able to achieve a few things, even though you were in pain? • Is there anything that you could do differently next time?
Reinforcer
• A reinforcer is a small treat that you give yourself for your own hard work in coping with pain

Without active involvement of the sufferers, and their realization that they are responsible for the outcome of therapy, these types of programs will not succeed.

14. How can psychologists and related therapists help?

- *"I see a psychologist regularly to deal with the emotions. Without the psychologist, I would be much less emotionally healthy than I am."*
- *"Another good reason for a psychologist is so I won't burden my family and friends."*

Cognitive behavior pain-management interventions tend to be multi-disciplinary, involving not just doctors, but also psychologists, physiotherapists, nurses, even occupational therapists. The reason all these professionals are involved is the wide ranging physical and emotional effect that pain can have on peoples' lives. These CBT programs can be run in a variety of ways, either on an individual basis or as group therapy. It is estimated that at least 6 sessions of one hour are needed, and it seems best if they run on a weekly basis. Some run more intensively and patients are admitted for a week-long inpatient pain management course.

Although not directly dealing with facial pain, the Stanford Patient Education Research Center has developed, tested, and evaluated self-management programs for people with chronic health problems. As they say on their Web site, "All of our programs are designed to help people gain self-confidence in their ability to control their symptoms and how their health problems affect their lives. Our small-group workshops are generally 6 weeks long, meeting once a week for about 2 hours, which are led by a pair of lay leaders with health problems of their own. The meetings are highly interactive, focusing on building skills, sharing experiences and support."

It would be extremely useful to work with such a group in order to develop a program for patients with facial pain. The mission statement of the Stanford center states, "We only develop and offer programs that we test for effectiveness with randomized, controlled trials that are funded by research grants and span two to five years. The aim of all of our programs is to improve the physical and emotional health of participants while reducing health care costs."

15. WHAT IS COMPLEMENTARY AND ALTERNATIVE MEDICINE?

This section is excerpted from a National Institutes of Health USA (NIH) publication, and dissemination of it has been encouraged. It stresses that this is for information only and is not an endorsement by the NIH, and that none of these therapies are a substitute for medical care.

There are many terms used to describe approaches to health care that are outside the realm of conventional medicine as practiced in the United States. This fact sheet explains how the National Center for Complementary and Alternative Medicine (NCCAM), a component of the National Institutes of Health, defines some of the key terms used in the field of complementary and alternative medicine (CAM). Terms that are underlined in the text are defined at the end of this fact sheet. Complementary and alternative medicine, as defined by NCCAM, encompasses a group of diverse medical and health care systems, practices, and products that are not presently considered to be part of conventional medicine.

Conventional medicine is medicine as practiced by holders of an M.D. degree (Medical Doctor) or D.O. (Doctor of Osteopathy) degrees and by their other health professionals, such as physical therapists, psychologists, and registered nurses. Other terms for conventional medicine include allopathy, Western, mainstream, orthodox, regular medicine, and biomedicine.

Some conventional medical practitioners are also practitioners of CAM. Other terms for complementary and alternative medicine include unconventional, non-conventional, unproven, and irregular medicine or health care. While some scientific evidence exists regarding some CAM therapies, for most there are key questions that are yet to be answered through well-designed scientific studies—questions such as whether these therapies are safe and whether they work for the diseases or medical conditions for which they are used.

The list of what is to be considered as CAM changes continually, as those therapies that are proven to be safe and effective become adopted into conventional health care, and as new approaches to health care emerge.

Are complementary medicine and alternative medicine different from each other?

Yes, they are different.

> **Complementary** medicine is used **together with** conventional medicine. An example of a complementary therapy is using aromatherapy to help lessen a patient's discomfort following surgery.

Alternative medicine is used **in place of** conventional medicine. An example of an alternative therapy is using a special diet to treat cancer instead of undergoing surgery, radiation, or chemotherapy that has been recommended by a conventional physician.

What is integrative medicine?

Integrative medicine, as defined by NCCAM, combines mainstream medical therapies and CAM therapies for which there is some high-quality scientific evidence of safety and effectiveness.

What are the major types of complementary and alternative medicine?

NCCAM classifies CAM therapies into five categories or domains:

1. **Alternative Medical Systems**

   Alternative medical systems are built upon complete systems of theory and practice. Often, these systems have evolved apart from and earlier than the conventional medical approach used in the United States. Examples of alternative medical systems that have developed in Western cultures include homeopathic medicine and naturopathic medicine. Examples of systems that have developed in non-Western cultures include traditional Chinese medicine and <u>Ayurveda</u>.

2. **Mind-Body Interventions**

   Mind-body medicine uses a variety of techniques designed to enhance the mind's capacity to affect bodily function and symptoms. Some techniques that were considered CAM in the past have become a part of mainstream medicine (for example, patient support groups and cognitive-behavioral therapy). Other mind-body techniques are still considered CAM, including meditation, prayer, mental healing, and therapies that use creative outlets such as art, music or dance.

3. **Biologically Based Therapies**

   Biologically based therapies in CAM use substances found in nature, such as herbs, foods and vitamins. Some examples include dietary supplements, (Some uses of dietary supplements have been incorporated into conventional medicine. For example, scientists have found that folic acid prevents certain birth defects and that a regimen of vitamins and zinc can slow the progression of an eye disease called age-related macular degeneration) herbal products, and the use of other so-called natural, but as yet scientifically unproven therapies (for example, using shark cartilage to treat cancer).

4. **Manipulative and Body-Based Methods**
   Manipulative and body-based methods in CAM are based on manipulation and/or movement of one or more parts of the body. Some examples include chiropractic or osteopathic manipulation, and massage.
5. **Energy Therapies**
   Energy therapies involve the use of energy fields. They are of two types:
   Biofield therapies are intended to affect energy fields that purportedly surround and penetrate the human body. The existence of such fields has not yet been scientifically proven. Some forms of energy therapy manipulate biofields by applying pressure and/or manipulating the body by placing the hands in, or through, these fields. Examples include qi gong, Reiki, and Therapeutic Touch.
   Bioelectromagnetic-based therapies involve the unconventional use of electromagnetic fields, such as pulsed fields, magnetic fields, or alternating-current or direct-current fields.

What is NCCAM's role in the field of CAM?

NCCAM is the federal government's lead agency for scientific research on CAM. NCCAM is dedicated to exploring complementary and alternative healing practices in the context of rigorous science, training CAM researchers, and disseminating authoritative information to the public and professionals.

Definitions

Acupuncture ("AK-yoo-pungk-cher") is a method of healing developed in China at least 2,000 years ago. Today, acupuncture entails a family of procedures involving stimulation of anatomical points on the body by a variety of techniques. American practitioners of acupuncture incorporate medical traditions from China, Japan, Korea, and other countries. The acupuncture technique that has been most studied scientifically involves penetrating the skin with thin, solid, metallic needles that are manipulated by the hands or by electrical stimulation.
Aromatherapy ("ah-roam-uh-THER-ah-py") involves the use of essential oils (extracts or essences) from flowers, herbs, and trees to promote health and well-being.
Ayurveda ("ah-yur-VAY-dah") is a CAM alternative medical system that has been practiced primarily in the Indian subcontinent for 5,000 years. Ayurveda includes dietary and herbal remedies and emphasizes the use of body, mind and spirit in disease prevention and treatment.

Chiropractic ("kie-roh-PRAC-tic") is a CAM alternative medical system. It focuses on the relationship between bodily structure (primarily that of the spine) and function, and how that relationship affects the preservation and restoration of health. Chiropractors use manipulative therapy as an integral treatment tool.

Dietary supplements. Congress defined the term "dietary supplement" in the Dietary Supplement Health and Education Act (DSHEA) of 1994. A dietary supplement is a product (other than tobacco) taken by mouth that contains a "dietary ingredient" intended to supplement the diet. Dietary ingredients may include vitamins, minerals, herbs or other botanicals, amino acids, and substances such as enzymes, organ tissues, and metabolites. Dietary supplements come in many forms, including extracts, concentrates, tablets, capsules, gel caps, liquids, and powders. They have specific requirements for labeling. Under DSHEA, dietary supplements are considered foods, not drugs.

Electromagnetic fields (EMFs, also called electric and magnetic fields) are invisible lines of force that surround all electrical devices. The Earth also produces EMFs; electric fields are produced when there is thunderstorm activity, and magnetic fields are believed to be produced by electric currents flowing at the Earth's core.

Homeopathic ("home-ee-oh-PATH-ic") **medicine** is a CAM alternative medical system. In homeopathic medicine, there is a belief that "like cures like," meaning that small, highly diluted quantities of medicinal substances are given to cure symptoms, when the same substances given at higher or more concentrated doses would actually cause those symptoms.

Massage ("muh-SAHJ") therapists manipulate muscle and connective tissue to enhance function of those tissues and promote relaxation and well-being.

Naturopathic ("nay-chur-o-PATH-ic") **medicine**, or naturopathy, is a CAM alternative medical system. Naturopathic medicine proposes that there is a healing power in the body that establishes, maintains, and restores health. Practitioners work with the patient with a goal of supporting this power, through treatments such as nutrition and lifestyle counseling, dietary supplements, medicinal plants, exercise, homeopathy, and treatments from traditional Chinese medicine.

Osteopathic ("ahs-tee-oh-PATH-ic") **medicine** is a form of conventional medicine that, in part, emphasizes diseases arising in the musculoskeletal system. There is an underlying belief that all of the body's systems work together, and disturbances in one system may affect function elsewhere in the body. Some osteopathic physicians practice osteopathic manipulation, a full-body system of hands-on techniques to alleviate pain, restore function, and promote health and well-being.

Qi gong ("chee-GUNG") is a component of traditional Chinese medicine that combines movement, meditation, and regulation of breathing to enhance the flow of qi (an ancient term given to what is believed to be vital energy) in the body, improve blood circulation, and enhance immune function.

Reiki ("RAY-kee") is a Japanese word representing Universal Life Energy. Reiki is based on the belief that when spiritual energy is channeled through a Reiki practitioner, the patient's spirit is healed, which in turn heals the physical body.

Therapeutic Touch is derived from an ancient technique called laying-on of hands. It is based on the premise that it is the healing force of the therapist that affects the patient's recovery; healing is promoted when the body's energies are in balance; and, by passing their hands over the patient, healers can identify energy imbalances.

Traditional Chinese medicine (TCM) is the current name for an ancient system of health care from China. TCM is based on a concept of balanced qi (pronounced "chee"), or vital energy, that is believed to flow throughout the body. Qi is proposed to regulate a person's spiritual, emotional, mental, and physical balance and to be influenced by the opposing forces of yin (negative energy) and yang (positive energy). Disease is proposed to result from the flow of qi being disrupted and yin and yang becoming imbalanced. Among the components of TCM are herbal and nutritional therapy, restorative physical exercises, meditation, acupuncture, and remedial massage.

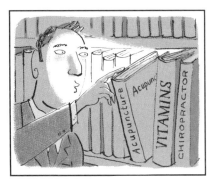

There is a very wide variety of material available for sufferers of pain, and these resources need to be used with caution.

What is the role of complementary and alternative medicine in trigeminal neuralgia?

A report, published in 2005 in the USA, estimates that up to 42 % of American adults use complementary and alternative medicine, spending more than $27 bn (£15bn) a year. Only 40 % of patients using CAM will tell the doctor that they do so. However, it is estimated that in the UK up to 50 % of doctors may refer patients for complementary and alternative medicine.

Even in 1990 it was estimated that there were more visits paid by adults to complementary and alternative medicine practitioners than to primary care doctors. The growth of complementary and alternative medicine has been enormous and its use by mainstream health care practitioners has increased, so the dividing line is becoming more blurred. However, concerns about it remain, as shown in Table 10 below.

Table 10

FEARS ASSOCIATED WITH USE OF COMPLEMENTARY AND ALTERNATIVE MEDICINE
• Diagnosis or treatment may be delayed • Treatments may cause harm • Poor quality goods • Misleading health claims • Feeling that if complementary and alternative medicine is ignored, it may delay improvement • Feeling of abandonment when complementary and alternative medicine does not bring improvement • Waste of money

If so much complementary and alternative medicine is being used, it is essential to ensure that it is both safe and effective. As Toby Murcott (2005) has pointed out in his book, **The Whole Story: Alternative Medicine on Trial,** few complementary and alternative medicine practitioners are helpful. He looks for the evidence as to whether "a billion dollar industry is based on nothing but good old- fashioned tender loving care (TLC)."

Murcott goes on to argue that even much of mainstream medicine is unproven, and that there is a need for improved scientific evaluations of all treatments. Although we have ample proof that conventional medicine has improved not only our quality of life, but also our life expectancy, there are signs that there is more to complementary and alternative medicine then just TLC. The environment, patients' expectations, practitioners' charisma, the "placebo" effect, and some as yet undiscovered mechanism, play a role in the success of these treatments.

It is difficult to conduct **randomized controlled trials** in this field because:

- complementary and alternative medicine modalities are gentle and slow-acting and therefore outcome measures are difficult to determine
- subjective effects are important and desired
- application is highly specific to an individual
- practitioners have variable approaches

More innovative techniques need to be found to evaluate these therapies. It is also important to set up a priority system for their evaluation. Doctors need to be open to new evidence, accept it and change their practice not just in conventional medicine, but also in the area of complementary and alternative medicine.

The public needs to be protected. Dietary treatments, herbal medications and supplements should be under strict quality control. Labeling of content should be accurate and comprehensive to ensure that misleading health claims are not made. These products must be standardized and reliable if they are to be evaluated scientifically.

There is a vast literature on complementary and alternative medicine and its relationship to main stream medicine, and numerous arguments have been put forward for both sides. I have just picked out an article by University of Florida Professor Allen Neims, M.D., Ph.D., who suggests that complementary and alternative medicine should be evaluated under two main questions:

- Does the therapy represent both diagnosis and treatment and can it be integrated with conventional medicine or are the two mutually exclusive?
- Is the therapy based on a relationship between sufferer and provider or not, e.g. taking herbs?

Neims argues that the two systems should be evaluated and practiced separately. He points out that conventional medicine has become more technological and places less attention on spirit and mind. These aspects, however, remain important, since patients do want their stories to be heard and attention paid to them, and they want a healing relationship to be established between them and the physician.

If the only thing that the patient expects from the treatment is the establishment of a healing relationship, then it may well be that a relationship-centered complementary therapy is the best treatment. We also need to remember that sometimes patients will sacrifice some efficacy if it is associated with less toxicity. Thus, to achieve a positive outcome based on a more holistic approach, it may be necessary to consider many different forms of treatment.

George Weigel, in his book, provides further information on complementary and alternative medicine for the treatment of trigeminal neuralgia, including a rating scale for the different types of therapy and how to look for reputable practitioners.

There are some published reports, mainly from China, on the use of acupuncture in patients with trigeminal neuralgia, but they are not well-conducted studies. They do suggest that many sessions are needed and that it is not a long-term cure. Acupuncture is not totally free of side effects and can cause bruising, infections, skin rashes and, if dirty needles are used, hepatitis B. Here are some reports from trigeminal neuralgia sufferers:

- *"I had acupuncture as well, and I went to a Chinese doctor. I've tried everything. They put needles and left them with me. I had five all around this area and just stayed with them all the time, and then when the pain came you just press on them. I think it helped, so if it's a good acupuncturist it can help, but these are all just things that just help."*
- *" My trigeminal neuralgia responded well to acupuncture ... I continued my tri-weekly appointments until the middle of May. At best, the treatments kept the attacks muted and bearable."*
- *Acupuncturist – a course of eight treatments, no help."*

Chiropractors appear to be popular, but again there is no scientific evidence and again side effects need to be guarded against, since injury to vital blood vessels can occur during the procedure. For their success or otherwise, here are some comments from sufferers:

- *"Chiropractor – recommended by TN for axle manipulation, three treatments, no help. "*
- *"I decided to try chiropractic with a practitioner who is trained in doing the upper cervical procedure claimed by some TN patients to be helpful. After about 10 weeks of 2-3 treatments a week, I concluded that it made no difference in the level of pain and I stopped the treatments."*
- *"I have to go to the chiropractor at least once a week, sometimes as many as three times, which gets very expensive and is not covered on my medical coverage. But this hope of having some relief has helped me immensely."*

- *"I truly believe that the combination of chiropractic and acupuncture/traditional Chinese medicine has helped me have so many remissions and to keep the pain at a minimum during my last bout."*

There has been considerable interest in the role of Vitamin B12 and many patients with trigeminal neuralgia report effects of its use. This should be a priority area for further research. Here are a couple of patients' comments:

- *"I have found by taking large doses of Vitamin B1, B6 have helped get the pain under control."*
- *"After I started injecting myself with vitamin B12 and taking vitamins daily, most of the pain is gone."*

MRS. G CASE STUDY
Mrs. G has had three recurrences of her pain and her last one was the most intense, since she had to use higher doses of her medication than before. Yet after her remission she said it was not as bad as previous episodes.
Why did Mrs. G report less distress from her last episode of pain?
Discussion   After her second episode, Mrs. G had been referred to a specialist facial pain clinic. Here she was seen by experts who have had years of experience in dealing with trigeminal neuralgia. They taught her how to take her medication and keep a pain diary so she could evaluate its effect, both in terms of pain relief and side effects. She now knows how much medication to take and how best to space it out during the day. She has begun to practice tai chi on a daily basis to help her relax and is aware of stresses that make her pain worse. This has led to careful goal setting and pacing so that in her enthusiasm she does not overdo things. When the pain comes she takes a rest, some gentle exercise and prioritizes her tasks carefully. She has her favorite picture and music selected so she can use these for distraction purposes if the pain threatens to overwhelm her. A leaflet on how to cope with flare-ups proved to be very useful, as did the trigeminal neuralgia support group with their contact details. Mrs. G has been able to explain trigeminal neuralgia to her family and friends so they now know what to do when she is having an attack of pain and she is able to ask for help. When everything had settled down, Mrs. G and her husband went out for a romantic meal to a restaurant along the riverbank. Mrs. G has lost her fear of the pain, has learned to control it, and knows where to go for help and so the pain causes her less distress.

16. WHAT DENTAL CARE IS NEEDED?

When in severe pain, it becomes very difficult to carry out routine oral and dental hygiene. However, attention needs to be paid to the teeth, since these can develop disease and cause pain in their own right, thus adding to the burden of pain. Patients need to find a dentist they can trust whom they visit regularly, especially when free of pain or under good control. Remember that a dentist can give a local anesthetic to provide pain relief from trigeminal neuralgia for a few hours while the medication kicks in. It is important, if going to a dentist during a pain period, that the medication is optimized, and this can mean raising the dose for a few days.

Table 11:Key facts

TRIGEMINAL NEURALGIA AND DENTAL CARE
• Brush your teeth regularly, especially at times when pain-free or when the medication is working at optimum conditions • Use a soft brush if necessary; an electric toothbrush may be easier • If brushing is impossible, use a chlorhexidine mouthwash to keep the mouth free of infection • Consider using fluoride rinses if you have a high decay rate • Chewing sugar-free gum can keep the mouth clean and stimulate more saliva • If your mouth is dry, drink plain water or use a form of saliva substitute • Visit your dentist regularly and tell him/her you have trigeminal neuralgia

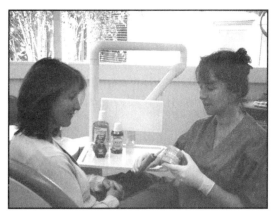

Here is Dr. Helen McFarland, one of the illustrators, discussing oral hygiene with one of her patients.

17. WHAT FUTURE RESEARCH IS NEEDED?

- It is crucial to develop pain-management programs that will suit patients with facial pain and trigeminal neuralgia. It would be important to assess which are the important elements that would lead to an improved quality of life. Collaboration with the Stanford University self-help pain management programs would be an excellent start.
- More attention needs to be given to this aspect of care, and physicians and surgeons need to adopt a **biopsychosocial** approach to care. This would need to be done through courses and publications.
- More research into the role of art and narrative in pain diagnosis and management would open up new avenues of communication, both with health care workers and also with the sufferer's family and the wider public.
- One of the major questions that needs to be answered is, "How can complementary and alternative medicine help sufferers with trigeminal neuralgia?" The priority for the relationship-type treatments would be to evaluate the roles of acupuncturists and chiropractors. The role of vitamins, and in particular Vitamin B12, needs to be determined through a large multi-center study.

SUMMARY

- Not only do sufferers need medications and surgery; they also need attention to the emotional aspects of the pain.
- Every sufferer needs to take the ten steps to move from being a patient to being a person.
- Relaxation, pacing, goal setting, improved sleep habits and managing stress are some ways to reduce pain distress.
- Complementary and alternative medicine may have a role to play in management of trigeminal neuralgia, but there is no scientific evidence as yet.
- Research is needed in this area.

FURTHER READING AND REFERENCES

Web sites
Checked April 2005

The following sites provide information on self-help programs:

The Neuropathy Trust, www.neurocentre.com
The British Pain Society, http://www.britishpainsociety.org/
The American Chronic Pain Association, http://www.theacpa.org
The Stanford University Research,
http://patienteducation.stanford.edu/
Mayo Clinic has an article on "Chronic Pain : Managing Your
Emotions", http://www.mayoclinic.com/invoke.cfm?id=PN00013
The US and UK TNA support groups also have their more specific
information at http://www.tna-support.org/ and http://www.tna.org.uk/

Sources of NCCAM Information provided by NIH:

NCCAM Clearinghouse
The NCCAM Clearinghouse provides information on CAM and
on NCCAM. Services include fact sheets, other publications, and
searches of federal databases of scientific and medical literature. The
clearinghouse does not provide medical advice, treatment recommen-
dations, or referrals to practitioners.
Toll-free in the U.S.: 1-888-644-6226
International: 301-519-3153
TTY (for deaf and hard-of-hearing callers): 1-866-464-3615
E-mail: info@nccam.nih.gov
Web site: nccam.nih.gov
Address: NCCAM Clearinghouse,
P.O. Box 7923, Gaithersburg, MD 20898-7923

Sources of Information on Dietary Supplements
ODS supports research and disseminates research results on dietary
supplements. It produces the **International Bibliographic Information
on Dietary Supplements (IBIDS) database** on the Web, which contains abstracts of peer-reviewed scientific literature on dietary supplements.**Office of Dietary Supplements, NIH**
Web site: ods.od.nih.gov
E-mail: ods@nih.gov

U.S. Food and Drug Administration (FDA)
Center for Food Safety and Applied Nutrition
Web site: www.cfsan.fda.gov
Information includes "Tips for the Savvy Supplement User: Making Informed Decisions and Evaluating Information" (www.cfsan.fda.gov/~dms/ds-savvy.html) and updated safety information on supplements (www.cfsan.fda.gov/~dms/ds-warn.html). If you have experienced an adverse effect from a supplement, you can report it to the FDA's MedWatch program, which collects and monitors such information. (1-800-FDA-1088 or www.fda.gov/medwatch).

Books and Booklets

Here are some examples of self-help materials:

Daniel C (2004) **Neuropathic Pain – Quality of Life Under the Spotlight** Available from the Neuropathy Trust, PO Box 26, Nantwich Cheshire CW5 5FP, UK.

Pollard J (2003) **Understanding and Managing Pain: Information for Patients.** The British Pain Society, 21 Portland Place, London W1B 1PY. The Society has compiled a reading list of books concerned with the relief of pain. These books have been found useful by other pain sufferers and should be available from most major bookshops.

Murcott T. (2005) **The Whole Story: Alternative Medicine on Trial** Macmillan ISBN 1-40394-500-4.

Newton John T and Zakrzewska JM. (2002) **Assessment and Management of Orofacial Pain.** Edited by Zakrzewska JM and Harrison SD. Volume 14 in series on Pain Research and Clinical Management Elsevier chapters 3, and 9 ISBN 0-444-50984-4.

Nicholas M, Molloy A, Tonkin L, Beeston L. (2003) **Manage Your Pain** Souvenir Press London ISBN 0-285-63679-0. An excellent book for patients.

Padfield D (2003) **Perceptions of Pain,** Dewi Lewis ISBN 1-904-58702-X. Features photographic images of patients' pain.

Weigel G., Casey K. (2004) **Striking Back! The Trigeminal Neuralgia and Face Pain Handbook.** Trigeminal Neuralgia Association, Gainesville, Florida ISBN 0-9672393 -2-X. Includes extensive section on complementary and alternative medicine and its evaluation.

References

Harrison S D, Glover L, Feinmann C, Pearce SA, and Harris M. (1997) A comparison of antidepressant medication alone and in conjunction with cognitive behavioral therapy for chronic idiopathic facial pain. In Jensen TS, Turner JA, and Wiesenfeld-Hallin Z. *Proceedings of the 8th World Congress on Pain, Progress in Pain Research and Management.* Seattle, IASP Press **8** : 663-672.

Keefe FJ (2000) Can cognitive behavioral therapies succeed where medical treatments fail. In Devor M, Rowbotham MC and Wiesenfeld-Hallin Z *Proceedings of the 9th World Congress on Pain, Progress in Pain Research and Management* IASP, Seattle **9**: 1069-1084

Neims AH. (1999) Why I Would Recommend Complementary or Alternative Therapies: a Physician's Perspective. *Rheumatic Disease Clinics of North America* **25**: 845- 853.

Morley S, Eccleston C and Williams A (1999) Systematic Review and Meta-Analysis of Randomized Controlled Trials of Cognitive Behaviour Therapy and Behaviour Therapy for Chronic Pain in Adults, Excluding Headache. *Pain* **80**:1-13.

Williams AC (2003) Cognitive behavioral Treatment. In Dostrovsky JO, Carr DB and Koltzenburg M *Proceedings of the 10th World Congress on Pain, Progress in Pain Research and Management,* IASP Press, Seattle **10**: 825-837

Vlaeyen JW, Morley S. (2005) Cognitive-behavioral Treatments for Chronic Pain: What Works for Whom? *Clin J Pain* 21:1-8.

CHAPTER 8

DECISION MAKING

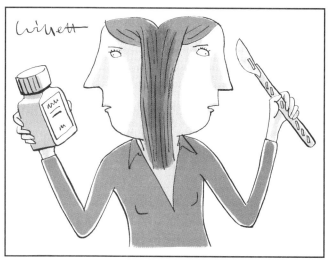

Trigeminal neuralgia can be treated both medically and surgically, and it can be very difficult to make this decision.

- *"As soon as you find out if you have TN or a related disease, do your homework and find out as much as you can about it."*

- *"Do your homework, and if you should have to have surgery, what type of treatment you want, what surgery if you need it and by whom. Make your family aware of what you want; if they won't listen, write it down."*

- *"Finally, I am very upset about the information that is available to TN patents that DO not have a computer. Where are the articles in the magazines, TV, talk shows, etc?"*

Some decisions about treatment are relatively straightforward, but this is not the case in trigeminal neuralgia. Thus the following questions need to be asked:
- What is the natural course of this disease?
- What would happen if we did nothing?
- What treatment options are there?
  For each treatment option you need to ask:
- What is the probability that I will benefit?
- How great is the benefit that I can expect - complete cure or simply a reduction of symptoms?
- What is the probability that I will he harmed?
- How severe are the harmful side effects? Is there a chance of dying?

For both benefits and harms, you could ask how good the evidence was on which the clinician bases his advice. There are additional questions that require more confidence, such as:
- How many microvascular decompressions have you done?
- Have any of your patients died as a result of surgery or had a serious complication?

Decision-making lines up the options and sorts out the values and then comes the difficult task of decision taking. This can be likened to a journey that benefits from a guidebook, which can include guidelines as described in Chapter 5. For any journey there are stages to go through, which involve getting ready, looking ahead, gaining perspectives and moving forward.

A sufferer making a decision has to think about the likely end of the journey, and the health care professional must make sure that the sufferer is aware of the end of the journey before it begins. Do you need an MRI if you are sure you do not want to undergo microvascular decompression surgery?

1. WHAT DO WE MEAN BY SHARED DECISION-MAKING?

"I went to four surgeons because we were going to do it privately and spoke to them all, and when I got to it, I'm afraid I just didn't feel confident. I finally found one who explained it very, very thoroughly, exactly what he would do, and I knew what he would do and what I would go through, so I wasn't frightened in the end, and it was exactly as he said, and I didn't have any surprises and shocks. There it was; it might not be for everybody. But it was for me."

Decisions require both thought and action. You can have thoughts, e.g. dreams and fears that do not lead to action. You can have actions without thoughts, e.g. impulsive behaviour such as making an immediate decision to have a microvascular decompression. In some decisions, the thought process is difficult. There are many choices as, for instance, in the surgical choices available for trigeminal neuralgia. On the other hand, the action can sometimes be more of a problem, since there are no resources to carry it out, e.g. you have no insurance coverage for a major operation.

Shared decision-making (SDM) between clinicians and patients increases involvement of the individual patient in decisions about clinical management. Facilitating patient choice is an important element in respecting the autonomy of patients. As Muir Gray points out in **The Resourceful Patient**, doctors can no longer maintain a paternalistic attitude toward their patients and need to identify and explain the treatment options available.

For SDM to work successfully, the patient needs to be confident that the doctor is focused on which treatments will generate the greatest benefit to him/her. This could be difficult for the doctor who, for a variety of reasons, may not inform the patient of all options. These include the unavailability of the treatment in some circumstances, e.g. no gamma knife, or the patient may make the choice without any consultation with the practitioner.

Familiarity with a clinical condition by both doctor and patient increases the desire for a shared role and relies on a trusting patient-physician relationship as discussed in Chapter 5. SDM requires longer consultation times and therefore is more costly.

Some definitions used in the next sections are provided in Table 1 below.

Table 1: Key Facts

Definitions to describe Practitioner – Patient Relationships – based of Trevena and Barratt 2003
Shared decision-making (SDM) – decisions characterized by the sharing of information by both parties and a discussion about the preferred management
Evidence-based patient choice – provision of research evidence on the pros and cons of one or more treatment option, along with promotion of active patient involvement in the clinical decision
Informed decision-making – provision of information to patients in order to permit the patient to make his or her own clinical decision; this can be done outside the health care system. *Continued...*

...*Continued*

Informed shared decision-making - decision made in context of a partnership between physician and patient. The options are discussed and the clinical decision is negotiated in partnership. Very similar to SDM

Equipoise – the point in decision-making where a number of options are possible, including no treatment. The practitioner has no clear preference and presents the options in a non-directive open manner, informed where available by research evidence.

Although patients' ability to participate in SDM varies in the ideal world, all patients should be afforded the opportunity of SDM. Charles et al (1999) proposes that doctor-patient partnerships for making decisions about treatment can take three main forms: the paternalistic (doctor led), the shared (patient shared), and the informed (patient-led). Most clinical consultations use elements of all these forms and, as the interaction proceeds, these elements may also change. Table 2 below summarizes these approaches.

Table 2: Key Facts

MODELS OF DECISION-MAKING			
Stages	doctor led	patient shared	patient led
Flow of information	One way (largely)	Two way	One way (largely)
Direction of information exchange	Doctor to patient	Doctor to patient to doctor doctor listens and reflects	Doctor to patient
Type of information	Medical facts with use of direct and closed questions	Medical and personal Doctor offers observations, seeks patient's views, encourages, clarifies, shows understanding	Medical
Deliberations	Doctor alone or with other doctors, instructs patient	Doctor involves patient (plus potential others)	Patient (plus potential others)
Who decides on treatment	Doctors, patient expected to be passive, ask few questions, does not influence consultation	Doctor and patient is expected to be active, ask questions, influence consultation	Patient has made the decision and does not ask doctor for advice

The paternalistic model – doctor-led

In the purest form of this model, the patient passively acquiesces to professional authority by agreeing to the doctor's choice of treatment. The doctor assumes that he/she can make the best treatment decision for the patient and needs neither the personal information from the patient, nor the involvement of the patient in the decision. Since no sharing has occurred, it could be said that no doctor–patient partnership exists. However, it could be argued that if the patient and doctor had agreed to this approach, then some form of partnership had been, at least tacitly, accepted.

Informed model – patient-led

In this model both parties contribute to the decision, but there is no partnership. The doctor provides all the information, including assessment of benefits and risks, that the patient requests. The patient then uses all this information to make a decision, but does not discuss this in any way with the doctor, as expressed in this patient comment: *"I want all the facts so I can make an informed decision."*

Shared model – patient-shared

In this model the doctor and patient share the decision-making process at all stages, and information flows between the two parties. The patient has to feel comfortable enough to express their preferences even when it may not be the doctor's preferred choice, e.g. doing nothing. This approach requires a considerable investment of time. In this model the patient is truly giving **informed consent** and this model is fundamental to high quality patient care.

Although it might appear that all patients would prefer a patient-centered approach, this is not necessarily the case. Some patients who are very sick may prefer a more paternalistic approach, and equally in a different situation, the same patient may opt for a different approach. A study of patients with breast cancer showed the following preferences among the patients: 22 % wanted the patient-led model, 44 % wanted patient-shared model and 34 % wanted doctor- led model. Patients need to match up with doctors who will enable them to use their preferred style, since there is evidence to show that patients who have participated in the decision-making process are better informed and their decisions match up with their values. This leads to improved compliance and satisfaction with treatment.

2. WHAT IS INFORMED CONSENT?

The definition is very difficult, but can be summarized as the process of communication between doctor and patient and is greatly improved if SDM has taken place. **Informed consent** has developed rapidly since it was introduced in the 1950s, reflecting changes in the practice of medicine that respect the increase of patient autonomy. Informed consent is an important symbol of the doctor-patient relationship that is based on medical ethics. In order for informed consent to occur, the doctor has to ensure that the following topics have been addressed:
- the procedure being done
- its purpose
- the risks associated with the procedure
- the benefits of the procedure
- the availability of alternatives to the proposed procedure
- the patient's concerns and values.

There are some exceptions when informed consent does not need to be carried out and these include an emergency and incompetence.

Prior to any major treatment being carried out, patients will be asked to sign a consent form. The purpose of the written consent form is to document that a process of informed consent has taken place. It is generally agreed that all surgical, as well as research procedures, require written consent. For certain non-surgical procedures, the decision regarding obtaining written consent will vary. The process of SDM facilitates informed consent, since it will have provided all the required information.

3. WHAT ARE THE BARRIERS TO SHARED DECISION-MAKING?

For SDM to occur, the patient must be well informed, and it can take time for the patient to acquire this knowledge. Studies have shown that patients remember only 50 % of a consultation, even less if it involves breaking bad news. Therefore, patients need to be given time to assimilate the information; it needs to be repeated and patients need to be encouraged to ask for it to be repeated. It is also important to remember that patients with lower educational achievements need more help to understand and remember information.

Patients with chronic conditions are more likely to be able to engage in SDM, since they are increasingly knowledgeable, not only about their medical conditions, but also about traditional, complementary and alternative treatment options. They understand their illness, their response to previous treatments, and their lifestyle preferences. Patients with chronic conditions are often used to making multiple and repetitive decisions, with variable outcomes, about how they will live with their condition. Despite this knowledge, chronically ill patients may still not have the confidence to share this knowledge with their practitioner, or they may not have the time.

A recent survey of patient postings on the Brain Talk epilepsy support group Web site, published in the British Medical Journal, provided the following facts:

- At their last visit to the doctor, 39 % had not been given the chance to fully explain the reasons for their visit.
- 40 % said the provider did not listen completely to what they had to say.
- 72 % felt that they had not received a complete explanation of the potential side effects of the drugs prescribed for them.
- 53 % had not been able to discuss the questions they had about their treatment for the following reasons:
  - provider did not have time – 47 %
  - patient forgot to bring up the question – 37 %
  - patient did not have the time to bring up the question – 29 %
  - patient was too embarrassed about bringing them up – 21 %

Some doctors still wish to retain the imbalance of power between themselves and their patients, and patients may be reluctant to share their preferences if they regard their doctor as more powerful and knowledgeable. Doctors may not have the appropriate communication skills. Risk communication is particularly challenging. Paling (2003) draws attention to the fact that virtually all doctors are faced with the need to communicate risk to patients and yet many do not have the training to do this. This may be made more difficult by the lack of good quality evidence and the lack of evidence-based guidelines. Doctors may be reluctant to discuss the more affective and emotional aspects of decision-making, thereby further preventing patients from overcoming those issues.

Patients' experiences are as important in the decision-making process as information from the medical viewpoint. Patients' experiences can be accessed through TNA support groups, patient meetings, E-mails and chat rooms. However, it must be remembered that this information can be biased and sufferers may get a distorted picture depending on whom they speak to. It is with this in mind that the charity DIPEx – database of individual patient experiences, was formed. The aims of the organization as published on their Web site are:

- to share the experience of illness or a health problem and to provide support for patients and caregivers who may feel that they are on their own

- answer the questions and problems that matter to people when they are ill or have a health-related problem and to help them make informed decisions about their health care
- provide reliable, evidence-based information about illnesses or advice on health problems
- be an educational resource for health professionals
- promote better communication between patients and health professionals

The data is provided in the form of interviews, videos and text and is very carefully researched using an experienced team of research workers. There are currently modules on depression and chronic pain, but funding has not been found to prepare a module on trigeminal neuralgia.

4. What factors influence decisions about treatment?

Although specific knowledge of the disease and the interventions that are possible is vital in decision-making, this information does not address a range of other issues that are taken into account when we make decisions. These may include:

- general health beliefs – influenced by satisfaction with interaction with health care professionals
- specific health beliefs - relates to severity of the disease and what effect it can have both now and in the future
- motives – why a certain treatment or outcome is desirable
- knowledge – previous health behavior and resultant health outcomes
- meaning of the decision on future quality of life
- experience – how previous health care has been experienced
- social interaction- supervision by others, social networks – support groups
- sociodemographic factors – age, gender, income, education, health insurance

Modern medicine has opened up new avenues of treatments and has enabled patients to have choice, but this in some ways makes it all tougher. It is further complicated by the varied data on the effectiveness of various treatments available. Making a decision means that options are lost and worries can then creep in about whether the right choice has been made. Someone has to make a decision about which option to take and accept the loss. Ideally the decision should be made by the patient, but it can be made by others. If made by others, then the person making the decision may not have the patient's best interest at heart – they may be making decisions based on convenience or cost. It may not be any easier for the doctors to make the decisions, especially if they are attempting to take into account individual patient preferences.

At the end of the day, it is the patients' perceptions that count more than the real risks and benefits, and patients must weigh the perceived barriers and benefits.

When making decisions about uncertain treatments, everyone takes a gamble and how large this is varies with every individual. In the management of trigeminal neuralgia it is inevitable that risks are taken and the consequences of making a particular decision have to be faced.

Figure 8.2 below lists some of the decisions that need to be made in the treatment of trigeminal neuralgia.

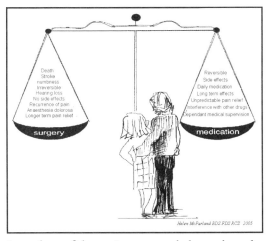

It can be useful to write out on a balance sheet the consequences of each treatment to gain a better idea of what the options really are.

5. WHAT IS INVOLVED IN THE MAKING OF SHARED DECISIONS?

In order for decision-making to take place, four basic steps need to occur:

1. Both the patient and the doctor need to be involved.
2. Both parties share information.
3. Both parties take steps to build a consensus about the preferred treatment, as illustrated by this patient's comment: *"I like to know it all, and you did it exactly right for me; you gradually eased me into it, and within six months I was quite prepared to have that operation, which I was petrified when you first started talking about it."*

4. An agreement is reached on the treatment to implement.

There is increasing interest in this important aspect of care. There are now several journals addressing these issues, which are listed at the end of the chapter. There is also a Web- based organization called The Foundation for Informed Medical Decision Making (FIMDM) that aims to:

- Provide patients with the perspectives and information they need when they face decisions about medical testing and treatment
- Improve the quality of decisions patients make in collaboration with their physicians
- Foster research to learn how best to help patients who face health care decisions."

There is also a very useful book written for the lay public by Cole Giller, a neurosurgeon, called **Port in the Storm – How to Make a Medical Decision and Live to Tell About It**. I will attempt to summarize some of the main points, but suggest you read the whole book. Details are provided at the end of the chapter. In Table 3 below I list the key steps in making a decision as suggested by Cole Giller.

Table 3: Key facts

THE SIX STEPS OF MEDICAL DECISION-MAKING BASED ON COLE GILLER'S BOOK PORT IN THE STORM
1. Identify your options, know all your possibilities without judging them
2. Identify the trade-offs, what are the pros and cons
3. Find the best medical data
4. Interpret the data, especially the numbers
5. Determine what your beliefs are
6. What does the decision you have made really means to you?

It is important that in going through each step, you write things down so you can go back through the steps and even add things in as you gather more information. You can put things side by side so that comparisons are easier. It is crucial that you keep your mind open and do not make any judgements in the earlier steps. It takes time to make decisions, since your subconscious will also be working and sifting through the evidence. This is why it is so important to consider all the options well before your pain becomes so suicidal that you cannot think clearly and will agree to any treatment that is offered. As this patient chronicles in her E-mail:

"The doctor came in and said something about surgery, and I said, 'I don't care if you cut off my head,' and I signed the papers."

The intensity of your pain will affect your decision, but it will be easier if you have done some background work during a period when you have less pain, since decisions come more easily to a prepared mind. It is inevitable that the pain intensity and its effect on your quality of life will alter some of your earlier decisions, and your doctors will accept this.

One of the difficult processes is gathering all the data, understanding it and interpreting it. Paling (2003) stresses that information is "considered to be data (facts) presented in a context that allows them to be meaningful to the listener." This is where the trigeminal neuralgia support groups can be helpful, since they attempt to do some of this for you and provide you with more help, as this patient describes:

"Tim is the lay neurologist-on-call. Through the years, he has collected information, and through his fantastic support network, he makes people, literature, facts, you name it, all available for the asking. He put me in touch with many wonderful people suffering from TN as I am."

6. WHAT ARE DECISION AIDS?

These are interventions that help people make specific and deliberate choices between two or more treatment options. A decision aid has two components:

a. provision of information together with choices and probabilities of outcomes associated with each choice, and
b. clarification of values, attitudes towards risk and time trade-offs.

The latter will often be a visual representation of risks, benefits and consequences of all decision options relevant to the person's health and an explicit discussion of the person's values, motives, beliefs about the decision options and consequences. They may also include information about costs associated with each option, information on others' opinions and some guidance on the steps in decision-making. Some will include a worksheet, and these require input from both doctor and patient.

Two reviews have shown that decision aids increase patients' desire to participate in SDM without increasing anxiety. They also increase knowledge, thus helping uncertain patients make decisions and reduce decisional conflict. However, they do not all lead to high quality decisions. The problems arise when the decision aids provide an option that cannot be carried out due to providers' or patients' lack of motivation, confidence or resources. Decision aids should ideally provide lists of providers who can carry out the treatment.

For patients new to this approach, some form of counselling may be beneficial. Early work shows that these aids are helpful, but more research is needed to develop high quality aids in a range of areas. Table 4 below shows a possible template.

Table 4: Key Facts

PATIENT DECISION TEMPLATE FOR TREATMENT OPTIONS		
Required element	Key patient questions	Information provided
Clinical condition	What are the characteristics of my trigeminal neuralgia?	Details on what is classical trigeminal neuralgia, atypical trigeminal neuralgia, symptomatic trigeminal neuralgia or other forms of facial pain that mimic trigeminal neuralgia
Patient decision situation	What are the different ways trigeminal neuralgia can be treated?	Options include drug therapy, complementary and alternative medicine, watchful waiting, surgery
For each treatment option		
Treatment process	What kind of treatment is it? How much time does it involve? What do I have to do to undergo this treatment?	Mode and duration of treatment. Nature of patient involvement
Outcomes and probabilities	What are the chances of improvement over the next few weeks/ months/ years?	Rates for the different outcomes over time, absolute number improved, improvement rate
	What are the side effects and what are the chances of each of them occurring?	Rates for each side effect
Value tradeoffs	What are the trade-offs between length of life and quality of life that apply mainly to microvascular decompression?	Material for clarification of values
	What are the trade-offs among the inconveniences, costs, chances of side effects, etc., in order to gain pain relief, long-term or short-term?	
	Where can I get descriptions of other patients' experiences?	

7. WHAT IS INVOLVED IN FOLLOWING COLE GILLER'S SIX STEPS?

STEP 1 Identifying your options and knowing all the possibilities

"Thank God I had discovered the Internet and the powerful search engines of the time. I entered a few key words (electric, stabbing, face, pain), and viola! I had a name for my facial shocks: trigeminal neuralgia."

This involves a number of supplemental steps, which you can work your way through using this scenario in the box below.

SCENARIO HOW TO SET ABOUT TRYING TO MAKE A DECISION

You have had left-sided trigeminal neuralgia for 7 years and this last attack has been the most severe you have ever had. You are now on very high doses of carbamazepine and are getting side effects from it. You have tried a variety of other medications, but they have not helped control your pain. You feel your quality of life is poor and you are unable to go out and socialize. Your neurologist tells you there is little else that he could do to help you. He suggests you go and see a neurosurgeon. You are 55 years old, fit and well, but have a metal implant in your right eye after you lost it in an accident 15 years ago.

---

a. Are **you sure you have the right diagnosis?**
   Check through what the criteria are for trigeminal neuralgia – see Chapter 1.

b. **Have you had a sufficient number of tests?**
   • Do you need an MRI?
   • Can I have an MRI given that I have a metal implant? The answer is no, which means I will not know whether I have a blood vessel in contact with the trigeminal nerve.

c. **Are there any other options that you could try medically, which perhaps your neurologist is not aware of?** Is anyone carrying out randomized controlled trials? The high quality ones will be registered on the registry of controlled trials.

d. **The neurologist has suggested seeing a neurosurgeon. What questions do you ask yourself?**
   • Do I really need to undergo surgery now because the results may be better? There is a suggestion in the surgical literature that after 8 years, outcomes after microvascular decompression may not be as good. This data is not well validated. I did not find this in a series of 300 outcomes I assessed after microvascular decompression and hence not all neurologists will believe it. The epidemi-

ological data shows that trigeminal neuralgia does not get better with time and the periods between attacks get shorter. The fitter you are medically, the less likely you are to get operative complications like deep vein thrombosis, pulmonary embolus. It also means neurosurgeons will be able to offer the full range of procedures. If you are on many drugs, these can complicate an anesthetic (the drugs used to put you to sleep) and recovery.

- Do I stay with a local neurosurgeon? It may be easier to get to the hospital, both for you and the family. Not all neurosurgeons operate on patients with trigeminal neuralgia, it depends on their specialization

- Do I go further afield to a more prestigious center where the surgeons may be more competent? A survey of US hospitals between 1996- 2000, reported by Kalkanis and colleagues(2003), showed that the risk of death and serious complications after microvascular decompression was lower in those hospitals that had higher throughputs of patients and were doing more operations. They suggested five or more microvascular decompression operations a year were associated with better results.

- So does the neurosurgeon I have chosen perform all the options? If only some, which ones does he perform?

- Is the surgeon knowledgeable? Search the medical literature and see which surgeons are writing papers; they are likely to be auditing their results and should be able to tell you the results of their work. Sweet showed in a questionnaire sent out to neurosurgeons that those who did not publish their data had more complications.

e. **How do I decide which type of surgery to choose? Here are some suggestions:**
   - Discuss this with your neurologist.
   - Discuss it with other patients – beware they may lack some understanding of the issues and may have had poor outcomes.
   - Contact your support group and discuss it with them.
   - Go through the high quality literature and write out all the pros and cons. See Chapter 9

STEP 2 Identify the trade-offs and pros and cons and interpret the numbers

Understanding the meaning of risk is essential when evaluating different treatment options. It is a complex phenomenon that everyone, including doctors, finds difficult to understand. Common errors that occur when assessing risks include:

- the tendency to overestimate small risks and underestimate large ones
- overestimation of the accuracy of the available knowledge
- patients' tendency to believe that they are at less risk of an adverse outcome than people similar to them

Numerical information is difficult to understand, and Paling therefore suggests the use of visual aids. He stresses that different methods are needed for individual patients. Differences in education, culture, age and experience will also affect patients' understanding of risk.

It is important that everyone understands that virtually all treatments are associated with some risk of possible harm. The language used by the doctor must be carefully chosen and the use of descriptive terms, such as low risk and high risk, are inadequate, since everyone has a different perception of what this means. When using these terms, it is important to define them.

The European Union has been trying to standardize the use of words such as common, uncommon, rare, etc. When expressing the odds of a possible outcome, it is helpful to use a common denominator. If you look at the table on the following page, you see that a variety of denominators have been used and it is more difficult to compare. Some may think that 1 in 400 is a bigger risk than 1 in 40 just because the numbers are larger.

Outcomes can be presented in positive and negative ways, and it is important to look at them in a positive way. It is better to say 70 % of patients will be pain-free for 10 years after microvascular decompression than 30 % of patients will have a recurrence. Statements such as "you have a six times higher risk of getting side effects if you use treatment A than treatment B," which expresses relative risk, are more difficult to interpret than the statement that "treatment A causes side effects in 60 % of patients and treatment B in 10 % of patients," which defines absolute risk.

Visual aids can help people understand the numbers in context. Florence Nightingale used the pie chart to describe risks. The example on the following page in figure 8.3 shows the number of patients who develop numbness after different types of surgical procedures.

Table 5

RISK ASSESSMENT	
Some familiar risks	The chance they will happen
Dying on the road over 50 years of driving	1 in 85
Transmission of measles	1 in 100
Dying of any cause in the next year	1 in 100
Annual risk of death from smoking 10 cigarettes per day	1 in 200
Needing emergency treatment in the next year after being injured by a can, bottle, or jar	1 in 1,00
Death by an accident at home	1 in 7,100
Death by an accident at work	1 in 40,000
Death playing soccer	1 in 50,000
Death by murder	1 in 100,000
Being hit in your home by a crashing aeroplane	1 in 250,000
Death by rail accident	1 in 500,000
Drowning in the bath in the next year	1 in 685,000
Being struck by lightning	1 in 10,000,000
Death from new variant Creutzfeldt-Jakob disease	1 in 10,000,000
Death from a nuclear power accident	1 in 10,000,000

Number of patients reporting sensory loss after diffrent surgical procedures .

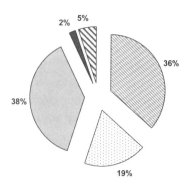

radiofrequency themorhizotomy   glycerol rhizotomy   microcompression ganglion
microvascular decompression   gamma knife surgery

Chart showing the likelihood of numbness after different surgical procedures for trigeminal neuralgia.

Below are a couple of examples of visual aids devised by Paling:

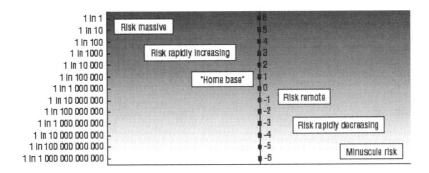

Risk language as proposed by Paling, published in British Medical Journal, 2003.

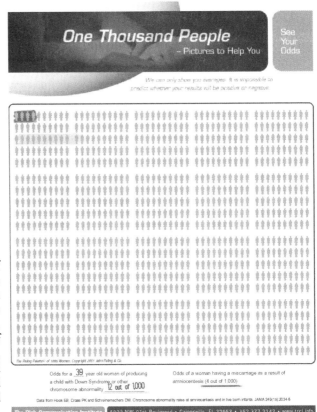

Another method of explaining risk where the chance of a risk per 1000 people is shown graphically. For the prevalence of trigeminal neuralgia, one figure only would be shaded. Published in British Medical Journal, 2003.

Every surgical procedure used in trigeminal neuralgia has trade-offs and these vary between the procedures. In the pie chart above, you see the chance of sensory loss is lowest after microvascular decompression, but if you look at the risk of dying during the operation, then it is highest for microvascular decompression. Each complication must be looked at individually, then the pros and cons of each procedure can be assessed. This is further complicated by the lack of good quality evidence, and a study we have just completed on decision analysis shows it is very difficult to predict the probability of a given complication, since there are insufficient studies providing the data needed for such analysis. Thus not only is the patient uncertain, but the doctor also has to make assumptions. It is important to ask your surgeon not only for the data, but also to help you interpret it. This needs time and may require several appointments.

First you will need to know the pros and cons of each of the possible surgical treatments. These are questions you need to ask about each procedure, which are discussed in Chapter 9:
- What are the risks of dying?
- What are the potential complications?
- What are the risks of serious complications, such as stroke?
- How long will it take you to get over the operation?
- When can I come off my medication?
- Which complications are likely to be permanent?
- Which complications are likely to be temporary?
- How long will the pain relief be?
- What happens when the pain comes back?
- Does the operation give equally good results in those with classical trigeminal neuralgia as with those with atypical trigeminal neuralgia?
- Does it make a difference if I delay having the operation?
- Does it make a difference which part of my face is affected by trigeminal neuralgia?
- Are there any medical reasons why I may not be eligible for the operation?

The answers you get to these questions unfortunately vary because different neurosurgeons use different data, either only their own or from a chosen set of studies. It is for this reason that we have tried to systematically review all the literature on surgery using strict quality criteria and attempting to remove bias by being clear why we selected to review the studies that we did. We hope future reports will adhere to the guidelines we suggest. See Table 6 on the following page.

For some questions, there are no data. For instance, not a single unit has published an audit of how long it takes to recover from a microvascular decompression operation. Many will quote some figures, but they are not based on a systematic review of every single patient going through a unit. There is no data published on what you should do with your medications after surgery and so it is difficult to be precise and it will be up to each individual neurosurgical unit to decide what they do.

Table 6: Key Facts

CHARACTERISTICS OF HIGH QUALITY REPORTS ON SURGICAL MANAGEMENT OF TRIGEMINAL NEURALGIA

- It is clear what type of study it is — **prospective, retrospective, case controlled**
- Independent observers were used to assess outcomes
- Diagnostic criteria of patients are cleared stated
- Differentiation is made between idiopathic trigeminal neuralgia and other forms of trigeminal neuralgia
- Details are provided of age at onset, site of pain, gender, duration of disease, age at operation
- Details of previous treatments are provided and the data is analyzed in relation to this
- Pain intensity, physical and emotional functioning were assessed pre treatment and post treatment
- Gross assessment of sensation in distribution of trigeminal nerve is reported pre- and postoperatively
- If available, results of MRI or other investigations are provided
- Brief description of operative technique is provided, and findings include report of technical failures
- The report states the number of surgeons performing the procedures
- Definitions are provided of what is classified as a recurrence of pain, failure of treatment, **dysesthesia, paresthesia, anesthesia dolorosa**
- Details are provided on patients lost to follow-up, including how they may differ from the reported patients and why they may be lost to follow-up
- Follow-up time, including mean and range, is crucial and ideally should be at least five years
- **Kaplan Meier** actuarial analysis using pain outcome for a minimum of three groups excellent, partial relief, no relief (see details in Chapter 5)
- Results are provided for the first-time treatment, rather than after multiple treatments
- The report includes details of any deaths and how they came about
- Complications that may occur around the time of surgery are reported
- The report describes complications in relation to time and severity, showing which are transient and which are permanent
- The report includes patients' own assessment of outcome using standardized questionnaires, which include psychosocial and quality-of-life parameters

Step 3 Discover the data

"The lesson I learned is that knowledge can literally save your life. People need good, balanced, fair and accurate information to make their own decision on what's best for them. There are lots of ways to deal with TN, but if you don't know what they are, they have no chance of helping."

Find as much medical literature as you can, using the TNA support groups, since they usually filter through the best. As this patient stresses:

"Information is more than just a guide to deciding on which therapy to try. It's hope. As long as we have hope, we'll keep trying. And we'll ultimately find an answer of some sort. But if we lose hope, we waste options that might have given us our lives back."

Use the checklist in Table 6, on things to look for when reading surgical papers. Discard low quality papers, which often are biased. Remember that few people like to publish negative results.

Step 4 Interpretation of numbers

Look at how the data is produced. When looking at a pain-free period, you need to see a **Kaplan Meier** plot as shown in Chapters 5 or 9. Depending on the scale used, the graph should not start at a 100 % or 1, since it is inevitable that some patients will not benefit from the procedure and thus will be a failure immediately. You need to ensure that most of patients have been followed for a minimum of 2 years, but 5 years is best. Use the information in Chapter 5 to evaluate the literature that you do find. Ask your doctor or neurosurgeon to help you understand the data. You particularly need to look at the risk(s) of different operations. For example, **radiofrequency thermocoagulation** can cause loss of sensation in the eye. If the eye has lost sensation, it is more likely to get infected and, in some cases, patients may even lose their sight. If you already have a problem with your other eye, you will not want to take a risk with your one functioning eye.

Many neurosurgeons will also evade the question of recurrences and failures, yet we know these occur and it may be difficult to force the neurosurgeon to give you an answer. You need as much data as possible and you need the neurosurgeon to be honest, since this increases trust. You will know from having read the literature that complications occur with every procedure, so you would like your neurosurgeon to admit that these occur.

It can take time to discuss all these issues with your neurosurgeon and it is helpful if they give you a leaflet with their local information, including frequently asked questions.

Step 5 Gathering Your Beliefs_

Beliefs are powerful and are an important part of who we are. They have been shaped by our experiences and what we have learned over the years and enable us to confront difficult situations. What risks we are prepared to accept are dependent on our beliefs and this is why one sufferer will accept a risk of 0.5 % death from a microvascular decompression, whereas others will not. It is important, however, to challenge your beliefs and ensure that they are based on good evidence; otherwise you may become over confidant and make the wrong decision.

Before you make a decision, make sure you have reflected on it and what it really means to you. For example, if you develop a numb face after surgery, do you really know what it will be like living with it? Consult with others and take time to make a decision. It may be useful to write down your subjective thoughts and feelings as you go through the processes. You will be able to come back to them to see if things have changed as a result of further events.

You may have thought very differently about the consequences of a microvascular decompression when your pain levels were low than when it is so intense that you feel you could commit suicide. Here is the comment of a patient who needed time:

"I like to know it all, and you did it exactly right for me; you gradually eased me into it, and within six months I was quite prepared to have that operation, which I was petrified when you first started talking about it."

Once you have made your decision, do not agonize over it. Think about the personal issues. These include questions such as the following:

- Which types of medical information will you believe?
- Whom will you trust?
- Is it really true that your trigeminal neuralgia can only be controlled by surgery? Are there other ways of learning to control your pain?
- Do you want to face a major neurosurgical procedure like microvascular decompression without knowing that you have a blood vessel compressing the nerve?
- Are you prepared to trust the surgeon when he /she tells you he does not need an MRI to make a decision to do a microvascular decompression once he/she has ruled out you do not have multiple sclerosis or a tumor?
- Have you had successful surgery before?
- Is your family willing to support you after surgery, especially if you should have side effects?
- Can you afford it and will your insurance cover all the costs?

Step 6 Contemplation of Meaning

In this final but very important step, you need to think through the consequences of your decision, not only if everything goes well, but also if you develop problems.

- What would happen if you were to die having the operation?
- What would it mean if you were left with a stroke?
- What would it mean to you to lose hearing on a permanent basis?
- What would it mean if you lost the sensation to your eye and had to take extra precautions to avoid infections?
- Would you be able to live with a numb face such as you would experience after having a dental injection? If you are not sure, ask a dentist to give you a local anesthetic and see how this feels.
- How badly has the quality of your life been affected?
- What would you be able to do if you were free of pain?
- Would you prefer a longer period of pain relief or could you cope with a recurrence of pain?

MRS. G CASE STUDY

Mrs. G has had trigeminal neuralgia for six years and is 62 years old. The time interval between the attacks has become shorter and the attacks themselves last longer. She is now on her fourth drug. The current drug has provided excellent pain relief, but trying to stop it results in a return of pain. After careful review Mrs. G decided to have an MRI scan and continue with medication. She decided that if the pain returned again with the same severity, she would undergo microvascular decompression. Over the last few months the pain has again become more severe and she is now re-thinking her options, since the neurologist has told her he would like her to see a neurosurgeon. The MRI has shown a small vessel in contact with the trigeminal nerve. In her medical history Mrs. G had suffered three deep-vein thromboses and is still taking an anticoagulant. She was also being investigated for a possible stomach ulcer. Otherwise, she is fit and takes regular exercise. She still works part-time at a local supermarket. Her children have grown up and her husband still has a fulltime job. She often baby sits her grandchildren, which she enjoys.

She has had a long and open discussion with her neurologist, who has told her clearly about the medical options and his concerns about his ability to provide further effective drugs. He suggests that she have a discussion with a neurosurgeon in the same way she has been talking to him. He reassures her that the diagnosis is correct and that the MRI does show a blood vessel lying in contact with the trigeminal nerve with no tumor or MS being present. He gives her a list of possible neurosurgeons and details of the TNA support group and encourages her to get more information.

Continued...

What should Mrs. G do now?

Discussion

Mrs. G has already made several important decisions about her care and each time has had to take a gamble and hope she made the right decision. She feels that she has done the right thing to this point in time,, but now faces an important new decision, since she believes surgery may be the real option. Utilizing the data she has from her neurologist and from what she has found out herself, she needs to identify a suitable neurosurgeon. Once Mrs. G has found a suitable neurosurgeon, she needs to ensure that he/she become involved in her care and that they both share information they have gathered. Mrs. G then needs to discuss each of the options with the neurosurgeon so they can both see what may be the preferred option. She will need to take into account her previous medical history and decide with a doctor whether it does reduce her chances of having a microvascular decompression. It may be that she no longer needs to take the warfarin, which would make everything simpler. The discussion will not only take into account the factual data, but also Mrs. G's emotional needs. She has never had surgery before and is worried by this. Death after microvascular decompression is less of a concern then the small chance of a stroke. She plays an important role in helping her daughter with her children and does not want to be a burden to her family. On the other hand, she realizes that her frequent pain attacks have made her useless at times and have affected the quality of life. She has to warn the grandchildren not to touch her face and sometimes cannot baby sit. She will need to take time off work to recover if she has microvascular decompression.

She needs to read through a book such as Cole Giller's **Port in the Storm** about making medical decisions, and go through each of the steps he suggests. She is then ready to return to the neurosurgeon to make the final agreement on which surgery to have done. In doing this she will have been through the process known as shared medical decision-making. Patients who go through this process are more likely to be satisfied with the outcomes of their treatment and to be more compliant in carrying it out.

8. WHAT RESEARCH IS NEEDED?

"Why can't they do their best research for me?"

The whole process of SDM is not possible for trigeminal neuralgia because of lack of high quality information, which would provide the facts on which decisions are made and a lack of tools for risk assessment. Research in several areas is needed.

- It is essential that more trials are performed, especially randomized trials. When these have begun, they should be registered so that duplication is avoided. Details of results can be quickly obtained when they are completed and patients can ask to be enrolled in them if they are taking place near their residence.

- The data on treatment outcomes, trade-offs, etc. that are needed for the decision-making template are nationally, if not internationally, agreed upon so patients get exactly the same information. This will then enable them to add their beliefs, etc. to make an individual decision.

• The quality standards Zakrzewska and Lopez (2003) have suggested for reporting of surgical results should be adhered to, and editors of journals can do much to enforce this standard.

• Reliable patient experiences would be a great advantage and add a further dimension to the information-gathering process. Funding would be needed to work with organizations like DIPEx to generate videos, interviews and reading materials on trigeminal neuralgia.

The whole area of risk assessment needs considerable research, which should include:

• innovative methods of training for doctors in risk management, including communication

• development of visual aids to describe risk of complications after surgery and methods of testing their validity

• assessment of how culture, age, gender, education affect the perception of risk

• objective evaluations of the effects of SDM on patient outcomes both in terms of satisfaction and quality of life

• doctors committed to involving their patients in decision-making should be supported and given consultation times that are commensurate with this activity

There is an urgent need to provide markers for high quality information and this includes:

• assessment of Web sites and encouragement of the use of those that meet the quality standards

• provision of uniform patient information, which has been evaluated by a range of stakeholders and been awarded kite marks so they can be easily identified

• development of Decision Aids for patients with trigeminal neuralgia, which would involve preparation of visual material that could be done with an organization such as the Foundation for Informed Medical Decision Making, which is dedicated to providing "a balanced presentation of each option, from both clinical and patient experience perspectives. Our goal is never to encourage any one treatment approach over the others, but rather to explain fairly and clearly the pros and cons of each option - and let patients, working with their doctors, decide which is best for them."

SUMMARY

Shared decision-making (SDM) are decisions in which there is sharing of information by both physician and patient and a discussion about the preferred management.

In order for SDM to take place, four steps must take place :
- **Both the patient and the doctor need to be involved**
- **Both parties share information**
- **Both parties take steps to build a consensus about the preferred treatment**
- **An agreement is reached on the treatment to implement**

SDM improves informed consent and leads to improved health outcomes.

In order to take part in SDM, patients must:
- be fully informed of all the options available and this will involve accessing medical literature, Web sites and patient information data
- understand the pros and cons of all the procedures, including the trade-offs and be able to interpret the data, including the assessment of risk
- take into account their own beliefs
- ensure that they understand the meaning of their decision

- **Risk assessment is difficult and can be improved by the use of visual aids, which need to be developed**
- **Considerable research is needed if SDM is to be made possible for trigeminal neuralgia sufferers**

FURTHER READING AND REFERENCES

Web sites

There are a vast number of Web sites to access, and the selection given below are just some personal ones, all of which were accessed early in 2005.

Health on the Net Foundation (HON) (www.hon.ch) and Health Internet Ethics (www.hiethics.com), which have promoted a voluntary code of conduct on the quality of Web sites.

National Institute of Neurological Disorders and Stroke is part of the National Institutes of Health (NIH). US Web site gives its mission statement as follows: *"Helping to lead the way toward important medical discoveries that improve people's health and save lives. NIH scientists investigate ways to prevent disease, as well as the causes, treatments, and even cures for common and rare diseases. The NIH translates research results into interventions and communicates research findings to patients and their families, healthcare providers and the general public."* http://www.ninds.nih.gov/disorders/trigemin/trigemin.htm

Foundation for Informed Medical Decision-making. Their mission statement as found on the Web site is: *"to strengthen the role patients play in selecting treatments for their medical conditions. Medical research on practice variation indicates that patient preferences are often less important in treatment decisions than factors having little to do with patients or their illnesses, such as geography, economics or supplier-induced demands."* http://www.fimdm.org

DISCERN is a brief questionnaire that provides users with a valid and reliable way of assessing the quality of written information on treatment choices for a health problem http://www.discern.org.uk/

DIPEx Personal Experiences of Health and Illness shows you a wide variety of personal experiences of health and illness. You can watch, listen to or read their interviews, find reliable information on treatment choices and where to find support. http://www.dipex.org/ there is nothing on trigeminal neuralgia at this site, but there is a module on depression and chronic pain.

Current Controlled Trials allows users to search, register and share information about randomized controlled trials.
http://controlled-trials.com/

Patient Decision-making / Patient Choice Initiative – this reading list can be downloaded from the Kings Fund
http://www.kingsfund.org.uk/library.

The Centre for Health Information Quality (CHIQ),
http://www.hfht.org/chiq/partners.htm

Patient UK information leaflets and details of support groups
http://www.patient.co.uk/

Developing Patient Partnerships provides innovative, relevant, accessible and practical information that benefits the public, patients and health providers, and promotes partnership between them.
http://www.dpp.org.uk/

The Centre for Health Information Quality (CHIQ). Their mission statement is:
  "We work with information producers and providers to raise standards in the production of consumer health information. .. a clearing house on all aspects of patient information, providing practical advice to the NHS and others on the production of good quality information for patients."
http://www.hfht.org/chiq/partners.htm.

Patient information can be obtained on NHS direct at
www.nhsdirect.nhs.uk.

Patient UK information leaflets on a large number of diseases and illnesses, and an extensive directory of patient support and selfhelp groups. http://www.patient.co.uk/

Books and booklets

Duman M. (2003) **Producing Patient Information: How to Research, Develop and Produce Effective Information Resources** - a complete, step-by-step guide to each stage of the information process, from developing an information policy, to writing and disseminating print and electronic materials. ISBN: 1857174704 Can be ordered from the Kings Fund at **http://www.kingsfundbookshop.org.uk.**

Giller C. (2004) **Port in the Storm – How to Make a Medical Decision and Live to Tell About It.** Lifeline Press, Washington ISBN 0-89526-132-.

Muir Gray JA (2002) **The Resourceful Patient** eRosetta Press Oxford UK ISBN 1-904202-00-4, this is also an Internet book and toolkit for those wishing to address the problems of health care in the 21st century. http://www.resourcefulpatient.org/

References

Journals that contain regular articles on SDM include Patient Education and Counselling, Medical Decision Making, Health Expectations.

Bekker HL, Hewison J, Thornton JG (2003) Understanding Why Decision Aids Work: Linking Process With Outcome *Patient Education Counseling* **50**:323-329.

Charles C, Whelan T and Gafni A. (1999) What Do we Mean by Partnership in Making Decisions About Treatment? *BMJ* **319**:780-782.

Kalkanis SN, Eskandar E N, Carter B S and Barker F G (2003) Microvascular Decompression Surgery in the United States, 1996 to 2000: Mortality Rates, Morbidity Rates, and the Effects of Hospital and Surgeon Volumes. *Neurosurgery* **52**:1251-1261.

Paling J. (2003) Strategies to help patients understand risks. *BMJ* **327**: 745- 748 also accessible on www. bmj.com.

Sepucha KR and Mulley A G (2003) Extending Decision Support: Preparation and Implementation. *Patient Education and Counseling* **50**:269-271.

Stevenson FA, Barry CA, Britten N, Barber N and Bradley CP (2000) Doctorpatient Communication About Drugs: the Evidence for Shared Decision Making. *Social Science and Medicine* **3**: 829-840.

Sweet WH (1990) Complications of Treating Trigeminal Neuralgia: an Analysis of the Literature and Response to Questionnaire. In Rovit RL, Murali R and Jannetta, PJ **Trigeminal neuralgia** Baltimore: Williams and Wilkins ISBN 0-683-07393-1.

Trevena L and Barratt A (2003) Integrated Decision Making: Definitions for a New Discipline. *Patient Education and Counseling* **50**:265-268.

Zakrzewska JM and Lopez B C (2003) Quality of Reporting in Evaluations of Surgical Treatment of Trigeminal Neuralgia: Recommendations for Future Reports. *Neurosurgery* **53**:110-122.

APPENDIX

HOW TO SEARCH THE INTERNET FOR HEALTH INFORMATION

To help health consumers make informed choices about Web sites.
Based on the views of health consumers and support groups.
http://www.judgehealth.org.uk

Summary of "How to search the Internet for health information"

These guidelines aim to help health consumers make informed decisions about Web sites. This leaflet summarizes advice on how to search the Internet for health information.

• **Information searching**
Time spent searching is not wasted. It helps you develop your critical skills and identify sites you can trust. It helps many people adjust to their condition.
Support groups are important sources of help, e.g. they provide emotional and personal support; they provide information; they advice about information; they act as a link between the patient or caregiver and the professional; they fight the patient or caregiver's corner.
Professionals can also provide information, e.g. staff at your public library; your local Patient Advice and Liaison Service (PALS) in hospitals and health care staff.

• **Gateways - searchable catalogues to good quality health Web sites**
Try a health gateway first. Here are some examples of health gateways.
  • NHS Direct Online (http://www.nhsdirect.nhs.uk)
  • Contact a Family (http://www.cafamily.org.uk)
  • Patient UK (http://www.patient.co.uk)
  • Organizing Medical Networked Information (OMNI) (http://omni.ac.uk)
  • National Electronic Library for Health (NeLH) (http://www.nelh.nhs.uk)
  • MEDLINEplus (http://medlineplus.gov)
  • MEDLINE (http://www.pubmed.gov)

• **Search engines**

Use search engines if you cannot find what you want from the gateways. Here are some examples of search engines.
  • Google (http://www.google.co.uk)
  • AllTheWeb (http://www.alltheweb.com)
  • Yahoo (http://www.yahoo.com)
  • MedHunt (http://www.hon.ch/MedHunt)
  • Mirago (http://www.mirago.co.uk)

• **Search tips**

Unless your search is very simple, always use the 'advanced search' option provided by the search engine. This allows you to do things like:
  • Find results with all of the words you type in your query. This makes it much more likely to find relevant sites and to cut down on the number of results;
  • Find results with the exact phrase, by putting the words in quote marks "...". This is very useful when looking for names of diseases, organizations, people.
  • Choose the language, for example, English.
  • The Help pages will give you details about how to use the search engine and how to search more efficiently. When using other search tools like gateways and directories, look at their Help pages too.

• **Confidence building - learning how to search**

Look for taster sessions or short courses at local organizations like public libraries, the WEA (Workers' Educational Association), further education colleges or universities.

Public libraries provide free access to the Internet.

Here are examples of some sites that provide free online tutorials for developing Internet skills:
  • The Online Netskills Interactive Course - TONIC
    (http://www.netskills.ac.uk/onlinecourses/tonic/)
  • Resource Discovery Network (RDN) Virtual Training Suite
    (http://www.vts.rdn.ac.uk)

Author: Sue Childs, Research Fellow, the Information Society Research Community, School of Informatics, Engineering and Technology, Northumbria University. These guidelines were produced by Contact a Family, the Information Society Research Community, School of Informatics, Engineering and Technology, Northumbria University and the Center for Health Information Quality, through a project supported by the Health Foundation. Published February 2003. Last updated February 2005. Review date February 2006. Permission to reproduce this has been obtained.

How to judge Web sites

The following Web site helps health consumers make informed choices about Web sites: http://www.judgehealth.org.uk Based on the views of health consumers and support groups.

Summary of "How to judge the quality of a Web site"

These guidelines aim to help health consumers make informed decisions about Web sites. This leaflet summarizes the things to look for that will help you judge whether a Web site is of good quality.

• **Trust and reputation**

Look for sites of trustworthy organizations with a good reputation, e.g. well-known, reputable organizations; organizations you already know and trust; sites recommended by a health professional or a support group.

• **Who produced the site**

Find out which organization or individual has produced the site, e.g. professional organizations, support groups, government departments, commercial organizations, individuals.

• **Purpose of the site**

Find out the purpose of the site, e.g. its aims or mission, its audience, how the site was developed and whether health consumers were involved.

• **Funding sources**

Find out where the site gets its funding from, e.g. financial accounts, names of sponsors, and the types of adverts on the site.

• **Date**

Look for the date when the site was last updated or reviewed. Information on the site should also be dated, with an update/review date given.

• **How the information is written**

Look at how the information is written, e.g. discussing different sides of an issue; not sensational or extreme; with correct grammar and spelling; simply written and easy to understand if aimed at health consumers; in other languages if aimed at non-English speakers.

• **Descriptions of conditions and treatments**

Look for the following details that indicate that the information is likely to be reliable: the name of the author, their job title, place of work, qualifications, potential conflicts of interest; the date the information was written, with an update or review date; the sources of information the author used; the author's contact details; links to related resources; descriptions of quality checks or editorial processes.

Detailed assessment of the correctness of medical information requires help from a health professional or a lay expert. A lay expert is a member of the public, who has spent a lot of time reading and learning about a specific medical condition.

• **Medical research**

Medical research literature is very complex and needs specialized knowledge to understand it fully. Support groups often explain about research on their Web sites or in their newsletters.

• **Personal experiences**
Personal experiences of patients and their caregivers are important sources of information. Check that they are clearly marked as personal experiences. Be cautious about individual patient or caregiver sites. Check the medical information they give carefully.

• **Foreign sites**
Find out the country of origin of the site. Health information on non-UK sites can be different to that provided on UK sites, e.g. different health systems and cultural practices, use of different terminology, recommending different treatments, different availability of treatments and drugs.

• **Communication**
Look for ways you can contact the organisation to discuss issues, ask for advice or comment on the site, e.g. an E-mail address, a postal address, a phone number, electronic forms.

• **Links**
Assess links to other Web sites too. The site should explain why and how they have chosen these links. It should be made clear that you are linking to another site.

• **Disclaimers**
Look at the site's terms and conditions and disclaimers. These should cover issues such as, medical information, privacy, and copyright, responsibilities for accuracy of information and for any harm caused by using the site.

• **Kite marks**
Kite marks are signs or logos indicating that the site has been 'endorsed' in some way by another organization. They do not necessarily mean that the health information is correct. The absence of a kite mark is not a sign of poor quality. Only a minority of sites apply for them.

• **Design**
Look at how well the site is designed, e.g. personal information should be kept private and secure; the site should be easy to use; the site should be easy to access; adverts should be clearly marked as such, and discrete; the site should have an attractive appearance, without the need to use extra software.

• **Interactive facilities, e.g. E-mail lists, bulletin boards, chat rooms**
Assess the quality of interactive facilities too. Look for the presence of experienced members; requirement for rules of polite, supportive behavior; presence of people ensuring the rules are followed; requirement to register to use the facility.

Summary of guidelines produced by Contact a Family, the Information Society Research Community, School of Informatics, Engineering and Technology, Northumbria University and the Center for Health Information Quality, through a project supported by the Health Foundation. Author: Sue Childs, Research Fellow, School of Informatics, Engineering and Technology. Published February 2003. Last updated February 2005. Review date February 2006.
Permission to reproduce this has been obtained.

Key facts

CHECK LIST FOR PRODUCING AND MAINTAINING PATIENT INFORMATION ON CONDITIONS AND TREATMENTS FROM CENTER OF HEALTH INFORMATION QUALITY CHIQ	
Theme	Objective
Accessibility	The information is in an appropriate format for the target audience.
Accuracy	The information is based on the best available evidence.
Appropriateness	The information communicates relevant messages.
Availability	The information is available to the widest possible audience.
Continuity	The information is presented in context with other resources.
Currency	The information is up-to-date.
Legibility	Written information is clearly presented.
Originality	Information has not already been produced for the same audience and in the same format.
Patient involvement	The information is specifically designed to meet the needs of the patient.
Readability	Words and sentences are kept short where possible. Jargon is minimized.
Reliability	The information addresses all essential topic areas.

CHAPTER 9

SURGICAL MANAGEMENT

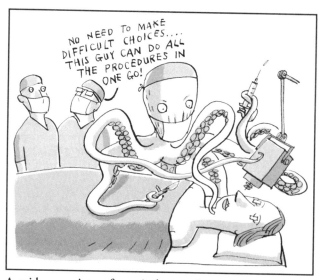

A wide a variety of surgical procedures are available for trigeminal neuralgia.

The procedure

Teflon, Ivalon, muscle, fat,
the MVD is where it's at.
Non-invasive approach they say,
shoot that nerve with gamma rays.

If the surgeon has good aim,
glycerol is the way some claim.
Radiofrequency heats the nerve,
it works better if the electrode curves.

A little air is all it takes
for a balloon compression in that space.
Make up your mind, what will it be?
Tegretol is fine with me.
By Cynthia Ezell

Perhaps the most difficult choice a trigeminal neuralgia sufferer has to make is that of whether to undergo surgery. Once having decided on surgery, there is a range of options that need to be considered. If surgery becomes the choice, then Table 1 below lists what should be the ideal surgical solution.

Table 1

THE IDEAL SURGICAL PROCEDURE

The surgery should :
- be widely available in many centers
- be minimally invasive, i.e. no extensive surgery – day stay or short admission
- give immediate and complete relief of pain
- allow all trigeminal neuralgia medications to be stopped
- be curative or have low recurrence rate
- cause no **systemic** complications, e.g. hearing, stroke, double vision
- have no or few local (around the face) side effects
- restore quality of life
- require no longterm followup
- be repeatable with no added risks
- be cost effective

This is a vital chapter for anyone contemplating surgery; it provides information that all patients who elect to undergo surgery should be aware of. Nick Ross (2004), writing in The Lancet on improved surgical consent, contrasts the information patients get about any drugs they are taking with that obtained for surgery. Medicines are now dispensed with detailed information listing every obscure side effect and yet when patients sign a consent form for surgery, an irreversible procedure, few obtain written information.

Ross argues for a comprehensive consent form and information leaflet for every major surgical procedure. This should be no longer than four pages, and even if the patient does not wish to read it at the time, they have it for future reference. The information leaflets would be prepared in partnership with patients and could even be trailed. Their content is shown in the figure below.

Panel: Proposed contents of surgical information leaflets

1 Simple anatomical diagrams to show what the operation entails.

2 Expected success rates.

3 Usual diagnostic or planning procedures and what results (such as blood tests or scans) the patient should expect to be shown.

4 Description of what patients will experience after surgery, including any tubes they may find inserted into their bodies, or supports or callipers clamped onto them.

5 Description of the probable appearance of scars, stitches, and bruises.

6 The range of times (from least to longest) patients are likely to experience pain or discomfort, and the range of likely severity (from least to most);

7 The type of drugs patients are likely to be prescribed, and why.

8 The prospect of routine post-operative treatments, possible additional procedures, and any exercise or diet regimes that are commonly recommended.

9 Where surgery is photographed or video-recorded (as with endoscopic surgery) or where other recordings are made, patients should be told that unedited copies will be made available to them on request, perhaps for a fee.

10 In particular, patients should be aware of how long they may feel sufficiently unwell to cope with children, work, housekeeping, travel, sports, and other routine activities.

11 In the plainest terms possible, there should be warnings of plausible risks of harm with an indication of the likelihood that such adverse events might occur and of whether or how they are treatable. The dangers might be defined as major risk, medium risk, rare, and very rare, and also expressed as percentages where possible.

Required surgical information from Ross, 2004.

This chapter is based largely on my chapter in the book, **Assessment and Management of Orofacial Pain**. Other details can be found in George Weigel and Ken Casey's book, **Striking Back! The Trigeminal Neuralgia and Face Pain Handbook**. There are also several Web sites that provide detailed descriptions of the different operations.

1. WHAT IS THE QUALITY OF EVIDENCE WE HAVE FOR SURGICAL PROCEDURES FOR TRIGEMINAL NEURALGIA?

The literature on trigeminal neuralgia is large, but apart from a handful of studies in the field of peripheral surgery and one in gamma knife surgery, there have been no randomized controlled trials and so all the studies are of the cohort type. The vast majority of the data is retrospective, written by experts and very rarely with an independent observer and therefore constitutes the lowest level of evidence. There is no internationally accepted format for the reporting of these results, yet our review showed this to be essential. It has led us to produce a trigeminal neuralgia survey questionnaire we hope will be taken up by neurosurgical units and which we have used to report the largest UK series of patients who have undergone posterior fossa surgery (Zakrzewska et al 2005b).

Reviewing the studies, one is struck by the vastly varying data available and how the studies have been quoted and results compared (Zakrzewska and Lopez 2003). For this chapter, I use the high quality data as defined in the previous chapter and which was selected using pre-determined criteria, not just those studies that supported my views. It would have been best to only use data that has been produced from surveys carried out by independent observers, but that would leave very few studies. Mortality and major **morbidity** is reported in most studies and all studies were used for this data.

There is a large body of literature in Japanese and Chinese, including some large series, but the quality is extremely poor and none of the studies scored highly on our criteria. Table 3 on the following page lists the data that should be available in studies reporting surgical treatments that would enable meaningful comparisons to be made.

Sweet (1995) reported in Rovit's book on trigeminal neuralgia the results of their own personal survey conducted among some 200 neurosurgeons. They wrote to their colleagues asking for details of their operative complications when treating patients with trigeminal neuralgia. Of these, 140 replied, which covered 91 units, not just ones in the US. The details of how the survey was conducted are poorly described, but they do highlight how major morbidity and mortality occur and remain unreported. More postsurgical deaths were reported by them than are recorded in all the published data.

As I pointed out in Chapter 1, the diagnosis is crucial when it comes to evaluating surgical results and, although this was pointed out by Szapiro et al as far back as 1989, only one study has used **the McGill Pain Questionnaire** before surgery to determine different types of pain (Zakrzewska et al 1999).

Table 3

DATA THAT SHOULD BE AVAILABLE IN REPORTS OF SURGICAL TREATMENTS

- diagnostic criteria
- differentiation between idiopathic trigeminal neuralgia and other types
- basic data sets such as age at onset, site, length of time of disease, age at operation, previous treatments
- severity of condition based on some measurements of pain
- analysis of data depending on type of trigeminal neuralgia and previous surgery
- operative data
- skill of surgeon
- patients lost to follow-up and details of how they may differ from the other patients
- definitions, e.g. recurrence of pain, failure of treatment, sensory changes
- outcome data (Some divide patients into three groups only, i.e. excellent, partial relief, no relief, whereas others may put patients into five categories)
- criteria for partial relief vary, but are often defined as use of regular medication
- recurrence in some series is only reported if a patient has to undergo repeat surgery; in others it is any pain report
- details of follow-up time and numbers of patients available in each follow-up group
- Kaplan-Meier actuarial analysis, i.e. probability of pain recurrence. See Chapter 5
- reporting complications in relation to time, i.e how many have the complication at one year, two years
- reports of patients' own assessment of outcome
- qualityoflife assessments using validated questionnaires
- economic factors, costs of the procedure and of patients' time off work

Two other studies have attempted to show that their patients could be divided into typical and atypical trigeminal neuralgia (Yoon et al 1999 and Tyler-Kabara et al 2002) based on character and timing, but they use retrospective methods and provide no details of how their data was validated. This could be a major reason for variation in outcome and why some patients do not experience the expected results.

How you define a recurrence is crucial. A recurrence can be said to have occurred if there is any return of pain, even if controlled by medication, but some surgeons will say a recurrence has only occurred if repeat surgery was needed. This will produce very different outcomes, with the latter surgeons claiming better results. Recurrences should also be reported for first procedures and should not be based on a cumulative result where patients may have had a number of procedures done before becoming painfree. Data should be given separately on those who have had more than one procedure to render them painfree, since it could well be that these patients have a different cause for their trigeminal neuralgia. Recurrence rates may vary if the patient has had previous surgery or secondary trigeminal neuralgia, so this should be stated.

Kaplan- Meier methodology (see Chapter 5) enables all patients to be included in the analysis, regardless of whether they have been lost to follow-up, died or have not had a recurrence of pain.

Unfortunately, even with some reports using this methodology, patients who failed to respond to treatment at the onset are excluded from the analysis, whereas they should be included; beware of graphs that show 100 % results at the start. Some patients will need repeat surgery as indicated by this patient's story:

"1999 Balloon Compression (off Tegretol for 10 months), 2001 Knife Stereotactic Radiosurgery (no help), 2002 MVD, scar tissue removed and trigeminal nerve rubbed vigorously with instruments. Medication was slowly reduced to zero over several months. Pain free since August, 2003."

Each of the surgical procedures will be described under the same headings to allow for easier comparisons and you may also like to read them in conjunction with the book, **Striking Back! The Trigeminal Neuralgia and Face Pain Handbook** by George Weigel and Ken Casey. The headings include:
• Definition of the procedure
• Selection of patients for each of the procedures
• Description of the operative technique
• Recurrence of pain on a yearly basis
• Prognostic factors for outcome
• Complications

The indications and contraindications for each procedure will be discussed at the end of all the procedures.

Surgery for trigeminal neuralgia is done at three levels and some procedures are quick to do and involve minimal surgery. Only microvascular decompression can be said to be a non-destructive procedure, whereas all other forms of surgery are destructive (**ablative**) and aim to reduce transmission of painful stimuli as described in Chapter 3. This, therefore, results in loss of sensation over a varying part of the trigeminal nerve.You may want to refer to Chapter 3 for the anatomical points described later in this chapter. In Table 4 you have a brief description of the major types of surgery.

Table 4: Key facts

TYPES OF SURGERY USED FOR TRIGEMINAL NEURALGIA			
Name of procedure	Location of surgery	Type of anesthetic used	Type of procedure
Neurectomy	peripheral – trigger point	local anesthetic	Destructive, ablative
Cryotherapy			
Injections of alcohol, streptomycin, phenol, glycerol			
Jaw bone cavities curretage			
Laser			
Acupuncture			
Peripheral radiofrequency thermocoagulation			
Percutaneous radiofrequency thermocoagulation	Gasserian ganglion	heavy sedation	
Percutaneous glycerol rhizoloysis		heavy sedation or general anesthetic	
Percutaneous balloon microcompression		general anesthetic	
Stereotactic radiosurgery – Gamma knife	posterior fossa	local anesthetic	
Partial sensory rhizotomy		general anesthetic	
Microvascular decompression		general anesthetic	Non destructive

2. WHAT IS PERIPHERAL SURGERY?

Definition

Peripheral surgery aims to identify individual nerve branches that are acting as **triggers** and to deliver treatment directly to them. They all rely on some form of damage to the nerve, be it mechanical, chemical or thermal. The treatments have included cryotherapy, laser, neurectomy, alcohol, radiofrequency, acupuncture or removal of necrotising cavitation lesions. Most of the procedures aim to destroy peripheral nerve fibers, i.e. the section of nerve between the nerve ending and before the **Gasserian ganglion. However,** more central changes are likely as a result of these interventions. It was hoped that some of these procedures would be more selective and hence result in less sensory loss, e.g. cryotherapy, and that the area of loss would be smaller than after treatments at the level of the Gasserian ganglion.

In 1979 Ratner et al proposed that among cavities developed in the alveolar bone after dental extractions, many were infected or showed chronic inflammatory changes or abnormal osteoid tissues. These cavities are always found in areas where teeth have been extracted months or years ago and many are not visible on examination or on X-ray films. The cavities are enclosed by bone and they may be empty. This condition has been termed NICO, necrotizing cavitational osteonecrosis.

Ratner proposed that curettage of these cavities led to a diminution of the symptoms of trigeminal neuralgia. In total, 11 articles describing this condition and its treatment have been identified, but none of them contain the data set that is described in Table 2 above. There has also been one published abstract of some work on cadaver material, which showed that bony cavities did not appear to be unique to trigeminal neuralgia or atypical facial pain. However, studies have shown that patients with rare coagulation defects may develop problems after extraction of teeth due to decreased blood supply and hence necrosis (death) of bone.

Results after any peripheral surgery are very mixed and shortlasting, as this patient recounts:

"I had the cryosurgery, and it was an enormous success; in fact, they wanted me to go and speak to people about it. It lasted for 18 months, no medicine, no pain, completely forgot about it, very, very successful, and it came back, and then I saw the doctor who did the surgery and he said, 'I don't think you should do it again, it's just not going to keep working.'"

Selection for peripheral surgery

Since most of these procedures are done under local anesthesia, the medical condition of the patients is not crucial. Care, however, needs to be taken if patients have a blood disorder that increases their chances of bleeding or if they are taking anticoagulant drugs, since surgery could result in excessive bleeding or bruising. The procedures do not require a hospital stay and can be done in the office. Only short-term relief of pain is likely, so sufferers need to be aware that they will either need a repeat procedure or need to take their medications.

Operative techniques

The different techniques are described below, but they are now rarely used and no sufferer should be offered these as a first line of treatment unless they are medically unfit for any other procedure.

Neurectomy

This is probably one of the oldest techniques used, and there are several old reports of large series of patients undergoing these procedures. The **trigger** nerve branch is first identified by the use of a **local anesthetic**. This gives the patient an idea of the area of numbness they would expect to be left with after the procedure. Then, under local anesthesia, the peripheral nerve is exposed from inside the mouth as far as possible so that no scars will be left. The nerve is then cut. Some surgeons have reported early regrowth of the nerve and so suggest obliterating the foramen (hole) through which the nerve emerges. This has involved either sealing the foramen with wax or packing with fatty tissues or wood chips.

Alcohol injections

These are mainly given at the level of peripheral branches, again into the trigger points, but in the past surgeons would even put the alcohol as far as the Gasserian ganglion. Absolute alcohol 0.75-1 ml is injected after the trigger branch has been identified with the use of local anesthesia.

Streptomycin

This technique is one of the very few that has been subjected to randomized controlled trials. The involved branch is identified by the use of local anesthesia and then streptomycin 1 gm with lidocaine is injected. The injections need to be given once weekly over a period of five weeks.

Phenol

Once the involved branch is identified and local anesthesia inserted, then 10 % phenol in glycerol is injected. The total amount used varies between 0.5 and 1.5 ml.

Glycerol

After giving a local anesthetic to localize the trigger area, 0.5–1.5 ml of sterile glycerol is injected into the trigger area.

Cryotherapy

The trigger nerve branch or branches are exposed using, as far as possible, intraoral incisions. A cryoprobe is then applied using temperatures varying from - 30^0C to - 70^0C for two or three freeze- thaw cycles, each lasting two minutes.

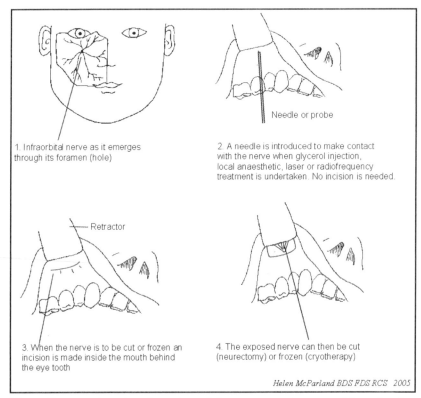

1. Infraorbital nerve as it emerges through its foramen (hole)

2. A needle is introduced to make contact with the nerve when glycerol injection, local anaesthetic, laser or radiofrequency treatment is undertaken. No incision is needed.

Needle or probe

Retractor

3. When the nerve is to be cut or frozen an incision is made inside the mouth behind the eye tooth

4. The exposed nerve can then be cut (neurectomy) or frozen (cryotherapy)

Helen McParland BDS FDS RCS 2005

These diagrams show how branches of the nerves can be exposed in order that peripheral techniques can be performed.

Laser

Only one report has been identified using this technique. A helium neon laser is applied on the face for 20 seconds. This is repeated three times a week for ten weeks.

Peripheral radiofrequency rhizotomy

This technique is the same as when performed at the Gasserian ganglion level, and lesions at temperatures of 70°C are made for 2-3 minutes.

Acupuncture

The basic technique involves the insertion of long slender needles into various pre-determined areas of the skin and typically leaving them for 20 to 30 minutes. The sites and number of needles vary, since there may be some 2,000 different points that can be used. The Chinese say this works because balance is restored to the body, whereas western doctors suggest it may work because of the release of pain-relieving chemicals called endorphins, or through a **placebo effect,** or as a means of distraction. This technique has been reported by Shuhan et al (1991), who used it on 1,500 patients. They perform acupuncture as a course of 10 sessions. The ten sessions are based on daily or alternate daily treatments. If the first course is not successful, an additional treatment is done 3-5 days later. On average, patients need 26 sessions, but the range is large (10-84).

Jaw bone cavity removal

Since it is difficult to locate the cavities on radiographs, the patient is asked to point to the trigger areas, and then a local anesthetic is given to try to eliminate the pain and hence find the cavity. To gain access to the bony cavity, the soft lining needs to be moved out of the way. When the cavity is found, it is thoroughly scraped clean and may be packed with gauze soaked in tetracycline, an antibiotic. This is repacked regularly until it heals over. For a month prior to the procedure and for a month after all pain is gone, the patients are put on antibiotics.

Peripheral surgery recurrences and prognostic factors

The results from all the better quality studies are shown in Table 5 on the following page. More detals are available in my book. In several of them, Kaplan Meier actuarial analysis was possible due to the provision of sufficient data, which are shown in the figure on the following page. The mean time to a recurrence is 9-18 months and it is interesting to note how consistent these changes are with all the techniques. Patients will also report similar results, such as:

"I went to see three maxillofacial guys and I was in such pain, they gave me injections of whatever it was and sent me home. They got sick of doing that and one of them suggested I have the nerve cut, which I did, but the pain started happening again so my GP put me on Tegretol."

There are no details on factors that may affect recurrence factors.

The randomized controlled trial (RCT) of streptomycin by Stajcic et al (1990) showed that initially more patients responded to the streptomycin injections than lidocaine alone, but at 30 weeks this effect was lost. Bittar et al (1993) showed no effects even in the initial follow-up time. Another group claimed that in their group of 157 patients, 64 % were still pain free at one year and that the mean time to recurrence was

Table 5

RECURRENCES AND COMPLICATIONS AFTER DIFFERENT PERIPHERAL TECHNIQUES DONE BY DIFFERENT GROUPS					
Intervention	Number patients / procedures	Average follow- up in years	% Pain Free one year	mean time to recurrence years	Complications
Cryotherapy – 70⁰C to - 30⁰C	181	3	61	Mean 0.9	Sensory loss locally 37 %, eating problems 14 %, taking anti-convulsants 49 %
Streptomycin 1gm/lidocaine weekly for 5 weeks versus lidocaine 2 different rcts	37	1	35 % for strepto-mycin and lidocaine and 38 % for lidocaine	Mean 0.9 for streptomycin Mean 0.8 for lidocaine	Swelling at site of injections, painful injection
Glycerol 0.5-1.5ml into nerve endings	157	Minimum 4 years	64	2-3 years	Mild dysaesthesia 14, local bruising
Alcohol 4 studies	766 patients	0.2- 8	52	Mean 0.9- 1.4	sensory loss 20 %, transient double vision 7 %, facial palsy 0.5% paresthesia 11 %, eye complications 4 %,
Neurectomy 4 studies	155 patients	2	60	Mean 1.9	Sensory loss 40 %, paresthesia 20 %, eye complications 8 %, dysesthesia 5 %, taking anticonvulsants 72 %
Peripheral radiofrequency thermocoag-ulation 70⁰C for 2-3 mins	71 patients	1.5	78	Mean 2.7, median 1.4	Mild numbness in all, trismus, minor bruising
Phenol injection 10% in glycerol 0.5 – 1ml	18	2	50*	Median 1 mean 1.6	Mild sensory loss, taking anticonvulsants 44 %
Acupuncture every day or other for ten times then another course ¾ days later	1500	1	46	Not possible to calculate	Difficulty opening mouth 6 %
Laser three times a week for 10 weeks rct	35 patients	10 weeks	Unable to ascertain	Significant improvement if had high baseline of pain, no numbers given	nil

rct = randomized controlled trial

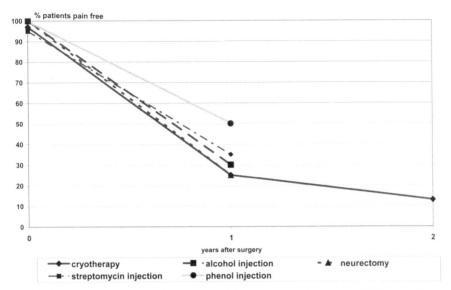

Probability of remaining pain free after peripheral surgery shows that 70 % of patients will have a recurrence within one year. Only the data on cryotherapy is totally reliable.

2-3 years. The patients had a very short history of trigeminal neuralgia, and it could be that these patients were going through a period of remission and this then yielded these good results. The small RCT on the use of laser reports very good results, but only short-term results (ten weeks) are given.

Complications after peripheral surgery

The complications from these procedures are summarized in Table 5. The only procedure that reported no complications was laser therapy.

- Peripheral surgery causes relatively few complications outside the trigeminal nerve, but eye complications can occur due to inadvertent injections. Alcohol injections have been reported to cause **diplopia**, (double vision), **facial palsy** and even loss of skin in the area of injection. Most procedures result in some local **edema** (swelling) and **hematoma** formation (bruising). The injections are all painful, even if initially local anesthetic is used. All procedures requiring direct access to the nerve, such as cryotherapy and neurectomy, can result in local infections as after any minor surgical procedure.

- An area of sensory loss and in some cases, **dysaesthesia** is reported after these procedures, although the area is less extensive than after Gasserian ganglion surgery and so will have less of an effect on overall satisfaction. It is more often reported after injections with alcohol and neurectomies than after cryotherapy.

- Many reports also state that up to 50 % of patients may need to continue to take anticonvulsants, although often in smaller doses that cause fewer side effects.
- Difficulty in mouth opening, due possibly to spasms of the muscles opening the jaw, is reported after acupuncture in up to 6 % of patients and in a small number undergoing peripheral radiofrequency thermocoagulation.

3. WHAT SURGERY IS DONE AT THE LEVEL OF THE GASSERIAN GANGLION?

Surgery at the level of the Gasserian ganglion was, until recently, the most frequently used treatment. The procedure involves reaching the Gasserian ganglion by inserting a needle through the foramen ovale, (a small hole in the skull through which the nerve passes) under radiographic (X-ray) control and then destroying all or parts of the nerve fibers. Initially the agents used, e.g. alcohol, were non-selective and, although good pain relief was obtained, it was at the risk of inducing not just sensory loss, but also **dysaesthesia**. All these techniques are called **percutaneous**, since they involve passing a needle through the skin of the cheek.

Procedures currently done at this level include percutaneous radiofrequency **rhizotomy** (gangliolysis, lesioning or thermocoagulation (RFT), percutaneous glycerol rhizoloysis (rhizotomy) (PGR) or percutaneous balloon compression (BC) (microcompression, gangliolysis).

Definition of procedure

RADIOFREQUENCY THERMOCOAGULATION

Electrocoagulation (destroying the nerve by use of heat) of the trigeminal nerve was first done by Kirschner in the 1930s. But the uncontrolled use of heat and lack of techniques to guide the surgeon to the exact location led to severe side effects, and this procedure did not gain widespread acceptance until it was modified by Sweet in the 1970s. The procedure of relies on selective destruction of nerve fibers by an electric current. Tactile (touch) sensations mediated by A alpha fibers and A beta fibers are preserved, while fibers carrying **nociceptive** sensation (A delta and C fibers) are destroyed (see Chapter 3 for further explanation). The temperature and time that are used can be altered in order to cause more or less sensory loss.

PERCUTANEOUS GLYCEROL RHIZOTOMY

In percutaneous glycerol rhizotomy the Gasserian ganglion is bathed in glycerol, a mild neurolytic (nerve-damaging) agent. The glycerol destroys the myelin and thereby stops transmission of impulses through the **myelinated** fibers. It causes less damage than alcohol. It was thought that it would produce less sensory loss than radiofrequency thermocoagulation and yet give equally satisfactory pain-relief periods. Altering the way in which the technique is done allows sparing or inclusion of the 1st or 3rd nerve divisions.

BALLOON COMPRESSION

In the 1950s it was found that compression of the nerve at the Gasserian ganglion level, especially if nerve injury occurred, seems to result in pain relief. This discovery led to the development of microcompression of the trigeminal nerve at the level of the Gasserian ganglion. The aim is to press the nerve against some bony tissue and, in so doing, damage it enough to stop transmission of painful stimuli through the large myelinated fibers, but not others. Less sensory loss and preservation of corneal reflex can be achieved, but often at the expense of shorter pain relief periods.

Selection of patients

Some procedures require a patient to receive a general anesthetic; others can be done under heavy sedation. Since a needle has to be passed through the foramen ovale for radiofrequency thermocoagulation and percutaneous glycerol rhizotomy, patients with any tendency to bleed should not be considered for these techniques. Blood pressure also tends to rise during these procedures, thus these procedures may not be suitable for patients with heart problems, especially high blood pressure.

Selection for radiofrequency thermocoagulation

Patients :
- need to be cooperative during the procedure
- with reduced vision should not be offered radiofrequency thermocoagulation in case they should develop corneal anesthesia (numbness of the surface of the eyeball) and possible eye complications
- must be ready to accept sensory loss
- who already have some numbness may sustain more severe sensory loss

- who want some control over the amount of sensory loss
- who are elderly, provided they have no bleeding problems
- with multiple sclerosis
- who do not want an MVD
- who have had a recurrence after other types of surgery

Selection for percutaneous glycerol rhizotomy

Patients :
- who are afraid of sensory loss and **anesthesia dolorosa**, since percutaneous glycerol rhizotomy causes less sensory loss than that predicted after radiofrequency thermocoagulation
- who have a medical history for whom a general anesthetic is contraindicated
- can have a general anesthetic if they wish
- with a possible allergy/adverse reaction to contrast medium or iodine should not have this procedure
- may not have an immediate result and need to be warned
- with jaw muscle weakness are good candidates for this procedure
- need to be ready to accept higher recurrence rates than for other procedures
- who do not wish to have an MVD
- who have had pain recurrence after other types of surgery

Selection for ballon compression

Patients :
- should have a CT scan or MRI to rule out abnormal arteries in the brain, since there is a suggestion that these patients do less well
- should have X-ray imaging done to assess the size of the foramen ovale in order to predict those patients whose foramen may be difficult to visualise or may be too small to allow penetration by a 14-gauge needle
- should have an ECG to identify those who may be at risk of arrhythmias (abnormal heart beats)
- who have pain in the first division of the nerve and in whom corneal anesthesia needs to be avoided
- who have weak jaw muscles on the opposite side should not have the procedure, since most patients sustain short-term jaw muscle weakness on the operated side
- who are elderly

- taking warfarin can have the procedure, provided the warfarin is stopped pre-operatively. There is a smaller risk of intracranial hemorrhage than with other Gasserian ganglion procedures, since the needle does not penetrate inside the skull as with the other techniques
- with multiple sclerosis
- who do not wish to undergo a MVD

Operative techniques

Some of these procedures require a full general anesthetic (microcompression), whereas others can be done under sedation using agents such as fentanyl and a local **anesthetic** to reduce the pain. Penetration of the foramen ovale by a needle (gauge 14 or under) is the most difficult part of the procedure and the point at which patients may experience pain and heart problems such as a decrease in blood pressure and extremely slow pulse rate. Monitoring is therefore very important. There are many excellent texts describing the procedures and these will be provided at the end of the chapter. A brief description will be given here. In all these techniques a special radiological device known as a **fluoroscope**, is needed to guide the needle into its correct position. Some patients may stay overnight after the procedure, but patients can often be discharged on the same day.

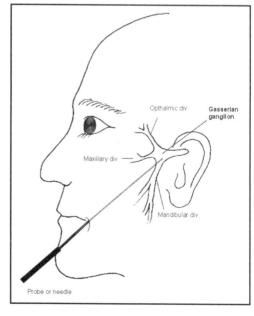

This diagram shows the general location of the instrument in the Gasserian ganglion.

Radiofrequency thermocoagulation

The full technique is well described by Taha and Tew in **Techniques in Neurosurgery** (1999) with diagrams to illustrate the various stages of the procedure. Use of different temperatures allows for variations in sensory loss.

1. The patient is given a short-acting anesthetic.
2. The procedure has to be done in a room with facilities for fluoro-scopic monitoring.
3. The patient is laid flat.
4. A hollow needle is introduced through the cheek using well-estab-lished landmarks. It is very important to ensure that the needle does not penetrate the mouth, since the needle becomes contaminated and spreads infection, which can result in bacterial **meningitis**.
5. Patients will often wince at the moment the surgeon penetrates the foramen ovale.
6. Localization of the needle now needs to be verified by fluoroscopy. The aim is to ensure that the needle lies in the retro-Gasserian area. Once the **stylet** is removed, free flow of **cerebral spinal fluid** (CSF) is often seen. Flow of CSF does not equate with correct placement, since CSF can be obtained from other places. If any blood vessel has been punctured inadvertently, blood will flow through the needle. Puncture of the carotid artery has been recorded in several studies.
7. Once precise localization has been achieved, the electrode is inserted. This electrode can either be curved or straight. It is at this point that patients are awoken so that they can verify whether the correct area is being stimulated. The patients are asked to indicate whether the area of numbness induced by the stimulation is in the same place as the original pain. This will feel like a tingling sensa-tion. The stimulation can normally be achieved using low temper-atures such as 40° C.
8. Once the desired effect has been achieved, a further amount of anesthesia is given so there is no pain during the lesion (heat) gen-eration. Lesions are made at temperatures from 60° C to 90° C in cycles of 45-90 seconds. A special machine is used to generate the heat and ensure the temperature is kept at the pre-set level. Many operators note an area of redness on the cheek in the division being treated.
9. The patient can then be awoken again and sensory testing carried out to check whether the correct amount of numbness has been

achieved. This normally means that a sharp pin is still felt, but not as sharply. Further lesioning can then take place until the appropriate sensory loss has been achieved. The aim is to reduce the sensory loss to a minimum.

10. The patients are then observed for an additional 15 minutes before returning to the ward from which they are discharged either later that day or the following day. The cheek may be slightly sore from the needle.

11. Before discharge, the extent of sensory loss needs to be established. Patients who are found to have lost or have a reduced **corneal reflex** must be warned about eye care, given safety glasses, and possibly, artificial tears. They should be advised to seek an ophthalmologist's opinion should the eye become red in appearance. If the jaw muscles have been damaged, the patient should be advised to eat a soft diet and do some jaw exercises for two weeks.

12. The medication is slowly stopped.

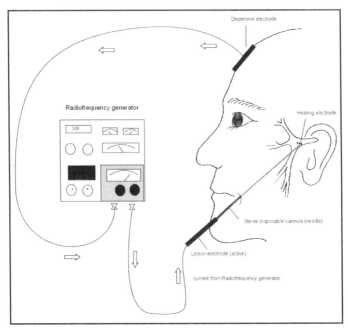

Radiofrequency generator

This diagram shows the procedure of radiofrequency thermocoagulation. Once the needle is correctly located, a lesion is created by the radiofrequency generator.

Percutaneous glycerol rhizotomy

Several variations have been introduced over the years, but none of them have been evaluated under controlled conditions. The procedure takes 25-40 minutes.

1. Patients are premedicated and a local anesthetic is used for needle penetration. Patients can be given an intravenous sedation with fentanyl. General anesthesia can be used, although it makes the technique more complicated.
2. The procedure has to be done in a room with facilities for fluoroscopic monitoring.
3. Patient is initially laid flat, but later the patient is brought up into a sitting position if **cisternography** is performed.
4. A hollow needle is introduced through the cheek using well-established landmarks. It is very important to ensure that the needle does not penetrate the mouth, since the needle becomes contaminated and spreads infection resulting in bacterial **meningitis**.
5. Patients will often wince at the moment the surgeon penetrates the foramen ovale.
6. Localization of the needle now needs to be verified by fluoroscopy. Correct placement of the needle is very important and aims to enter the trigeminal cistern in such a way that the **preganglionic** trigeminal rootlets become bathed in the glycerol. Passing the needle through the foramen ovale does not guarantee entry into the trigeminal **cistern**. The needle may need to penetrate further if divisions 1 and 2 are to be treated. Once the stylet is removed, free flow of **cerebral spinal fluid** (CSF) is often seen.
7. The correct placement of the needle and the size of the cistern can be estimated by injecting a known amount of **contrast medium** and ascertaining the amount it takes to achieve a cup shape, around 0.3- 0.9 ml . For this the patient is put into the sitting position. It is important to remember that a certain volume of contrast medium needs to be injected before it is visualized on X-ray films. Some operators do not do cisternography for one or more of the following reasons:
   • increases the cost of the procedure
   • increases chance of needle moving out of position while it is draining
   • need to change the patient's position
8. If cisternography has been used, it is important to remove the contrast medium, which can be done by flushing with sterile saline.

Some contrast medium (which is heavier than the glycerol) can be left if seeking to avoid the third division and wishing to only affect the first division.

9. The position of the needle must be checked again if cisternography has been used before the glycerol is injected with the patient in the sitting position. Placement of the glycerol outside Meckel's cave increases the chances of sensory change. It is important to ensure the glycerol is sterile to minimize the risk of meningitis and the **anhydrous** form seems to be the most satisfactory. Volumes injected in a range from 0.25 to 0.4 ml. More than this, and there is a risk of overfilling the cistern. Some will also add a small amount of tantalum dust so that the cistern can be visualised at a later date. Different positions of the head can result in some selectivity of nerve fiber injury.

10. After the injection, the flow of CSF should be checked, since this will confirm that dislocation of the needle has not occurred.

11. It is important to leave the patient in the sitting position for 2-3 hours after the procedure to avoid leakage of the glycerol out of the cistern.

12. Patients can be kept in the hospital overnight to ensure no complications develop. This is recommended for elderly patients.

13. Pain relief may not be immediate; it can be delayed for 5-7 days, so it is important that medication is continued until the patient is pain free.

The ganglion is bathed in Glycerol

This diagram shows how the glycerol is put into Meckel's cave so that it bathes the ganglion.

Ballon compression

The technique is well described by Brown and Gouda (1999) in a special supplement on trigeminal neuralgia in Techniques of Neurosurgery. The procedure lasts 30-60 minutes.

1. A general anesthetic is used, since the patient does not need to be awoken and the larger needle that is used can cause more pain.
2. The procedure has to be done in a room with facilities for fluoroscopic monitoring.
3. Patient is placed either in the semi-sitting or supine position.
4. Significant drops in blood pressure and heart rate occur at the time the needle is inserted, or the balloon catheter advanced and inflated, so it is crucial to monitor arterial blood pressure and heart rate. Some surgeons will even use a non-invasive temporary pacemaker, which responds rapidly to changes.
5. The needle is inserted through a point in the cheek using a No.14 needle or a liver biopsy needle just as in the other techniques. Fluoroscopy is used to visually guide the needle into position.
6. Often at the point the needle touches the emerging nerve, **bradycardia** (slowing of the pulse) occurs (called the pain reflex). It is crucial not to push the needle through the foramen ovale as is done with the other techniques.
7. A No.14 Fogarty balloon catheter without its stylet is then advanced through the needle. It is advanced beyond the needle in the aim of locating it in Meckel's cave. The balloon is fully distended and in the correct location if it assumes a pear shape. If not advanced far enough, it will miss the third division fibers.
8. Compression is then carried out. There have been no trials to estimate the optimal pressure to use or the duration of compression. If distended too much, the balloon may burst, and over distension leads to severe numbness and 4th cranial nerve **palsy**.
9. Compression at appropriate pear shape is maintained for one to one and a half minutes, although longer times have been recorded. The duration of compression does relate to sensory loss. If the balloon is well inflated frequently, bradycardia will occur, and this is considered a good sign.
10. The balloon is deflated and everything is withdrawn.
11. Pressure maintained at puncture site for 5 minutes.
12. Patient may be discharged the next day.
13. May get delay in pain relief of a few days.

Sometimes the procedure fails because the foramen ovale is too small or the blood pressure falls too low.

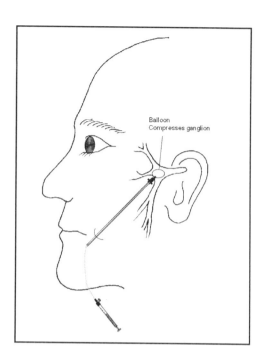

Balloon
Compresses ganglion

This diagram shows how the balloon on the Fogarty catheter is distended in the ganglion.

Gasserian ganglion surgery recurrence rates

General remarks on recurrence rates

Trigeminal neuralgia is one of the few neuropathic pains in which 100 % pain relief can be obtained. Most patients when questioned want at least no pain for five years. This would therefore preclude any peripheral therapies and even some of the Gasserian ganglion options. Figure 9.9 below shows the results from three forms of ablative surgery from reported data (Lopez et al 2003). These are based on the best quality studies that were selected according to strict criteria. Most recurrences of pain occur in the first two years, after which there is a more gradual decline in the number of patients who develop a recurrence. There are always a few times when there is difficulty penetrating the foramen and some in whom, despite a satisfactory procedure, no pain relief occurs.

Patients who are medically unfit are more likely to be offered peripheral techniques and this may affect results.

Radiofrequency thermocoagulation

The number of patients likely to be pain free at any one time is shown in the figure and Table 6 on the following page.

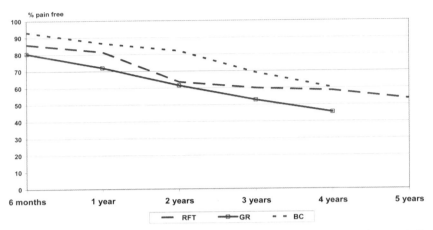

This graph shows the time for complete relief of pain (off all medication) for radiofrequency thermocoagulation (rft), percutaneous glycerol rhizotomy (GR) and balloon compression (BC) for trigeminal neuralgia. It shows that 50 % of patients will be pain free at 5 years.

Table 6

PROBABILITY OF A RECURRENCE AFTER RADIOFREQUENCY THERMOCOAGULATION										
No. of patients	Mean (range) follow up year	Failures (%) yrs	Rates of complete pain relief						Median time to recurrence	References
			.5 yr	1 yr	2 yr	3 yr	4yr	5yr		
96	5 (1-8)	6 (6)	88	77	65	61	60	53	Median 6	Latchaw et al 1983
185	8 (1-15)	NA	74	70	63	58	56	51	Median 5	Oturia 1996
31 TN	2.5 ± 1 (0.6-4.7)	0	94	90	64	64			Median 4.5	Zakrzewska et al 1999
17 ATN		0	87	80	64	54			Median 4	Zakrzewska et al 1999
1216	5.8 (1-25)	163 (2.4)		90	62	62	59	56	Median 6	Kanpolat 2001

NA - not available, TN - classical trigeminal neuralgia, ATN - atypical trigeminal neuralgia

In their 15-year follow-up of 154 patients, Taha and Tew (1995) showed that the rate of pain recurrence was higher in those with mild numbness as opposed to deep numbness. The degree of numbness relates to the extent of the lesion, i.e the temperature and length of time it is applied for. It is therefore possible to have a shallower lesion, but then patients need to accept an earlier recurrence of pain, as recounted in this patient's statement: *"After 18 months of having no pain, it came back again with a vengeance…it did not come as a real surprise."*

The existence of clear diagnostic criteria has been shown to be important in this technique. In our small cohort of 48 patients followed up for three years, we carefully classified patients into those with classical trigeminal neuralgia and those with atypical trigeminal neuralgia, i.e. a background pain, and have shown that those with classical pain had better results (Zakrzewska et al 1999). Further evidence for this can be seen in earlier data we published on 265 procedures (Zakrzewska and Thomas 1993). These procedures were done by the same surgeon, but patient selection was not as meticulous and at three years, only 31 % of patients were likely to be pain free as compared to 65 % in my later study. Yoon et al (1999) also had poorer outcomes in patients with atypical trigeminal neuralgia, but the data was analyzed retrospectively and little details are given regarding the criteria used to assign patients to the two groups.

Percutaneous glycerol rhizotomy

The number of patients estimated to be pain free at any one year is shown in the Table 7 below and the figure above. It shows that after two years, patients are highly likely to experience pain recurrence.

Table 7

PROBABILITY OF A RECURRENCE AFTER GLYCEROL RHIZOLYSIS								
No. of patients	Mean (range) follow up year	Failures (%)	Rates of complete pain relief				Median time to recurrence yrs	References
			.5 yr	1 yr	2 yr	3yr		
85	3 (0.5 – 4.5)	NA	78	68	60	54	3	North et al 1990
60	4.5 (4.5-9)	4 (7)	88	86	68	53	4	Slettebo et al 1993

NA - data not available

North et al (1990) showed how recurrence rates change depending on which end points are used, i.e. use of medication, or need for re-operation. These relatively high recurrence rates have led some clinicians to abandon this type of surgery. Multiple sclerosis does not appear to affect recurrence rates.

The pain can return suddenly as this patient describes: *"About three years later I was sunbathing in my backyard. I said something to my son and the pain shot through the whole side of my face."*

Balloon compression

There are only two studies that report longer-term outcomes and there is only one report that uses Kaplan Meier analysis shown in Table 8.

Table 8

PROBABILITY OF A RECURRENCE AFTER BALLOON COMPRESSION							
No. of patients	Mean (range) follow-up year	Failures (%)	Rates of complete pain relief				Median time to recurrence yrs	References
			.5 yr	1 yr	2 yr	3yr		
50	3 (1-7)	3 (6)	91	86	79	69	NA	Brown et al 1993

NA - data not available

The one report recording the largest number of procedures (496) contains insufficient data for analysis. When compared to other Gasserian ganglion data, the results appear promising, but these are based on a very small number of patients.

Prognostic factors for recurrence rates

There are several studies that analyze their results in terms of factors that may affect long-term outcome, but some of these are conflicting and the quality of the evidence is poor. This could be due to some of the factors mentioned above, i.e. lack of diagnostic criteria, including mixed cases, length of follow-up, definition of recurrence, and lost to follow-up cases.

Prognosticators for radiofrequency thermocoagulation

There are two studies that have looked at prognostic factors using actuarial data (Latchaw et al 1981, Yoon et al 1999). Both studies found classical trigeminal neuralgia cases did better. I also found that classical trigeminal neuralgia patients did better in terms of both pain-free intervals and complications (Zakrzewska et al 1999). Most would suggest that sensory loss increases the chances of a longer pain-free period. Duration of disease, response to medication, age, or the presence of multiple sclerosis made no difference to outcome (Latchaw et al 1981, Yoon et al 1999). Yoon et al (1999) showed that prior surgery other than radiofrequency thermocoagulation was a poor prognostic sign and multipledivision pain was probably also a poor prognostic factor.

Prognosticators for percutaneous glycerol rhizotomy

There is considerable discrepancy between the results and, again, it is related to small numbers and lack of clear criteria for recording of these. The type of glycerol used can affect results and has led to the use of an anhydrous form. Previous peripheral treatment made no difference to the outcomes, but posterior fossa surgery may make a difference. Patients with multidivisional pain experience better results than those with single- division pain in contrast to the radiofrequency thermocoagulation patients. The amount of sensory loss was a significant predictor; the more sensory loss, the more likely a low recurrence rate was found.

Prognosticators for balloon compression

Given the small numbers reported and the lack of Kaplan Meier analysis, there is no reliable data on prognostic factors.

Complications after Gasserian ganglion surgery

Some surgeons consider that sensory loss is a side effect of surgery and do not wish to call it a complication, but I think sensory loss affects quality of life and should be classified as a complication.

Complications can be divided into those that:
- occur around the time of the operation, some of which can be short-term in their effects, e.g. infection or long-term such as a stroke
- bleeding and bruising around the site of entry of the needle has been reported in many series
- relate to **cranial nerves** 4, 6 and 7, most of which are transient, i.e. one to six months (see Chapter 2 for an explanations of what functions these nerves perform.)
- relate to the 8th cranial nerve (the nerve of hearing), which can be mild and transient or can result in permanent effects
- relate to the trigeminal nerve itself; some may be permanent, others may be transient, such as difficulty with eating or temporary hearing problems
- eye problems

Oturai et al (1992) report a patient satisfaction survey among their patients who underwent peripheral alcohol injections, neurectomy or radiofrequency thermocoagulation. They were asked about quality of life as affected by the complications, and it was found that 36 % were unaffected by them, 51 % were slightly or severely affected, and 13 % reported a marked effect.

The figure below shows the percentage of patients likely to suffer from complications after surgery, which includes sensory loss. If sensory loss is included as a complication, then only 10 % of patients undergoing radiofrequency thermocoagulation have no complication, whereas 85 % of patients having gamma knife surgery, 74 % of patients undergoing a MVD, 45 % of patients undergoing percutaneous glycerol rhizotomy and 23 % of those having balloon compression are likely to have no complications.

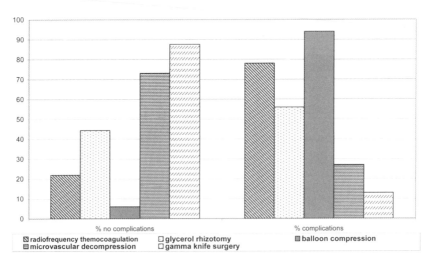

Likelihood of complications after different types of surgery

Complications reported from the main studies for the ablative procedures are shown in Table 9 and in the figure on the following page.

Very few complications around the time of the operation have been reported and yet Sweet (1990) notes there are significant low blood pressure and **bradycardic** episodes during placement of the needle. Cardiac arrests have been reported. The presence of abnormal anatomic features can also lead to puncture of the wrong foramen, as well as penetration of the inferior orbital fissure (Sweet 1990). Both aseptic and bacterial

meningitis have been reported. They result in headache, fever, neck rigidity, altered mental state within 6 hours.

A **lumbar puncture** needs to be done in order to culture the CSF to determine whether it is infective. The bacterial type will require treatment with antibiotics and the aseptic ones with steroids, and these usually resolve in 48 hours. Herpes labialis (cold sores on the lips) have been reported in many patients after these procedures. It is speculated that the presence of the herpes virus may increase the tendency to develop dysesthesia.

Table 9: Key facts

PERCENTAGE OF PATIENTS HAVING COMPLICATIONS AFTER ABLATIVE PROCEDURES								
	No. pts	Difficulty eating	Cranial nerve deficits	Meningitis	Troublesome dysaesthesia	Anesthesia dolorosa	Corneal numbness	Keratitis
RFT	4657	12	1	0.2	4	2	10	1
PGR	1252	3	0.2	1	8	2	8	2
BC	294	NS	2	3	10	0	0	0
Gamma knife	337	NS	0	0	9	0.3	3	NS

NS not stated

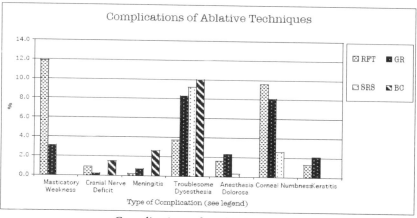

Complications after ablative surgery

Legend: Masseter weakness is usually transient. Rates of masseter weakness are not reported for balloon compression, since this nearly always occurs. Cranial nerve deficits (usually transient), meningitis and vascular injury resulting in arterial bleeding or arteriovenous fistula occur more frequently with balloon compression *RFT:* percutaneous radiofrequency thermocoagulation; *GR:* percutaneous glycerol rhizolysis; *SRS:* stereotactic radiosurgery; *BC:* percutaneous balloon compression of the Gasserian ganglion; *%:* percentage of patients with complications.

Sensory loss is very high after all Gasserian ganglion procedures, and is considered essential after procedures such as radiofrequency thermocoagulation, but many patients learn to cope with it as indicated by this quote: *"I wonder when the numbness is going away, but I can live with it."*

Overall sensory loss is reported as occurring in the following percentage of cases: 62 % after radiofrequency thermocoagulation, 38 % after balloon microcompression, 28.6 % after percutneous glycerol rhizotomy, 2.8 % after MVD and 8.7 % after GKS. The pie chart below shows the proportion of patients likely to get sensory loss after surgical procedures.

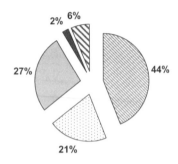

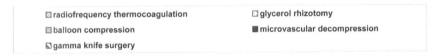

Proportion of patients reporting sensory loss after different surgical procedures.

Sometimes there is more than sensory loss and patients report pain in the numb area. Very few studies define what they mean by **dysaesthesia** and very few classify it as mild or severe enough to affect the quality of life as this patient describes: *"I had relief from the original pain, but had new symptoms. I had a cold burning sensation in the skin around my eye and an ache in the eye itself... The pain was tolerable, compared to the original pain, so I managed."*

Anesthesia dolorosa, which can be defined as pain in an area of numbness, is the most severe form of sensory damage that can occur, as this patient describes: *"whole half of my head from the top to my chin was experiencing it, tightness, nerves crawling and little stings on my tongue, eye, etc. Half of my tongue was numb and sometimes it felt as if I could itch my eye right out of my head and sometimes it felt as if a worm was crawling around in my nose."*

The rates of development of dysaesthesia or anesthesia dolorosa have been shown to be highest in those procedures that result in nerve destruction, i.e. ablative procedures. Anesthesia dolorosa can occur in up to 2 % of patients and has a profound effect on quality of life. The likelihood of these occurring after different procedures is shown in Table 9 and in Figure 9.13 below.

Some of these problems resolve over time, whereas others necessitate treatment with antidepressant drugs, as illustrated by this sufferer's comment: *"not having any more of the sharp, stabbing, explosive type pain, but only the numbness and the burning pain...am currently taking 300 - 400 mg of Neurontin and .25 mg of Klonopin twice daily and .5 mg at bedtime. The combination of these drugs help with the burning pain and also ease the tugging and pulling on my face."*

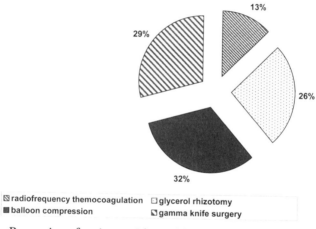

radiofrequency themocoagulation glycerol rhizotomy
balloon compression gamma knife surgery

Proportion of patients with troublesome dyseasthesia.

A variety of eye problems can occur for three main reasons: as part of the process of causing direct damage to the trigeminal nerve, incorrect placement of the needle during the procedure, or indirect effects of the treatment on surrounding structures. Eye problems can result in:
• corneal **anesthesia** and loss of **corneal reflex**
• neuroparalytic keratitis – infections in a numb eye
• ocular motor cranial nerve damage leading to double vision, which can be permanent or transient
• blindness - direct damage to the eye
• cataract formation related to radiation damage

Corneal numbness can lead to corneal scars and ulcer formation, which compromise vision. If severe, it can result in the need for a further operation to do a **tarsorrhaphy** (partial closure of the eye). Neuroparalytic keratitis leads to reduced corneal nerve supply, which reduces the vitality of the cornea, leading to decreased tear production and drying of the cornea with increased potential for damage. Many patients tolerate corneal anesthesia well, but it does require constant vigilance.

Patients with pain in the first division of the nerve are often not offered radiofrequency thermocoagulation, and a higher proportion of these patients may undergo balloon compression; thus comparison between different techniques can be misleading.

Complications after radiofrequency thermocoagulation

The complication rates after radiofrequency thermocoagulation are shown in Table 9. If sensory loss is excluded, then 29 % have some other type of complication. Fewer complications tend to be reported from the larger centers. Sweet (1990) describes a wide range of serious complications ranging from death to intracranial hemorrhages leading to strokes. Loss of speech, infections and blindness can occur, but are not reported. These are often due to intracranial or subarachnoid arterial hemorrhages and intracerebral haematomas (clots) often on the opposite side. Although radiofrequency thermocoagulation has a high rate of complications, these need to be evaluated carefully, since many of those occurring after radiofrequency thermocoagulation are relatively minor. Some of the complications that can occur are explained below:

Infective complications
- meningitis, although of the Gasserian ganglion surgeries, it is least likely to occur after this procedure

Changes in sensation of the face
Some sensory loss must be obtained for a good result as this patient describes:

"Where there was previously a trigger point around my jaw, it now was quite numb - quite a pleasant change. The numbness does not cause me any problems."

This complication is, to some extent, under the control of the operator; Tew and Taha suggest that this can be further reduced using the curved electrode. Sensory loss may be restricted to the area in which the pain was present, in around 68 % of patients. However, sensory loss may occur both in the pain area and outside it. **Dysesthesia** is more likely to occur in older patients. Although the incidence of anesthesia dolorosa is highest after radiofrequency thermocoagulation (up to 15 % in some series), the incidence of dysesthesia is the lowest for the three Gasserian ganglion surgeries. We showed that in patients undergoing radiofrequency thermocoagulation the quality of life was affected either slightly or markedly by sensory loss in over 60 % of patients, and it did not drop off significantly after time (Zakrzewska and Thomas 1993, Zakrzewska et al 1999). Some patients will need treatment, and antidepressants appear to be the drugs of choice. Coping strategies are going to play an important role in helping patients come to term with these complications.

Eye complications
• transient diplopia (double vision)
• reduction or loss of corneal reflex is around 10 % and is only slightly lower than after PRG. The comparison, however, may not be valid, since patient selection could bias the results. Patients with pain in the first division of the nerve are often not offered radiofrequency thermocoagulation, and percutaneous glycerol rhizotomy is recommended due to initial reports, which suggested that corneal reflex loss did not occur with PRG. Eye problems such as **keratitis** are rare, but one patient is reported as having lost his sight due to severe neuroparalytic keratitis
• blindness due to cranial nerve damage has been reported in 10 patients

Eating problems
• transient masseteric problems, around 12 % are reported. These can lead to difficulty in eating and wearing dentures. Patients may be embarrassed about eating in public, thus quality of life can be compromised. It is important to explain to patients that they need to be careful when eating and that they do not need new dentures. One patient described her experience this way:
"I came out with a really dead left side of my face, but mainly the cheek area. For the first month I had trouble biting my cheek, tongue and lower lip, but this has slowly subsided. I ate only soft food for a week or two."

Other facial pain
• facial pain other than trigeminal neuralgia has been reported in up to 37 % of patients, and this is higher in patients with atypical trigeminal neuralgia (Zakrzewska et al 1999). It may be postulated that the procedure may uncover other facial pain. It is crucial to take a careful pain history when patients return with pain after surgery, since it may not be trigeminal neuralgia, but this type of pain.

There is a significant reduction in the number of patients who report depressive symptoms after
surgery (as picked up on the Hospital Anxiety and Depression Scale), and anxiety is also significantly reduced (Zakrzewska et al 1999).

In our prospective study, we inferred patient satisfaction with treatment from a yearly questionnaire that asked patients whether they wished to have repeated surgery (Zakrzewska et al 1999). There was little change over time, and over 90 % of patients were prepared to undergo a repeat radiofrequency thermocoagulation if necessary. But patients with atypical trigeminal neuralgia, who experienced less pain relief and more complications, were less sure whether they would want to undergo the treatment a second time (12 % no, 43 % unsure).

Complications after percutaneous glycerol rhizotomy

Complications after this procedure are shown in Table 9 and described below:
• Two mortalities have been reported
• Aseptic meningitis may be due to the contrast medium or overfilling of the cistern
• Cranial nerve complications other than in the 5th nerve are very rare
• Sensory loss did not correlate with quantity of glycerol used, preoperative dose of carbamazepine, age or duration of disease, or the presence of multiple sclerosis. There was a tendency for higher recurrence rates in patients who experienced mild or no sensory loss. Some reports suggest an increased risk of developing dysaesthesia if patients had had previous surgery, but it was not related to whether they had sensory loss prior to the procedure. The type of glycerol used may affect sensory disturbance, sinces it depends on the amount of **arachnoiditis** that it induces; it is this that reduces the size of the cistern. The following quote is from a patient who developed problems after PRG:

"It was a complete failure. The pain became much worse, and a horrible burning, aching numbness developed."

- Periodic itchiness of the eye, as well as change in flow of tears, has been reported. This, as well as reduced corneal reflex, may contribute to the development of conjunctivitis reported in up to 40 % of patients in some series
- There does not appear to be any increased risk of corneal anesthesia after recurrent surgery
- Motor paralysis of the masticatory muscles is rarely reported

Complications after balloon compression

The complications reported in the higher quality studies are shown in Table 7. Two mortalities have been reported due to technical problems.
- Temporary 6th nerve palsy has been reported
- Dysesthesia does occur and can be severe, but as yet no cases of anesthesia dolorosa have been reported
- A very small number of cases have been reported with transient reduction of corneal reflex, but there are no reports of keratitis or other eye problems, and this is lower than after other Gasserian ganglion procedures
- Motor weakness is invariable for up to 3 months and is reported in most studies, and is more frequent than after other Gasserian ganglion procedures. Patients need to be warned that eating may be difficult and that dribbling may be a problem. Patients may do better if they eat a soft diet that requires less chewing; hence the risk of biting the inside of their cheeks

WHAT TYPES OF SURGERY ARE DONE IN THE POSTERIOR FOSSA?

Definition of procedure

Microvascular decompression (MVD) aims to decompress the trigeminal nerve from vessels or tumors that may be in contact with it without causing damage to the nerve. The rationale behind this operation lies in the hypothesis that vessels or tumors compressing the trigeminal nerve result in areas of **demyelination** and resultant **ephaptic transmission** or reverberating circuits (See Chapter 2 for explanations). The area particularly vulnerable to this compression is the root entry zone, which is a cone- shaped junction between central and peripheral **myelin** in the main sensory root of the trigeminal nerve located approximately 3 mm from the **pons**. In many instances the compressions can be visualized on **MRI scans**. If at operation no compression is found, some surgeons will perform a partial **sensory rhizotomy** (PSR) in which some of the trigeminal nerve fibers are cut in order to stop pain transmission. However, PSR also may result in sensory loss.

Selection for Microvascular decompression / partial sensory rhizotomy

- Since these procedures are classified as major neurosurgical procedures, patients need to be medically fit.
- Initially, patients over the age of 65 years were not considered good candidates, but with improved anesthetic techniques, the medical condition rather than age of the patient should be taken into account.
- Patients with MS can be considered if the MRI shows a compression and if there are no demyelinating plaques in the root entry zone, pontine tract and nuclei.
- Partial sensory rhizotomy is often done if patients are found not to have a compression; thus patients need to be warned that they may have some sensory loss if this procedure is done.
- Since hearing loss is a well-known complication, it is important to stress this, especially to patients who are musicians, dependent on hearing, or who may already be deaf on the other side. Some neurosurgeons will do a hearing test prior to the operation.

Operation

The following summary of the procedure of MVD is based largely on a study by McLaughlin et al (1999), which is based on observations after 4,400 operations. There are many other texts and books that describe variations of this technique, including the book by George Weigel and Ken Casey. The operation takes about two to three hours. Partial sensory rhizotomy is exactly the same, except that the surgeon will cut a small piece of the sensory part of the nerve.

1. **Informing the patient**. Providing information prior to surgery is essential, and it is preferable for this to be available in the written format. Patients must make it clear to the surgeon what they would like done if no compression is found – either a PSR or nothing.
2. **Positioning the patient**. Position is crucial for correct exposure. The lateral position is used with the patient's head placed at the foot of the operating table to enable the surgeon to have more room. The head is secured with a three-point fixation device after

the anesthetic is given. The hair is shaved behind the ear on the side of the pain. The patient is carefully taped in the correct position to prevent movement.

3. **Surgical incision.** The aim is to minimize the length of the incision, but at the same time allow adequate exposure for the burr hole. The position and size of this incision is dependent on the size and thickness of the patient's neck.

4. **Bone removal.** A small piece of bone, about a half-dollar size is drilled. During this procedure, some partial removal of **mastoid** air cells may occur. These air cells need to be immediately protected with wax or muscle after exposure to reduce ear complications.

5. **Exposure of the trigeminal nerve.** One of the most intricate steps of the procedure is the exposure of the nerve. Once the **dura** is sutured back, an operating microscope with a 250 millimeter objective lens is brought into the operating field. Draining **CSF** helps to expose this area and reduces the amount of traction that may be necessary.

6. **Looking for the compression.** It is important to bear in mind that the route entry zone can be very variable in length and can extend fairly distally. Several reports stress the importance of exploring the full length of the nerve. The use of a small-angled **endoscope** to inspect the whole area may be a useful adjunct to the microscope. There may be more than one compression.

7. **Monitoring** with the use of what are called brainstem-evoked potentials is advocated in order to reduce damage to the auditory 8th nerve.

8. **Decompression.** This can be done in a variety of ways using a range of materials. There have been no controlled trials to assess the effectiveness of different materials. The materials used have ranged from resorbable ones such as muscle or dura, and hard materials such as Ivalon (polyvinyl alcohol foam) or Dacron, or softer materials such as gelatine sponge, Surgicel and Teflon in a variety of forms, shredded felt, tapes and woolen slings and glue. Reports on re-operations have shown that resorbable materials tend to cause adhesions, are lost and so lead to recompression. Teflon felt can cause **adhesions** and **granulomas,** but it tends to remain in place as do Ivalon sponges. Some neurosurgeons stress the importance of avoiding any contact of the nerve with any decompressant. Sindou et al (1991) have suggested that improved results are obtained if the offending artery is dislodged from the

nerve and then suspended by small tapes of Teflon. If the vertebral artery or basilar artery is causing the compression, then more manipulations are likely and hence more complications. Veins are difficult to decompress and so these are often sealed off. If no compressing vessels are found, most surgeons will then proceed to do a PSR. By careful sectioning; sensory loss can be reduced to a partial lower-face sensory loss.

9. **Closure.** Complete and effective hemostasis is essential to prevent strokes. The layers must be closed very tightly to prevent leakage. Some surgeons put in a titanium mesh plate to cover the defect where the bone was removed. Others put back the bone pieces, and still others do nothing and allow scar tissue to grow into the space.

10. **Post operative care.** Monitoring of blood pressure is crucial, and patients may spend one night in intensive care unit. Patients can be mobilized after one day and discharged within 48 to 72 hours. Patients may be given steroids after the operation to prevent swelling of the brain. Frontal and incision pain is expected, but should be controllable with mild narcotics. If mild narcotics fail to control the pain, then investigations need to be done to rule out hemorrhage or a CSF leak with the use of a CT scan. Medication can be tapered off slowly. Most patients are able to return to work after two weeks, but it can take 6 – 8 weeks to fully recover, as this patient reports: *"I awoke free of the TN pain. I fully recovered from the surgery in 6 to 8 weeks."* There is no reliable data on this, and our Bristol data suggest that 50 % of patients recover in 6 weeks. More details can be seen in Table 12.

What is meant by compression?

There is relatively good evidence to suggest that compression of the trigeminal nerve by a vessel is not normal. Although 16-40 % of people without trigeminal neuralgia may exhibit contact between a blood vessel and the nerve, no grooving or distortion of the nerve is found (Hamlyn and King 1999). The vessels involved in order of frequency are:
- superior cerebellar artery (SCA)
- anterior inferior cerebellar artery
- basilar artery
- superior petrosal vein
- inferior petrosal vein
- petrosal vein

It is considered that compression by an artery is likely to be more significant than by a vein. The presence of compression or contact between vessels and the trigeminal nerve is not always easy to establish and many neurosurgeons do not define their criteria. A range of descriptions is used to describe the relationship between the vessels and the nerve. Grooving or distortion of the nerve, once the vessel has been lifted off, is considered by most to indicate compression. Mild compression where contact is seen, but with no grooving or distortion, is also described.

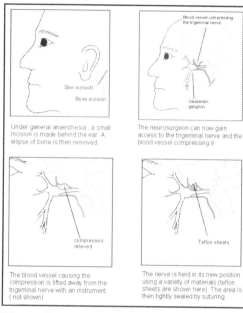

Under general anaesthesia, a small incision is made behind the ear. A ellipse of bone is then removed

The neurosurgeon can now gain access to the trigeminal nerve and the blood vessel compressing it

The blood vessel causing the compression is lifted away with an instrument (not shown)

The nerve is held in its new position using a variety of materials (teflon sheets are shown here) The area is then tightly sealed by suturing.

These schematic diagrams show the basic steps of microvascular decompression.

This photograph shows the trigeminal nerve compressed by a blood vessel.
(courtesy Prof H. Coakham)

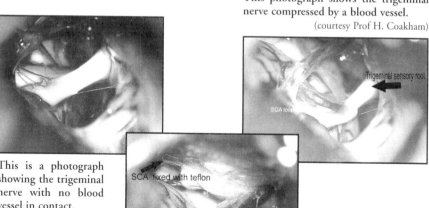

This is a photograph showing the trigeminal nerve with no blood vessel in contact.

(courtesy Prof H. Coakham)

This photograph shows the decompressed trigeminal nerve; Teflon pieces separate the nerve from the blood vessel. (courtesy Prof H. Coakham)

Hamlyn (1999), based on his anatomical and clinical work, proposes the following definitions that he considers to be feasible when using an operating microscope with binocular vision: *"vessels are or are not in contact; they either do or do not lie within half of their diameter from the brainstem or nerve, and there either is or is not a groove left after the vessel is dissected free."*

Posterior fossa recurrence rates

The probability of being pain free at any particular time is very similar in all the major centers and the following figures and Table 10 provide some of this data. These graphs can be compared with those for the ablative procedures, which have been constructed in the same way.

Table 10

No. of patients	Mean follow-up years	Immediate Failures	% pain free			Reference Year
			1 year	5 years	10 years	
104	5	2	83	71		Piatt & Wilkins 1984
41	8.5	2	95	88		Burchiel 1988
35*	6.2	NA	82	66	60	Pollock et al 1988
10*	6.2	NA	100	78		Pollock et al 1988
252	5	13	88	84		Bederson 1989
94	4.8	3	87	75	59	Cutbush et al 1994
61	6	3	88	85		Sun 1994
133	5.3	NA	87	81	80	Mendoza et al 1995
1185	6.2	24	84	78	70	Barker 1996
146	3.2	11	78	73		Broggi et al 1999
225	10.9	0	82	70	85	Tronnier et al 2001
245	5	17	82	79		Zakrzewska et al 2005
2531			86	83	71	Combined

PROBABILITY OF REMAINING PAIN FREE EITHER WITH NO MEDICATION OR MEDICATION AFTER MICROVASCULAR DECOMPRESSION

* Pollock et al (1988) did 45 operations on 35 patients and the results on 10 patients who had bilateral procedures are reported separately NA – not available

The rate of recurrence changes over time, being 2 % at five years, but becoming 1 % by 10 years. The highest rate of recurrences is in the first year. Patients with MS appear to have poorer results after an MVD, but there are very few reports on this group of patients.

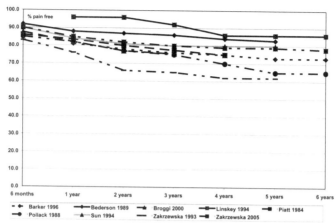

Probability of remaining pain free after microvascular decompression, based on some of the higher quality studies.

There is little data on PSR alone, and most of the data is included in the MVD data. We recently completed a study of 245 patients who had an MVD and 60 who had a PSR done by the same surgeon and followed up for a mean of 5 years. The figure below shows the probability of a recurrence of pain for the two procedures (Zakrzewska et al 2005a) . This shows that at five years 79 % of patients who have had an MVD are likely to be painfree, whereas the comparable figure for PSR is 72 %. There is therefore little difference, and this has been noted by other centers (A probability of 1 = 100 %).

Probability of being pain free after microvascular decompression (245 patients) or partial sensory rhizotomy (60).

Legend: survival = pain free, probability of 1 = 100%

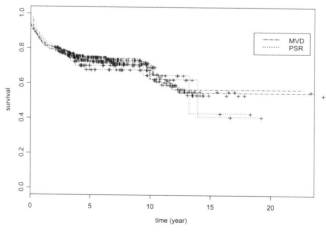

Patients' reports also show there are some with excellent results. Examples include:

- *"I have been pain free for ten years."*
- *"He found a very large artery that had snaked itself around my right trigeminal nerve and was squeezing it at several points. He skillfully dissected it and padded it away. It's been nearly 12 years and I haven't had any pain attacks. I take no medication. The surgery was a godsend."*

But there are also those in whom the procedure works for a very short time, as this patient notes:

- *"I felt no pain and was sent home with the idea that all the pains were gone...forever. A month later while brushing my teeth, the pains gradually returned, a little more each day."*
- *"The surgery went great. I could eat a hamburger again. It was September 2002. My son was born May 2004, and two weeks later it hit me again".*

Prognosticators for MVD

Unfortunately, the available data is not of the highest quality and it is still impossible to predict which patients are likely to do better. Some of the data is conflicting. It all begins with diagnosis. Szapiro et al (1985) stress the importance of dividing the patients into two groups before doing any analysis i.e. those who have only paroxysmal pain (pure pain) and those who have paroxysmal and background pain (mixed group), since this was a major predictor for outcome. When they did their further analysis on the separate groups, they had very small numbers and so did not get statistical significance. They found more compression in those with pure pain and were unable to explain why patients with mixed pain did not show a correlation between sensory loss and degree of compression. They were also at a loss to explain why, despite decompressing a definite compression, patients still reported background pain.

Prognostic factors that may need to be taken into account include:

- type of pain
- length of duration of trigeminal neuralgia
- age at onset
- distribution of pain – side and divisions
- pre-operative sensory changes
- gender
- type of compression
- previous treatment

• sensory loss
• type of material used to decompress
• blood pressure

The current data is conflicting and these issues will only be resolved if data is collected prospectively, combined from many centers and collected independently of the surgeon.

A very important factor for patients is whether timing of the operation affects results. According to two studies, patients having an operation within eight years of developing trigeminal neuralgia did better, but four other studies did not find early treatment to correlate with longterm success, and our Bristol data also did not find any correlation. Again, this will not be resolved until clear criteria are laid down for what constitutes the first symptoms. This should be achievable, given that over 85 % of patients remember their first attack.

It may also be important to assess whether prior ablative surgery influences outcome. In the Bristol data we divided patients into so-called primary and non-primary groups: primary group – patients who had not undergone any previous surgery, and non-primary group - patients who had a previous ablative procedure. A few differences are then seen, as in the primary group 84 % of the patients after a MVD are likely to be pain free, whereas in the PSR, this is 70 %. However, there is less of a difference between those having a MVD and PSR who have had prior surgery as seen on the following graphs.

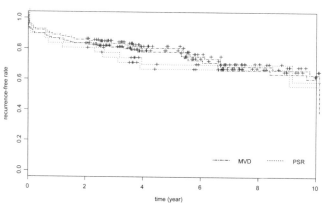

Probability of being pain free after microvascular decompression (primary procedure 169, or partial sensory rhizotomy (primary procedure 21). It shows that for the primary group, though statistically non-significant, recurrence-free rates for MVD group are consistently higher than that for PSR group. At 5 years the mean recurrence-free rates were 84 % for MVD and 70 % for PSR.

Legend: Primary group = patients who have never had any surgical procedure for their trigeminal neuralgia. Probability of 1 = 100 %

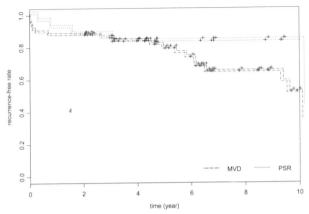

Probability of being pain free after microvascular decompression (non-primary, 76 patients) or partial sensory rhizotomy (non-primary, 39 patients) shows that for the non-primary group, recurrence-free rates for the two surgical groups were similar by 5 years. The different rates shown after 5 years are not stable due to the small sample size and thus we do not attempt to interpret the differences.

Legend : survival non primary=patients who had some form of Gasserian ganglion surgery prior to present operation. Probability of 1 = 100 %

Complications after MVD

With more than 8,000 procedures reported in the literature, it is now possible to gain a much better picture of the types and rates of complications. Overall, around 30 % of patients are reported as having complications, of which only 15 % are likely to be permanent, as shown in Table 11 and the following figure. A review of the poorer quality studies shows similar types of complications, but fewer of them 12.5 % (370/2958). I suspect that some series collect their data more meticulously and so report in greater detail all their complications, including such relatively minor ones as herpes infections. Others only report the more major ones. Yet if surgeons are to obtain fully informed consent from their patients, they need to be able to give them substantial information on complications and how these change over time.

Some reports stress that complications are transient, but few give any indication of the length of this transient period. The only reports that give details of change of complications over time are those dealing specifically with hearing changes and sensory features. Not a single study reports all their complications at different time periods. Some reports classify complications as major or minor, but none specify what criteria they use to place them in these categories. I consider that only the patients can decide whether a complication is major or minor, since they need to judge how the complication affects their quality of life.

Table 11

COMPLICATIONS REPORTED AFTER MICROVASCULAR DECOMPRESSION (TOTAL QUALITY DATA)													
pts	AM	BM	CSF	I	H	PE	Ataxia	4th	5th	6th	7th	8th trans	8th perm
2711	268	9	51	6	8	6	9	17	75	9	57	42	60
%	9.9	0.4	1.9	0.2	0.3	0.2	0.34	0.6	2.8	0.4	2.1	1.5	2.2

Legend: AM aseptic meningitis BM bacterial meningitis CFS – CFS leaks, I – cerebellar infarcts, H – hematomas PE – Pulmonary embolus, 4th, 5th, 6th, 7th, 8th – cranial nerve palsies/dysfunctions, trans – transient, perm - permanent

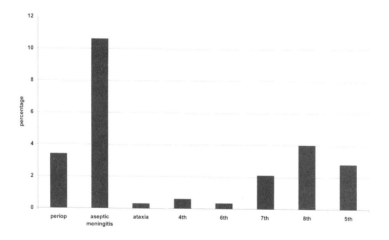

Complications after microvascular decompression as reported in the literature.
Legend: Peri-operative refers to those complications in the immediate operative period, ataxia –unable to walk straight, 4th, 5th, 6th, 7th and 8th th refer to the cranial nerves, some of these are transient and resolve after a few weeks or months.

Attention to detail during the operation, including the use of auditory evoked potentials (tests to check hearing), as well as surgical experience, does affect the number of complications. A major survey of outcomes after microvascular decompression has been done in the US, which suggests that complications are fewer in those centers where 4-5 microvascular decompression procedures are done a year (Kalkanis et al 2003). Modifications have been introduced, which appear to have further reduced complications.

But many patients will put up with complications provided they are painfree as suggested by this patient: *"Took a little time to get over walking problems, permanently lost hearing in right ear, and have dry eyes, but worth it."*

Mortality

Early reports quoted a 1 % mortality rate for this operation. This has now dropped and in the total literature of over 5,000 reported cases that quote their mortality data, there have been 26 deaths, giving a percentage of 0.46. If we look onlyat the top studies, then the mortality rate is 0.41 %, while in the poorer reports it is 0.5%. The deaths are either those to be expected after any major surgery, which occur at distant sites, e.g. lung embolus, or at local sites due to technical problems. The most common causes of death are either cerebellar **infarct**s (death of a vital part of the brain tissue) or hemorrhage (bleeding) and is more likely to occur in patients with tumors.

Complications occurring in the immediate period after surgery

The most common complication is that of an **aseptic meningitis** and can occur in up to 11 % of patients. **Cerebellar infarct** and **hematomas**, which are not lethal, could leave patients with a significant disability such as **ataxia** or strokes. Some of these patients may need to be re-explored. Other complications are those associated with any neurosurgical operation and are not specific to posterior fossa surgery. Epilepsy, headaches, postoperative nausea and vomiting, wound infections, postoperative confusion, heart attacks, **pulmonary emboli**, or stomach bleeding are reported, and I suspect some of these are under- reported because they are considered non-specific. Herpes infections (cold sores) on the lips often occur and may be due to manipulation of the nerve. The commonest one I have come across is leakage of cerebrospinal fluid.

Complications involving cranial nerves except the auditory nerve

Many of the complications involving the 5th, 6th and 7th cranial nerves are transient and the percentages of reported complications are low. (See Chapter 2 for an explanation of their functions). Complications within the trigeminal nerve are low compared to the Gasserian ganglion procedures and are either mild sensory loss or at the most, dysaesthesia, but with no reports of anesthesia dolorosa as this patient reports: *"I had an MVD and since then I have had no pain whatsoever, just some numbness in half my cheek and tongue."*

Many of these sensory changes may have been present pre-operatively, since few reports give details of sensory changes before the operation. Other sensory changes may be too mild to pick up on gross testing. Careful testing after the operations shows that up to 30 % of patients may have some sensory loss. It has also been suggested that patients with vertebrobasilar artery compression are more likely to have sensory complications than are patients with other compressions due to the need for manipulation.

Table 12 on the following page shows the complications reported by the Bristol patients, who were surveyed independently of the surgeon using a very detailed questionnaire and is the only data of its kind that we have at present (Zakrzewska et al 2005a and b). The results were not validated by an examination, e.g. testing hearing loss. They do not include the immediate post-operative complications that had resolved by the time of the survey. All patients had there surgery done at least six months prior to the surgery. The high response rate to the questionnaires means that it is highly representative of the sample, which is the largest in the UK. When comparing the data in Table 11, you will see more complications being reported and this is related to the method of collection of the data. Some of the complications, such as numbness, may have been due to prior surgery, but again pre-operative sensory testing had not been done in order to assess these.

Hearing complications due to auditory nerve damage or local complications

The most serious and frequent complication after MVD is hearing loss as reported by this patient: *"The operation left me with ringing in right ear and significant loss of hearing."*

Hearing loss is reported as transient or permanent and either complete or partial. Some also distinguish between hearing loss that is picked up on audiometry and not reported by the patient. Very few centers report that they do audiometry pre-operatively, so the accuracy of the postoperative findings must be questioned. Some studies report on eighth nerve damage separately from transient middleear effusions or **otitis media,** which occur immediately after surgery. Middle-ear effusions occur probably due to lack of application of bone wax to the mastoid air cells. Hearing complications occur less frequently if auditory evoked potentials have been measured during the operation. A very rare case of delayed hearing loss was reported three years after a MVD which, on re-operation for recurrence of pain, found scar tissue and progressive thinning of the auditory nerve.

Table 12

DETAILS OF BRISTOL PATIENTS WHO UNDERWENT THEIR FIRST POSTERIOR FOSSA SURGERY – COMPLICATIONS		
	MVD	**PSR**
Response rate	90% (220/245)	88% (53/60)
Gender	131 female, 89 male	37 female, 16 male
Mean age at operation	59	57
Mean duration of TN	6.7	7.0
Mean followup in years	5.3	5.7
Types of previous surgery	19 peripheral surgery 20 Gasserian ganglion 37 do not know	3 peripheral surgery 15 Gasserian ganglion 3 do not know
Patients who needed further surgery	28 of these 18 currently pain free	4 of these 2 currently pain free
Patients with both prior surgery and repeat surgery after posterior fossa surgery	9 of these 6 currently pain free	0
Patients reporting any form of facial pain at time of survey	40	16
Numbness	5%	48%
Headaches	13%	14%
Burning sensation	5%	24%
Hearing problems	13%	16%
Unsteadiness	11%	18%
Dizziness	8%	20%
Eating problems	3%	27%
Eye problems	5%	22%
Any complication	26%	62%

Effects of MVD on quality of life and satisfaction with surgery

There is remarkably little in the literature about patients' satisfaction with surgery and only our recent publication of the Bristol data has made it the center of a report (Zakrzewska et al 2005a). The results are shown in Table 12. In the patients' "stories" I received, there was also a lack of report of success, probably because these patients no longer remain active members of support groups, but here are a couple of comments after MVD surgery:

- *"I have now been pain free for two years; I laugh again, I run again, I dance as I please. If you feel like giving up, don't !!! The surgery saved my life. I would do it again if I had to stay 3 days in ICU and 3 days in hospital. It was worth it ... not the end of the world, but the end of torture."*
- *"I can actually enjoy a glass of ice cold water again. My life is back to normal. I thank God for the miracles of modern medicine, for I have regained the quality of my life."*

We have previously reported that the incidence of depression and anxiety in patients after this type of surgery is low. The recent Bristol data have shown similar results with only 3 % of MVD patients showing evidence of depression on the Hospital Anxiety and Depression Scale. But depression occurs more often in the PSR patients, in 17 %, and is probably related to some extent to the sensory loss, although this is still only slightly higher than that in the general population where one would find around 15 % of patients with depression.

Many felt that the operation should have been done earlier, as shown in Table 13 on the following page. Patients who had a complication, mainly related to sensory loss among the PSR group, were statistically less likely to express satisfaction with the operation and report that it did not meet their expectations. This suggests it is very important for patients to know before surgery what the likelihood of a PSR being done are; some patients will give surgeons specific instructions not to proceed with this procedure.

Table 13: Key facts

PATIENTS' VIEWS ON THEIR SURGICAL OUTCOMES AFTER MVD OR PSR, BRISTOL DATA				
	Primary Group		*Non-primary Group*	
	MVD 144 pts	PSR 32 pts	MVD 76 pts	PSR 21 pts
Looking back now, how would you consider the timing of your surgery? *				
Should have been earlier	78%	65%	71%	52%
About right	22%	31%	29%	48%
Could have been delayed	0%	4%	0%	0%
How long did it take you to completely get over the operation?				
Mean (weeks)	10.7	14.5	11.1	7.5
Median (weeks)	6	6	7	4
Range (weeks)	0-78	2-52	0-52	0-26
How well did this operation meet your expectation? *				
Better than expected	82%	60%	59%	52%
Just as expected	14%	16%	22%	30%
Worse than expected	4%	24%	19%	18%
Overall how satisfied are you with your current situation *				
Satisfied	96%	75%	76%	64%
Slightly dissatisfied	3%	4%	14%	14%
Dissatisfied	1%	21%	10%	18%
If you needed treatment again what treatment would you choose? *				
The same surgery	80%	59%	66%	52%
Other form of surgery	1%	11%	0%	5%
Drug therapy	2%	8%	2%	5%
Other	2%	0%	0%	0%
Unsure	5%	22%	32%	38%

Legend: * Statistically significant differences
primary =no previous surgery for trigeminal neuralgia,
non primary = some previous ablative type of surgery for trigeminal neuralgia

What is Gamma Knife Surgery (GKS) – radiosurgery?

Definition of procedure

This relatively new method of stereotactic surgery, using the gamma knife, enables lesions of the trigeminal nerve to be made in the posterior fossa without the need to do an open procedure, since it relies on high quality **magnetic resonance imaging**. New data is continually being published on this topic, and this is kept relatively up to date on the Web site of the National Institute of Clinical Excellence (NICE). The precise location of the target is achieved by the stereotactic guidance, hence the name stereotactic radiosurgery. It is a non-invasive method and therefore is potentially available to every patient, however medically unfit. The equipment needed is very expensive and at present there is limited availability.

The linear accelerator (LINAC) works on a different principal and is used more for cancer and vascular abnormalities. It has been used for trigeminal neuralgia but there is insufficient data to be able to compare it to other techniques.

Mechanism of action

Radiosurgery, i.e. the use of a radiation beam to perform non-invasive procedures, has been used since Laskell introduced it in 1950. The way it works has not been entirely clarified. Radiation results in both acute and delayed changes in the targeted tissues. Clinical reports record a considerable latent period (up to 12 months) before maximum pain relief is obtained and maximum sensory loss is noticed. It was hypothesized that irradiation of the trigeminal nerve would block **ephaptic** transmission, but not normal axonal conduction and thus its effects would be selective. However, it seems logical to assume that any treatment, be it chemical, thermal, mechanical or irradiation, will affect the integrity of the whole trigeminal nerve, and both myelinated and non-myelinated fibres will be damaged.

There remains controversy about the relative radiosensitivity of different cranial nerves, and some believe that sensory nerves are more radiosensitive than motor ones. To date, clinical studies have reported sensory loss in up to 17 % of patients, but there is only one case report of motor involvement in the form of jaw clenching by a patient who received repeat surgery to a total of 160 Gy.

Animal work on irradiated nerves has shown that **axonal degeneration** and edema affects all nerve fibers at doses of 80 Gy, and necrosis is observed at six months when nerves receive doses of 100 Gy radiation. These findings are supported by reports that patients who develop some loss of sensation (evidence of axonal damage) have a longer pain-free period than those without sensory loss. Longer pain-free periods are more likely to occur in those patients with higher doses of irradiation, and in those in whom a greater length of the nerve is irradiated.

It is now appreciated that exact location of the lesions may have a significant bearing on outcomes, both in terms of pain relief and complications. It has been postulated that the so-called **root entry zone** (REZ) is more radiosensitive. (See Chapter 2 for details.) However, this needs to be weighed against the fact that irradiating in the REZ inevitably leads to some irradiation of the brain stem.

When initially used in trigeminal neuralgia, the irradiation was aimed at the Gasserian ganglion and retro-Gasserian portion of the trigeminal nerve, rather than REZ. The results were not encouraging and did not appear to offer any advantage over other techniques. It was decided that results might be more reliable if the beam were to be directed more at the REZ, with the brain stem receiving up to 20 % of the dose, since this was considered the site of compression. Dosage, imaging methods, position and outcome measures needed to be addressed, and this was initially done through a multicenter study. Later, the position and length of irradiated nerve was determined in one of the first randomized controlled trials in neurosurgery for trigeminal neuralgia (Flickinger 2001).

Selection for Gamma knife surgery

Since this technique does not require a general anesthetic and does not involve major surgery, almost all patients are eligible. The following are some of the factors that need to be considered:
- patients who are medically compromised and/or very elderly
- patients who do not want an invasive procedure
- MRIs are used in the plotting of the fields and so patients who are not eligible for MRIs may be excluded although this can be circumvented with the use of **CT**. These will include patients with metal implants, including pacemakers and those who suffer from severe claustrophobia
- patients need to be able to lie flat and still for around one hour, so this may exclude patients with cardiac failure
- the finding of a compression on MRI does not exclude a patient from this procedure
- suited to patients with hemoglobinopathies, i.e bleeding disorders
- patients in whom penetration of the foramen ovale has proven difficult may be specially suited to this procedure
- patients need to be aware that results may not be immediate and this may be a major problem in patients who are in severe pain
- patients need to be warned that they may need to be on medication after treatment indefinitely if they only get a "good" result

• sensory loss also can occur and may be delayed up to two years
• patients need to be warned that radiation is cumulative
• the procedure is only available in a few centers and is very expensive

Operation

More details can also be found in George Weigel and Ken Casey's book, and more technical details on this technique can be found in Kondziolka's article in Neurosurgery Clinics of N America (1997). This procedure involves a whole team, which includes the neurosurgeon, radiation therapist, medical physicist and nurses. It takes four hours in total, but the actual treatment only takes around an hour.

1. **Frame fitting**. A halo frame is first fitted on the head using four screws, two on the forehead and two at the back of the head. Since this may be painful, **local anesthesia** and sedation may be used. This is necessary to ensure that the head is positioned accurately in the MRI machine and for the radiation beams to be aimed precisely where needed.

2. **Localization of the trigeminal nerve**. This is best done using MRIs, but CT can be used in those patients who have implanted metallic foreign bodies or those who do not have easy access to an MRI machine. Previous surgery can make this more difficult.

3. **Computer dose planning**. This process may take an hour or two, so the patient has time to relax during this period. The exact position (isocenter) to which the radiation will be directed is then calculated. The dose used has varied from 28 to 90 Gy. When treatment is planned for tumors, the dose is calculated based on tumor volume and proximity to radiosensitive structures.

4. **Treatment**. When the planning is completed, the patient lies on the Gamma Knife couch and the head frame is secured inside a larger helmet, which has 200 holes in it, as shown in the illustration. The patient's head is moved inside the globe and the radiation (radioactive cobalt) is delivered through the globe over periods varying from 20 to50 minutes. It is not known whether the dose rate is important for outcomes.

5. **Completion of treatment**. The frame is removed and the patient hospitalized overnight, although some may be discharged at the end of the day.

6. **Post-operative management**. Medication needs to be continued for at least 3-4 days and tapering down should only begin once pain relief is being achieved. Delays of up to 120 days have been

noted, but the mean is 14 days. Here is a patient's description of the process: *"He and an associate put the TEMPLATE over my head in the morning and left it there all day long. It has several screws, which were screwed into my forehead to hold the template in place while I was waiting to be treated. They got around to me late in the afternoon and gave me the Gamma Knife Treatment, which took all of 10 minutes. Dr. ...told me I would not begin to feel the relief or improvement until approximately six weeks had passed."*

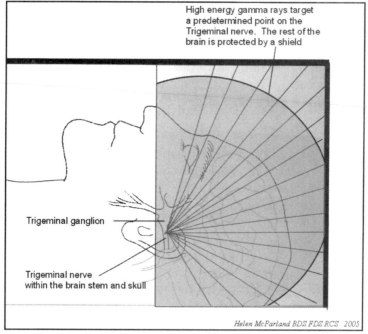

This is a diagrammatic representation of the gamma knife.

Recurrence rates after Gamma knife surgery

A systematic review of the use of GKS in trigeminal neuralgia has been carried out by the University of York Center for Reviews and Dissemination (Web site is listed in references and the details can be found on the NICE Web site also provided in references). When reading reports on GKS, it is important to remember the following factors:

• Some series contain patients treated with different doses and different number of isocenters.

- Reports with a very short follow-up may not pick up on patients who develop delayed effects of radiation.
- Pain relief can be considerably delayed and so patients need to continue on medications.
- The patient characteristics are variable in that some have had previous surgery, while others are new cases. Some have only recently been diagnosed and some have pre-operative sensory changes.
- Patients who already have a pre-existing numbness are at higher risk of developing further paresthesia and ultimately, a dysesthesia that comes to affect the quality of life.
- Fewer patients get complete relief of pain, as with other techniques. One patient reports. *"It was a blessing for me because the pain only happens on rare occasions. I still take Tegretol; however, the pain is manageable and no more electric shocks."*
- Many patients need to remain on low-dose medication to get full relief of pain.
- It has been suggested that GKS costs are 3.5 times greater than a percutaneous procedure, but 40 % less than a microvascular decompression procedure. However, this does not take into consideration long-term costs, such as repeated procedures of any types of surgery dealing with complications, etc.

Table 14 shows the recurrence rates from the best studies and the graph for recurrence rate is shown in Figure 9.9 in the section on ablative procedures. There can be considerable delay in the onset of pain relief, although most patients will get some immediate improvement. Actuarial analysis of delay in maximal pain relief after irradiation shows that 75 % of patients with partial or complete pain relief will achieve it within three months, and 90 % will have achieved it by six months. Only 5 % are likely to still get relief after six months. The mean time to maximum relief is eight weeks. At 5 years, one report shows that only 33 % of patients are pain free (Maesawa 2001). Considerable new data is being prepared, so this data may change as more careful analysis is carried out. Similar results seem to be obtained with the LINAC accelerator. The failure rate is highest after this procedure as seen on the table and reported by this patient:

"The end result, after all was done, is that there was no improvement in the TN pain at all. It was and is still there. The operation resulted in my having lost approximately 35 % of my hearing."

Table 14

PROBABILITY OF BEING PAIN FREE AFTER GKS						
Patients	% failed	% recurrence	% pain free 1 year	% pain free 2 years	Time to recurrence months	Report Author, Year
110	12	34	79	69	25 months mean previous surgery	Young et al 1998
			88	79	33 mean no prior surgery	
54	11	21	NS	64	6.7 months median	Rogers et al 2000
27 41	70 Gy 15 90 Gy 7	70Gy 26 90Gy 15	NS	NS	NS	Pollock et al 2001
220	15	17	60	59	15.4 months mean	Maesawa et al 2001
44 43	1 isocenter 16 2 isocenters 19	42	59		12 months median	Flickering et al 2001
68	14	20	65	58	5- 8 months median	Pollock et al 2002

Prognosticators for GKS procedures

Lower recurrence rates are found in:
• patients with classical trigeminal neuralgia
• those who achieve complete relief of pain with no medication
• have GKS as the primary treatment
• develop new numbness

The following figure illustrates how the results can vary depending on which groups of patients are used in the analysis. There is as yet insufficient data to determine whether the dose of radiation (80 or 90 Gy), the number of isocenters used, or the presence of a vascular compression and atypical features, affects pain outcomes.

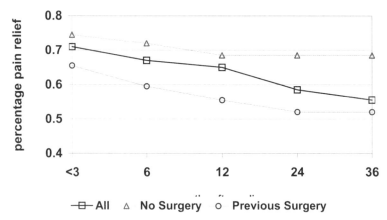

Probability of being pain free after gamma knife surgery depending on whether the patient has had some prior surgical procedure. It shows that patients who have had no prior sugery have a longer pain relief period.
Legend: probability of 1 = 100%

Complications after gamma knife surgery

No peri-operative complications or deaths have been reported. There remain concerns about the long-term effects of radiosurgery, both in its potential to induce cancer and in its effect on the eye, leading to increased risk of cataract formation. In contrast to all other surgical treatments, complications after GKS may be delayed for months or even years, thus it is crucial that these patients are carefully followed up and questioned about the possible development of late complications.

Complications are more likely to occur when higher doses of radiation are used or when the procedure is repeated, and these are shown in Table 15 on the following page. All reports acknowledge that the major complication after radiosurgery is of sensory loss, which can occur up to two years after treatment, as this patient describes:

"I have been free of side effects and pain since that day. Nine months later I have noticed slight tingling of my tongue and lips. I have no idea what this indicates."

In patients treated with 90 Gy, half of them may develop numbness, whereas this drops to 9-16% in those treated with lower doses. The numbness may not affect quality of life, as this patient states:

"The only side effect is a numb feeling on the left side of my face that might be from the radiation nerve damage. The numbness is better than the pain I had prior to the operation."

Taste may also be affected. When using higher doses, the motor division of the trigeminal nerve may be affected and can lead to jaw clenching. Corneal reflex loss has also been noted.

Whether radiosurgery causes structural changes to the trigeminal nerve is still debatable. As in patients who have undergone an MVD after radiosurgery, no consistent pattern emerges as yet.

Table 15

COMPLICATIONS AFTER GAMMA KNIFE SURGERY						
Permanent numbness %	Mild paresthesia %	Severe paresthesia %	AD %	Corneal reflex loss	Time scale Median	Reference year
3	0	1	1	0	9 months	Young et al 1998
9	NS	0	0	NS	NS	Rogers 2000
7- 18*	10	1	1	NS	Up to 2 years	Flickinger et al 2001
7	NS	0.4	0.4	0	8 months	Maesawa et al 2001
15 with 70Gy 54 with 90Gy	NS	4 with70Gy 13 with 90Gy	0	0 with 70GY 7 with 90Gy	NS	Pollock 2001
8	16	12	NS	2.6	8 months	Pollock 2002

*Depending on number of isocenters, NS not stated, AD anesthesia dolorosa.

No reports mention any psychological problems that the patients may have encountered during the procedure, especially while undergoing MRI. Reports have shown that up to 30 % of patients having an MRI may suffer from anxiety-related reactions. This can be allayed most effectively by the use of patient information, which also contains some hints on psychological preparation, the use of music, prone position, the presence of a relative, and distracting thoughts. In severe cases sedation may be needed.

6. HOW DO THE DIFFERENT SURGICAL TREATMENTS COMPARE?

It remains difficult to compare different techniques for the reasons given at the start of this chapter, and Table 16 on the following page can only provide some pointers and general guidance. As better data is published, the results may change.

Table 16: Key Facts

SURGICAL MANAGEMENT OF TRIGEMINAL NEURALGIA			
Procedure	% Probability of being pain free	Mortality	Complications
Peripheral _ neurectomy, cryotherapy, alcohol, injection, acupuncture	Two years – 22	Nil	Low, sensory loss, transient bruising, swelling
Radiofrequency thermocoagulation	Two years –68 Five years- 48	Low	62% sensory loss and 25% other complications mainly relating to trigeminal nerve, dysesthesia, anesthesia dolorosa, eye, eating problems
Percutaneous glycerol rhizotomy	Two years – 63 Five years – 45	Low	28% sensory loss and 27% other complications mainly relating to trigeminal nerve, dysesthesia, anesthesia dolorosa, eye, eating problems
Balloon microcompression	Two years –79 Five years – no data	Low	38% sensory loss and 38% other complications mainly relating to trigeminal nerve, dysesthesia, eye, eating problems
Microvascular decompression (MVD)	Two years – 81 Five years – 76 Ten years- 71	0.5%	Overall 75% no complications, complications 14% peri-operative complications, 5% transient cranial nerve $4^{th}, 6^{th}, 8^{th}$ dysfunction, 2.2% permanent deafness, 3% sensory loss
Gamma Knife surgery (GKS)	Two years – 75 Five years – 58	nil	12% sensory loss up to two years post treatment

What are the advantages and disadvantages of each of the different types of surgery?

Indicators for use of peripheral surgery

Advantages of peripheral surgery:
- elderly and medically unfit can be treated
- immediate results and most can be done in the dental office
- least invasive of all surgical procedures
- relatively small area of sensory loss and no anesthesia dolorosa
- no mortality

Disadvantages of peripheral surgery
- very high recurrence rate, most within the year
- can only be done if there is a very discrete trigger area

- many patients need to continue to take drugs
- high incidence of transient side effects
- sensory loss occurs and some cases of dysesthesia have been reported

Indicators for use of Gasserian ganglion surgery

Advantages of radiofrequency thermocoagulation
- safe in medically compromised patients
- does not require a specially skilled surgeon
- highly specific and can avoid other branches
- can vary amount of sensory loss
- high level of initial success
- immediate pain relief
- low mortality
- relatively low recurrence rate
- few complications outside trigeminal area

Disadvantages of radiofrequency thermocoagulation
- patients with bleeding disorders not suitable
- co-operative patient needed - patients anxious about their ability to give accurate response
- expensive equipment
- tedious to do as need to keep waking the patient
- mortality has been reported
- sensory loss inevitable
- risk of anesthesia dolorosa
- risk of corneal damage, need to wear safety glasses
- risk of eating difficulties

Advantages of percutaneous glycerol rhizotomy
- suitable for the elderly
- more suitable for patients with first division pain
- can use sedation or general anesthesia for the procedure
- easier to carry out than radiofrequency thermocoagulation
- no sophisticated machinery required so is one of the cheapest procedures
- not necessary to do intra-operative sensory testing so causing less anxiety
- lower mortality and morbidity than after radiofrequency thermocoagulation
- less risk of anesthesia dolorosa and eye problems than radiofrequency thermocoagulation

- few problems outside trigeminal area
- easy to repeat

Disadvantages of percutaneous glycerol rhizotomy
- cannot use in patients with sensitivity to contrast medium
- very technique sensitive so needs a skilled operator
- higher recurrence rate than other Gasserian ganglion procedures
- may have a delay before get pain relief
- glycerol does induce **arachnoiditis** and this could lead to long-term problems
- difficult to do repeat procedures

Advantages of balloon microcompression
- suitable for most elderly as less likely to cause intracranial bleeding as needle not advanced all the way
- although it requires a general anesthetic, it is a quick one
- do not cause pain and anxiety while doing procedure as there is no need to wake the patient during the procedure
- less experienced surgeon than for radiofrequency rhizotomy; it is not necessary to be selective, since all fibers get the same amount of compression
- very low mortality
- immediate high success rate
- few complications outside trigeminal area
- no reports of anesthesia dolorosa
- less likely to cause loss of corneal reflex than other Gasserian ganglion procedures so useful for patients with first division pain

Disadvantage of balloon microcompression
- not suitable in patients who have **arrhythmias** due to risk of **bradycardia**
- requires general anesthetic with intubation
- recurrence rate as high as for any Gasserian ganglion procedure and higher than posterior fossa
- jaw muscle weakness can be a problem, especially if patients are trying to control their dentures. Patients with weakness on the opposite side should not undergo the procedure
- sensory loss is inevitable and can be a problem in patients who already have some sensory loss

Indicators for use of posterior fossa surgery

Indicators for MVD
Advantages of MVD
- longest pain-free intervals
- high initial success rate
- few patients will need a further surgical procedure
- small percentage of patients will have complications
- most complications are transient
- risk of sensory loss is very small
- no anesthesia dolorosa or **keratitis**

Disadvantages of MVD
- mortality rate of 0.5 %
- expert surgeons required
- need to be fit enough to undergo a surgical procedure with a full general anesthetic
- requires longest hospital stay and takes several weeks to get over it
- risk of strokes or bleeding higher than with other procedures
- permanent hearing loss in up to 3 % of patients
- initially expensive procedure

Indicators for gamma knife surgery (GKS)

Advantages of GKS
- can be done on medically unfit patients, elderly and those with heart problems
- suitable for patients with **acromegaly** or other bony disorders, which make entry through foramen ovale difficult
- no general anesthesia needed
- non-invasive with no operative complications
- rapid return to normal life
- lowest rate of complications
- especially useful for first division pain, since no keratitis
- at the most requires one overnight stay
- can be done on patients who have had previous surgery, although results may not be as good
- can possibly be repeated

Disadvantages of GKS
- patients who are claustrophobic may not tolerate the treatment
- not suitable for patients who cannot stay still or lie flat, e.g. some cardiac patients
- currently still lacks long-term results

- current 5-year data are poor, but may be related to early use of low doses
- need to continue medication after treatment for months or in some cases indefinitely
- can take over 6 months to get maximum pain relief
- difficult to decide when treatment has failed and what treatment should be used next
- side effects in the form of sensory loss can occur months after treatment
- other side effects may have not yet become apparent, e.g. vascular or increased risk of cancer
- patients with pre-operative sensory loss may be at increased risk of developing troublesome anesthesia
- corneal reflex loss has been reported
- although not reported, I postulate that anxiety may be high, even post-treatment, due to delayed effects and fear of the unknown
- concerns remain about the long-term effect of radiation
- availability is poor, costs are much higher than for Gasserian ganglion

---

MRS. G CASE STUDY

Mrs. G decided that she preferred to have a longer-term solution to her trigeminal neuralgia, since her pain was getting more severe and affecting all aspects of her life. She discussed her anticoagulant therapy with the hematologist, who agreed she could stop the warfarin for the time of her surgery. It was a risk Mrs. G was prepared to take.

Which surgery did Mrs. G choose to have and what result would she anticipate getting? How could you minimize her risk of getting another deepvein thrombosis or pulmonary embolus?

Discussion

Mrs. G is relatively fit and decided that she would like to have a microvascular decompression rather than an ablative procedure, which would give her relief for 45 years as compared to over 10 years. She was not keen to have numbness of her face, which she had a high chance of getting after these procedures. Mrs. G. enjoys many outdoor activities and did not want the risk of having corneal anesthesia and needing to wear glasses when outside. She was fully assessed by an anesthetist prior to the operation in view of her heavy smoking and her anticoagulant medication and put in the special program for patients who are at risk for **emboli**. At operation Mrs. G was found to have a superior cerebellar artery distorting her trigeminal nerve. This was lifted out of place. Mrs. G spent one night in intensive care and was discharged home after five days. She was immediately pain free, but slowly tapered off her medication over the next few weeks. Mrs. G felt she had fully recovered after six weeks. Apart from occasional headaches, she has not had any complications either in the immediate operative period or in the longterm. She does not have a numb face and has restarted her anticoagulant. Her quality of life has been totally restored and she is fully satisfied with her outcome.

8. WHAT RESEARCH IS NEEDED?

Here is one suggestion that a patient has proposed, which is very valid:

"Seventy five percent of people who have MVD get improvement, but I think there should be more research on the other 25 percent. I would like to know how many successful MVDs each neurosurgeon has done. So number one, why are the other 25 percent still suffering and number two, how many of the experts who treat trigeminal neuralgia have 75 percent of successful cases?"

Surgical information leaflets should be prepared for national use, which are written together with patients and then trailed as suggested by Ross (2004).

It is essential that data from all the centers are collected in the same way by independent observers and, if they were sent to one center, then a meta–analysis of the results could be done. Long-term data, covering a minimum period of 5 years, are needed. We have proposed an annual postoperative questionnaire (Zakrzewska et al 2005b), which we have modified subsequently and is produced in the appendix. Perhaps if the neurosurgeons do not collect the data, patients could do so themselves and the data could be analyzed through the trigeminal neuralgia support groups.

We need reliable and valid outcome measures, which include not only pain recurrence rates, but also rates of complications, their rate of resolution and the effect they have on quality of life. Better prognosticators would enable more accurate selection of patients.

Randomized controlled trials are needed, which take into account patient and surgeon preferences, since these would provide the answer to effectiveness of treatments.

There is a need to do economic evaluations of the various treatments and compare these to the cost of keeping patients on long-term medical care. The psychological costs must be taken into account; i.e does surgery result in fewer sufferers having depression than use of medication?

SUMMARY

- When medical management fails, surgery can be performed.
- There is no ideal surgical treatment and all have their advantages and disadvantages.
- The more peripheral the surgery, the faster the return of pain. Microvascular decompression (MVD) results in 70 % of patients becoming pain free at 10 years.
- Apart from MVD, all surgical techniques result in damage to the trigeminal nerve, since they are ablative procedures, most often manifested as sensory loss.
- The highest mortality is in the MVD group, but it also has one of the lowest complication rates.
- Gamma knife radiosurgery, is the latest procedure to be used and gives similar results to those of other ablative procedures without the need for needles or general anesthesia.

FURTHER READING AND REFERENCES

Web sites
Checked April 2005

The National Institute for Clinical Excellence works on behalf of the National Health Service and the people who use it. We make recommendations on treatments and care using the best available evidence. http://www.nice.org.uk/
(Typing in the words "trigeminal neuralgia" in the search engine will yield all the articles on gamma knife, including a leaflet for patients.)

Centre for Reviews and Dissemination contains a review on Gamma Knife Surgery. http://www.york.ac.uk/inst/crd/welcome.htm

An Interactive Animated TN Tutorial, developed by A. Kaufmann and M. Patel, is your userfriendly tool to understanding Trigeminal Neuralgia and its treatment options and has animated pictures. http://www.umanitoba.ca/cranial_nerves/trigeminal_neuralgia/tutorial.html

Kim Burchiel has put up a series of slides and presentations on trigeminal neuralgia, as well as his diagnostic quiz. http://www.ohsu.edu/facialpain/mvd-videos.shtml

The Surgical Treatment of Trigeminal Neuralgia and Hemifacial Spasm:A guide for You and Your Family, by University of Florida neurosurgeon A. Rhoton. This site includes other helpful papers. http://www.neurosurgery.ufl.edu/FacultyPage/TicBrochure.html

Books and booklets

Coakham H B (2000) The Microsurgical Treatment of Trigeminal Neuralgia, Hemifacial Spasm and Glossopharyngeal Neuralgia. In J T Robertson, H B. Coakham and J H. Roberstson (eds.), **Cranial Base Surgery**. London: Churchill Livingstone.ISBN: 0443056854

Fromm G H (1987) **The Medical and Surgical Management of Trigeminal Neuralgia**. New York: Futura Publishing Company; ISBN 0-87993-303-8

Rovit R L Murali R and Jannetta PJ (1990) **Trigeminal neuralgia.** Baltimore: Williams and Wilkins; ISBN 0-683-07393-1 especially chapter 13 by Sweet

Weigel G. and Casey K F (2004) **Striking Back! The Trigeminal Neuralgia and Face Pain Handbook.** Trigeminal Neuralgia Association, Gainesville, Florida ISBN 0-9672393-2-X patient handbook

Zakrzewska J M (2002) Trigeminal neuralgia In Zakrzewska JM & Harrison SD (Ed) **Assessment and management of orofacial pain.** Elsevier Vol 14 in Series on Pain Research and Clinical Management ISBN 0444509844 chapter 15

Hamlyn PJ. (1999) **Neurovascular Compression of the Cranial Nerves in Neurological and Systematic Disease.** Elsevier Sciences BV, Netherlands. ISBN 0-444 82977 6

References

Barker FG2, Jannetta P J, Bissonette D J, Larkins M V and Jho H D (1996) The Long-Term Outcome of Microvascular Decompression for Trigeminal Neuralgia. *N Engl J Med* **334**:1077-1083.

Bederson JB and Wilson C B (1989) Evaluation of Microvascular Decompression and Partial Sensory Rhizotomy in 252 Cases of Trigeminal Neuralgia. *J Neurosurg* **71**:359-367.

Bittar GT and Graff-Radford S B (1993) The Effects of Streptomycin/Lidocaine Block on Trigeminal Neuralgia: a Double Blind Crossover Placebo Controlled Study. *Headache* **33**:155-160.

Broggi G, Ferroli P, Franzini A, Pluderi M, La Mantia L and Milanese C (1999) Role of Microvascular Decompression in Trigeminal Neuralgia and Multiple Sclerosis. *Lancet* **354**:1878-1879.

Brown JA and Gouda J J (1999) Percutaneous Balloon Compression Treatment for Trigeminal Neuralgia. *Techniques in neurosurgery* **5**:232-238.

Brown JA, McDaniel M D and Weaver M T (1993) Percutaneous Trigeminal Nerve Compression for Treatment of Trigeminal Neuralgia: Results in 50 Patients. *Neurosurgery* **32**:570-573.

Burchiel KJ, Steege T D, Howe J F and Loeser J D (1981) Comparison of Percutaneous Radiofrequency Gangliolysis and Microvascular Decompression for the Surgical Management of Tic Douloureux. *Neurosurgery* **9**:111-119.

Flickinger JC, Pollock B E, Kondziolka D, Phuong L K, Foote R L, Stafford S L and Lunsford L D (2001) Does Increased Nerve Length Within the Treatment Volume Improve Trigeminal Neuralgia Radiosurgery? A Prospective Double-Blind, Randomized Study. *International Journal of Radiation Oncology, Biology, Physics* **51**:449-454.

Kalkanis SN, Eskandar E N, Carter B S and Barker F G (2003) Microvascular Decompression Surgery in the United States, 1996 to 2000: Mortality Rates, Morbidity Rates, and the Effects of Hospital and Surgeon Volumes. *Neurosurgery* **52**:1251-1261.

Kanpolat Y and Savas A (2001) Radiosurgery and Trigeminal Neuralgia. *Journal of Neurosurgery* **94**:1018-1019.

Kondziolka D, Lunsford L D, Habeck M and Flickinger J C (1997) Gamma Knife Radiosurgery for Trigeminal Neuralgia. *Neurosurgery Clinics of North America* **8**:79-85.

Latchaw JP, Jr., Hardy R W, Jr., Forsythe S B and Cook A F (1983) Trigeminal Neuralgia Treated by Radiofrequency Coagulation. *J Neurosurg* **59**:479-484.

Linskey ME, Jho H D and Jannetta P J (1994) Microvascular Decompression for Trigeminal Neuralgia Caused by Vertebrobasilar Compression *Journal of Neurosurgery* **81**:1-9.

Lopez BC, Hamlyn P J and Zakrzewska J M (2004a) Stereotactic Radiosurgery for Primary Trigeminal Neuralgia: State of the Evidence and Recommendations for Future Reports. *Journal of Neurology, Neurosurgery & Psychiatry* **75**:1019-24.

Lopez, B C, Hamlyn P J and Zakrzewska J M (2004b) Systematic Review of Ablative Neurosurgical Techniques in the Management of Trigeminal Neuralgia. *Neurosurgery 54* : 973-82; *discussion 982-3.*

Maesawa S, Salame C, Flickinger J C, Pirris S, Kondziolka D and Lunsford L D (2001) Clinical Outcomes After Stereotactic Radiosurgery for Idiopathic Trigeminal Neuralgia. *Journal of Neurosurgery* **94**:14-20.

McLaughlin MR, Jannetta P J, Clyde B L, Subach B R, Comey C H and Resnick D K (1999) Microvascular Decompression of Cranial Nerves: Lessons Learned After 4400 Operations. *Journal of Neurosurgery* **90**:1-8.

Mendoza N and Illingworth R D (1995) Trigeminal Neuralgia Treated by Microvascular Decompression: a Long-Term Follow-Up Study. *British Journal of Neurosurgery* **9**:13-19.

North RB, Kidd D H, Piantadosi S and Carson B S (1990) Percutaneous Retrogasserian Glycerol Rhizotomy. Predictors of Success and Failure in Treatment of Trigeminal Neuralgia. *Journal of Neurosurgery* **72**:851-856.

Oturai AB, Jensen K, Eriksen J and Madsen F (1996) Neurosurgery for Trigeminal Neuralgia: Comparison of Alcohol Block, Neurectomy, and Radiofrequency Coagulation. *Clinical Journal of Pain* **12**:311-315.

Pollock BE, Phuong L K, Foote R L, Stafford S L and Gorman D A (2001) High-Dose Trigeminal Neuralgia Radiosurgery Associated With Increased Risk of Trigeminal Nerve Dysfunction. *Neurosurgery* **49**:58-62.

Pollock BE, Phuong L K, Gorman D A, Foote R L and Stafford S L (2002) Stereotactic Radiosurgery for Idiopathic Trigeminal Neuralgia. *Journal of Neurosurgery* **97**:347-53.

Ratner EJ, Person P, Kleinman D J, Shklar G and Socransky S S (1979) Jawbone Cavities and Trigeminal and Atypical Facial Neuralgias. *Oral Surg Oral Med Oral Pathol* **48**:3-20.

Rogers CL, Shetter A G, Fiedler J A, Smith K A, Han P P and Speiser B L (2000) Gamma Knife Radiosurgery for Trigeminal Neuralgia: the Initial Experience of The Barrow Neurological Institute. *International Journal of Radiation Oncology, Biology, Physics* 47:1013-1019.

Sindou M, Amrani F and Mertens P (1991) Does Microsurgical Vascular Decompression for Trigeminal Neuralgia Work Through a Neo-Compressive Mechanism? Anatomical- Surgical Evidence for a Decompressive Effect. *Acta Neurochir Suppl (Wien)* 52:127-129.

Slettebo H, Hirschberg H and Lindegaard K F (1993) Long-Term Results After Percutaneous Retrogasserian Glycerol Rhizotomy in Patients With Trigeminal Neuralgia. *Acta Neurochirurgica* 122:231-5.

Stajcic Z, Juniper R P and Todorovic L (1990) Peripheral Streptomycin/Lidocaine Injections Versus Lidocaine Alone in the Treatment of Idiopathic Trigeminal Neuralgia. A Double Blind Controlled Trial. *J Craniomaxillofacial Surgery* 18:243-246.

Sun T, Saito S, Nakai O and Ando T (1994) Long-Term Results of Microvascular Decompression for Trigeminal Neuralgia With Reference to Probability of Recurrence. *Acta Neurochir (Wien)* 126:144-148.

Szapiro J, Jr., Sindou M and Szapiro J (1985) Prognostic Factors in Microvascular Decompression for Trigeminal Neuralgia. *Neurosurgery* 17:920-929.

Taha JM and Tew J M, Jr. (1995) Long-Term Results of Radiofrequency Rhizotomy in the Treatment of Cluster Headache. *Headache* 35:193-196.

Tronnier VM, Rasche D, Hamer J, Kienle A L and Kunze S (2001) Treatment of Idiopathic Trigeminal Neuralgia: Comparison of Long-Term Outcome After Radiofrequency Rhizotomy and Microvascular Decompression. *Neurosurgery* 48:1261-1267.

Tyler-Kabara EC, Kassam A B, Horowitz M H, Urgo L, Hadjipanayis C, Levy E I and Chang Y F (2002) Predictors of Outcome in Surgically Managed Patients With Typical and Atypical Trigeminal Neuralgia: Comparison of Results Following Microvascular Decompression. *J Neurosurg* 96:527-531.

Yoon KB, Wiles J R, Miles J B and Nurmikko T J (1999) Long-Term Outcome of Percutaneous Thermocoagulation for Trigeminal Neuralgia. *Anaesthesia* 54:803-808.

Zakrzewska JM, Jassim S and Bulman J S (1999) A Prospective, Longitudinal Study on Patients With Trigeminal Neuralgia Who Underwent Radiofrequency Thermocoagulation of the Gasserian Ganglion. *Pain* 79:51-58.

Zakrzewska JM and Lopez B C (2003) Quality of Reporting in Evaluations of Surgical Treatment of Trigeminal Neuralgia: Recommendations for Future Reports. *Neurosurgery* 53:110-120.

Zakrzewska JM and Thomas D G (1993) Patient's Assessment of Outcome After Three Surgical Procedures for the Management of Trigeminal Neuralgia. *Acta Neurochir (Wien)* 122:225-230.

Zakrzewska J M, Lopez B C, Kim S E and Coakham H B (2005a) Patient reports of satisfaction after microvascular decompression and partial sensory rhizotomy for trigeminal neuralgia. *Neurosurgery* 56: 1304-1311.

Zakrzewska J M, Lopez B C, Kim S E, Varian E A and Coakham H B (2005b) Patient satisfaction after surgery for trigeminal neuralgia - development of a questionnaire. *Acta Neurochir (Wien)* 147: 925-932.

APPENDIX

Proposed annual post operative questionnaire

ANNUAL TRIGEMINAL NEURALGIA SURVEY

This survey relates to the last operation you had for trigeminal neuralgia.

Name: Today's Date:

Name of last operation: Date of operation:

Age: Gender: Male   Female

Please *tick or circle* the most appropriate answer there may be more than one. This section is about any pain you may have experienced following your ***most recent operation*** for your trigeminal neuralgia.

QUESTIONS:	ANSWERS:
1. Have you had any type of facial pain since your last operation?	No *(please go to question 13)* Yes
2a. Does the pain you have now, feel the same as it did before your operation?	No Yes Not sure
2b. If it does NOT feel the same, please indicate how it is different.	A) Still 'shooting' but ii) Less severe ii) More severe B) It is dull/achy now C) Other: _____
3. Following your most recent operation, when did you first experience the pain?	Immediately 1- 6 months later 7-12 months later 1-2 years later 3-4 years later 5-6 years later 6-7 years later 8-9 years later Over 10 years later
4. Is the pain continuous?	No Yes *(please go to question 7)*
5. If it is not continuous but, as a rule, intermittent (comes and goes in short bursts), how long does a single incident of pain last?	Seconds Minutes Hours Days
6. How long do you usually go without any episodes of pain?	Minutes Hours Days Weeks
7. How intense does the pain feel? 0= no pain	0 1 2 3 4 5 6 7
8. Where is the pain?	Same area as before the operation Different area than before the operation
9. Do any of these activities set the pain off?	Washing face Brushing teeth Wind Cold Touch Laughing Talking Eating Other:_____
10. Have you taken any medication for the facial pain since the last operation?	No *(please go to question 13)* Yes: Now and then as needed Regularly
11. Roughly how often in the past month have you been taking medication?	Daily 2-3 times a week Less than once a week Other: _____
12. What drugs are you taking, and how many tablets a day?	Drug(s): Dose per day (in milligrams):

*This section is about complications you may have had as **a result of the most recent operation** for your trigeminal neuralgia. scales 0 = none, 7 = very severe. You may circle more than one answer.*

13a. If you had numbness **before** this operation has it changed as a result of this operation?	No Yes : Worse than before Same as before
13b. Following the operation, does any part of your face feel numb that was not numb before?	No (*please go to question 17*) Yes
14. If yes, how soon after the operation did the numbness begin?	Immediately 1-2 months later 3-5 months later 6 or more months later
15. How severe is the numbness (compared to stages of a dental injection wearing off)?	0 1 2 3 4 5 6 7
16. How painful is it to touch this area of numbness?	0 1 2 3 4 5 6 7
17. What degree of burning or other altered sensation do you have on the same side of your face as the operation site?	0 1 2 3 4 5 6 7
18. Did the operation result in any hearing loss?	No Yes: cannot use phone with that ear
19. If yes, has the hearing loss changed in any way?	Lasted 1- 6 months but now it's gone Lasted 6 + months but now it's gone It's still the same It's still there, but has improved It's getting worse
20. Do you feel unsteady on your feet as a result of the operation?	No Yes
21. Do you suffer from more dizziness than usual following this operation?	No Yes
22. Do you suffer from more headaches than usual following this operation?	No Yes
23. Following the operation do you have any difficulty with eating that you didn't have before?	No Yes, difficulty with: Chewing food Controlling dentures Dribbling Excessive biting of cheek Muscles going into spasm other _____
24. Have you got any problems with your vision that you didn't have before this operation? (please tick all that apply)	No if yes please complete below Blurred Bits floating Watering a lot Seeing double Eyes do not focus well Eye infections Other:_____
25. Have you got any other complications that we have not mentioned? If yes, please list.	

26. Please state how the complications
    (from questions 13-25) currently affect
    the quality of your life, if at all:

Numbness	Not at all	Slightly	Moderately	Severely
Burning sensation	Not at all	Slightly	Moderately	Severely
Hearing loss	Not at all	Slightly	Moderately	Severely
Unsteadiness	Not at all	Slightly	Moderately	Severely
Dizziness	Not at all	Slightly	Moderately	Severely
Headaches	Not at all	Slightly	Moderately	Severely
Trouble eating	Not at all	Slightly	Moderately	Severely
Trouble with vision/eyes	Not at all	Slightly	Moderately	Severely
Other: _____				

This section deals with your general views about the surgery, please circle the most appropriate answer

27. Looking back now, how would you consider the timing of your surgery?	Done at the right time Should have been earlier Should have been later Should have never been done
28. Overall how satisfied are you with your current situation in comparison to before the operation?	0=Very unsatisfied 7 = Extremely satisfied 0 1 2 3 4 5 6 7
29. In the last month have you felt a lack of pleasure in life?	No Yes
30. In the last month have you felt depressed?	No Yes
31. Have you had any treatments other than medications for your trigeminal neuralgia in the past year? Please give details if yes.	No Yes: Microvascular decompression Posterior sensory rhizotomy Radiofrequency thermocoagulation Glycerol injection Balloon compression Gamma knife Laser Acupuncture Cryosurgery Other:_____

If you are in pain or if you have any complications, please complete the **Brief Pain Inventory and the McGill Pain Questionnaire attached.**

Any other comments, any other things you feel we should know about? (Please feel free to use the back of the paper)

Would you like a review appointment?   No   Yes

THANK YOU for completing this questionnaire. Please send it back in the envelope provided. Your replies will ensure that we offer all our patients an improved service.

Prof Joanna Zakrzewska
Neurosurgery Team

CHAPTER 10

RECURRENCES AND MANAGING SIDE EFFECTS AND COMPLICATIONS FROM TREATMENT

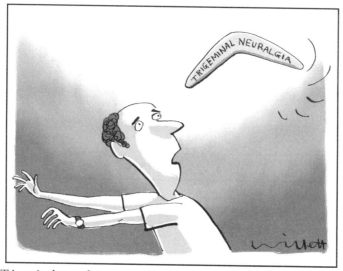

Trigeminal neuralgia can recur after apparently effective treatment.

"I am a 76-year-old TN patient. In spite of a variety of procedures (radiofrequency thermocoagulation, MVD, glycerol injections and a combination of glycerol and radiofrequency thermocoagulation), I continue to have occasional bouts of considerable discomfort (as I am having currently, which affect my speaking and sometimes my swallowing.

I do not anticipate a cure. Some of the above procedures have helped for periods of up to three years. In addition, and lately, I have been able to manage my discomfort with modest amounts of medication, most recently carbamazepine. There are some irksome side effects. If the current discomfort turns into significant pain, I will seek some lesser form of surgical intervention.

I believe the TN disorder and remedies taken for it act differently for different patients. What works for one patient may do nothing for the next patient. For me, I believe I will be 'managing' an irregularly chronic condition for the rest of my years, while always on the lookout for more effective treatments."

1. WHAT TO DO WHEN PAIN RECURS AFTER MEDICAL TREATMENT?

The pain can come back slowly or suddenly. It is possible to have a different cause for pain, and it is therefore very important to go back to the beginning and assess the features of the pain in terms of intensity, character and location. Details of this can be found in Chapter 1. It is worthwhile to assess the circumstances in which the recurrence occurred, since stress often plays an important role in a recurrence. It is important not to panic and to think carefully how to manage the pain. Once the diagnosis has been established, and it is the same as the original one, then re-start the last medication that was successful. Table 1 below summarizes the steps in managing a recurrence.

Table 1: Key Facts

WHAT TO DO WHEN THE PAIN RECURS
• Analyze it:
• **Is it the same type of pain?**
• **Is it in a different place?**
• **Is it as severe as previously?**
• Re-start the medication slowly
• If still on medication, raise the dose
• Do not take too much; take as directed
• Do not mix too many different medications
• Get medication in liquid form if necessary
• Keep a diary of the response to medication

It is important to keep a diary of response to medication, since the sufferer can take this record to his or her doctor to assess further management. If the medication is effective, the sufferer needs to ensure the use of an adequate amount and continue with it until the pain settles. Once the pain has been controlled well for a month or so, it is worthwhile to assess whether the pain has in fact settled. Slow reduction of the medication can then be tried. Sometimes it is worth changing to a slow-release form of medicine as described in Chapter 5.

However, if the pain does not settle, it is important to re-assess the diagnosis, and this should be done by a specialist. Another medication could be used either as an add-on or in place of the original medication. However, no more than two drugs should be used. There is some evidence that drugs like lamotrigine and baclofen can work well with carbamazepine. Table 2 below summarizes these details.

Table 2: Key facts

How to re-assess medication
If responding to medications,
• remain on medication at the dose that gives control
• if no pain after one month, then consider slow reduction
• consider stopping the medication
• consider using a slow-release form (retard)
• inform the doctor about the recurrence and medication if not responding to medication
• consider the diagnosis may have changed
• consider change of medication
• avoid adding on more than two medications
• reconsider repeat surgery

Psychological management as detailed in Chapter 6 must also be considered. If the pain still does not settle, then it may be necessary to look at possible surgical options as outlined in Chapter 9.

2. WHAT COMPLICATIONS CAN OCCUR FROM THE USE OF LONG-TERM MEDICATION?

These are discussed in Chapter 6. Side effects from drug therapy are common and some patients gradually get used to the drugs and no longer notice any side effects, Sometimes it is not until the drugs are stopped that patients realize they have had side effects. Most of the side effects are dose related, and so a reduction in daily amount may help, as well as spreading out the medication dosage more evenly. At night the side effects are less noticeable; thus it is better to take the larger doses at this time.

Regular monitoring by blood tests is important in those taking higher doses. Most of the medications were designed for continuous long-term use, thus complications rarely arise from length of use. The side effects are thus reversible on stopping the therapy. It is a good idea to reduce or stop the therapy when the pain goes into remission.

Slow-release (retard) medication can sometimes help reduce side effects, since the drug is released in slower and lower dosage levels into the bloodstream. On the other hand, taking a greater number of medications increases the risk of side effects and drug interactions.

3. CAN PAIN RETURN AFTER SURGERY?

As shown in the previous chapter, pain can recur after surgery. The timing of the recurrence will to some extent depend on the level at which surgery was done. The highest chance of a recurrence is likely in the first two years, as shown on the graphs in Chapter 9. When the pain recurs after surgery, the first thing to determine is whether it is of the same type as that before the operation. It is important to re-assess the pain using the criteria given in Chapter 1. The patient's medical history needs to be reviewed, since changes in general health may occur and these could then affect subsequent management.

Medical management is the first line of treatment and has been outlined above. It can sometimes be sufficient and in some sufferers only needs to be used for a short period of time.

If surgery is to be contemplated, then the whole decision process begins again, as outlined in Chapter 8. This time it is necessary to bring into the equation any complications that occurred after surgery and what effect they, and side effects, may have had on the quality of life. These factors can sometimes determine what repeat procedure is to be done, if it is necessary at all. If **dysethesia** is already present, then the risk of developing **anesthesia dolorosa** is greatly increased.

The data on management of recurrences is poor, although there are a number of studies reporting exclusively on this aspect of management. Overall, it appears that sufferers tend to go back to having the same surgery that they had the first time. Among the few studies dealing with an analysis of recurrences, Oturai et al (1996) showed that among their 316 patients, 72 % had one surgical procedure, 19 % required two surgical procedures and 9 % had more than two different types of procedures.

How are recurrences after peripheral surgery managed?

Many patients who have had surgery on peripheral nerves, such as cryotherapy, neurectomy or alcohol injections, are highly likely to experience a recurrence within a year. Sometimes the recurrences are in a different branch. Among patients who underwent cryotherapy, we found some 38 % of the recurrences were in a different nerve branch. However, this has little significance for the sufferer who still experiences pain, albeit in a different position. Repeat surgery appears to give similar results again; therefore it may be important to rethink the role of peripheral surgery in long-term management.

How are recurrences after Gasserian ganglion surgery managed?

There is only one study in which researchers looked in depth at recurrence rates after radiofrequency thermocoagulation. Latchaw et al (1983) showed that the time elapsing before a recurrence of pain was similar to that after the initial procedure, and that 70 % of patients experienced the same complication in a repeat surgical procedures as in the primary.

Here is the account of a patient who has had numerous repeat surgeries:

"I have had Gasserian blocks in recent years that seem to take the pain level down for about six months after I have three blocks in a row, each a month apart. With the Gasserian blocks working, I can eat even more things and can talk and keep up a busier schedule without as much pain. However, this year, after three years of help from the Gasserian blocks, they seem not to be working well."

However, if sensory loss is still present at the time of a recurrence pain, then deeper sensory loss, and potentially the development of anesthesia dolorosa, is more likely.

Glycerol rhizotomy can be repeated, but sometimes the procedure is more difficult to do again because of local irritation to the nerve coverings, which reduces the size of the cistern. The chance of more sensory loss and dysesthesia is increased, especially if patients have had prior radiofrequency thermocoagulation.

Patients who have undergone a balloon microcompression do not appear to have any different results after repeated surgery. However, the number of patients who have been reported after a repeat of this surgery is small.

How are recurrences after posterior fossa surgery managed?

Recurrences after microvascular decompression are most likely in the first two years. Some recurrences are classified as minor and others as major. The criteria used to classify patients in these two groups are vague and often relate to whether the pain responds to medication or needs to be treated surgically. There is very little detail on the character and severity of the pain recurrence. Barker et al (1996) report on a larger series of recurrences after microvascular decompression, which have been analyzed using Kaplan Meier survival data. In 132 patients, this showed that recurrences were higher than after primary surgery, with the probability of being pain free at one year of 57 %, falling to 52 % by five years. Recurrences may be higher if no compression is found.

Several authors suggest reasons for pain recurrences include:
- continuing elongation of vessels
- change in arterial position due to aging
- recanalization of divided veins
- missed compressions
- changes in the implants themselves

Some patients will undergo a repeat microvascular decompression, and there are a number of reports dealing with these. Barker et al (1996) do not report any negative explorations, but found a high number of small unidentified veins and arteries. In some cases, the material used to separate the blood vessel from the artery has slipped or even induced changes, such as **fibrosis** and **adhesions**. These scars can therefore act as a compression (of the nerve) in their own right.

The following is a patient's reaction to her recurrence of pain:

"A month later while brushing my teeth, the pains gradually returned, a little more each day. I confronted Dr. M with this and she said, 'Well, the sling must have slipped. We can go in there and see what happened.' I told her, "No thanks!", I mean, how many times does it take to get it right? Within weeks the pain became worse than ever before. I knew something had to be done, and I didn't want another MVD. I had read about the "Gamma Knife Surgery" that was the buzz in various newsprints, etc. I asked to be scheduled for a Gamma Knife Surgery..... The end result after all was done is there was no improvement in the TN pain at all. It was and is still there."

Most reports also show an increased number of complications after re-operation. This has, therefore, led some surgeons to suggest that a recurrence of pain after microvascular decompression should be managed with a procedure at the level of the Gasserian ganglion.

When all else fails, a few other procedures may be done, which are described in more detail in George Weigel and Ken Casey's book, but the evidence for their use is very low. Nashold developed an operation called the **DREZ** (dorsal root entry zone) or trigeminal tractotomy, but this is a major procedure that can have severe side effects in its own right.

One of the latest procedures being used is that of motor cortex stimulation. Two small electrodes are placed on the surface of the dura over the cortex region of the brain, which controls movement of the face. A low-grade current is then passed through these electrodes to stimulate the thalamus and counteract the pain.

This is a patient's description of his experience with motor cortex stimulation:

"I was his eleventh case and it was a difficult ordeal for us both. It reduced the burning pain in my eye and the rest of may face. I'd estimate it eliminated 50-66 % of my pain. I'm still disabled, but am able to taper off the opioids."

How are recurrences after gamma knife surgery managed?

Data from gamma knife use is still very limited, and some patients have had a repeat of gamma knife surgery. The doses of radiation, however, are often reduced, since it must be remembered that these are cumulative. It appears that sensory loss is more likely to occur after repeat gamma knife surgery. This risk has led to many patients tending to choose another form of surgery, including microvascular decompression and surgery at the level of the Gasserian ganglion.

Table 3: Key Facts

EFFECT OF REPEAT SURGERY
• Results from repeat surgery may not be as good. • Currently insufficient evidence is available to be able to advise which form of surgery is best • If you have unpleasant numbness, there is an increased risk that repeat surgery (except MVD) can make it worse

How are complications after surgery managed?

There are very few reports that provide guidance on how to manage complications dealing with this aspect of care. A summary is provided in Table 4 below.

Table 4: Key facts

MANAGING COMPLICATIONS AFTER SURGERY	
Effect	Management
Sensory loss, dysesthesia and anesthesia dolorosa	Severely affect quality of life and should not be managed with surgical methods – antidepressants may help
Oral problems, difficult eating, ulcers	Eat slowly, inspect the mouth, visit the dentist regularly
Other facial pain	Psychological, antidepressants
Eye problems	Wear protective glasses, daily inspections of the eye, visit specialist if the eye becomes red or tears
Hearing problems	Little can be done, but some are transient
Depression	Psychological, antidepressants

Sensory changes

Abnormal sensations after surgery, especially those done at the level of the Gasserian ganglion, are common, and most sufferers are likely to develop a loss of light touch sensation. On its own, this causes relatively little disability. However, if combined with a painful sensation, then the quality of life can be affected.

These two patients provide typical descriptions:

- *"Currently, I have some burning pain around the right side of my lips and mouth area, as well as my tongue. The right side of my face, from my chin to above my right eye, is numb and I frequently experience a 'crawling' sensation on the right side of my face and scalp. Also, my face has quite a bit of pressure and feels as though it is being pulled or tugged, as if in a vise. My right eye has pressure sensations and, sometimes feels as though an insect is buzzing around inside the wall of this eye. At times, I feel a bit sorry for myself, but I usually try to go on with my life as though I had no problem. If I choose not to dwell on my problems, I seem to get along much better. I lead a very busy life. I am 65 years old, and work every day and certainly more than 40 hours per week this time of the year. I feel really fortunate that, at least for now and, I hope for the rest of my life, the horrible stabbing pain is gone."*
- *"Although I have numbness in my chin and part of my lower face, it often feels like something is crawling along my chin or like I'm drooling, even though I'm not always. I do sometimes drool without realizing it."*

The worse form of sensory loss is that of anesthesia dolorosa. This is most likely to occur after radiofrequency thermocoagulation, but has been noted in all the ablative procedures. The condition develops weeks or months after surgery and progresses over several years, after which it becomes static. It is a continuous burning, stinging, stabbing or aching pain localized in a numb part of the face, most commonly around the eye and mouth.

This patient describes his pain after a radiofrequency thermocoagulation:

"I had relief from the original pain, but had new symptoms. I had a cold, burning sensation in the skin around my eye and an ache in the eye itself. The skin on the left side of my face was numb from my eye to the middle of my scalp."

Its constant nature causes sufferers more distress than the initial severe trigeminal neuralgia. Changes in temperature, especially cold, can aggravate the pain. It can, therefore, result in various psychological side effects. There are very few guidelines on how to manage this form of pain. Treatment with tricyclic anti-depressants can sometimes be helpful, otherwise non-medical management needs to be instituted as discussed in Chapter 7.

Other forms of facial pain

Sufferers who have a less typical type of trigeminal neuralgia may still complain of facial pain after surgery. Often this pain no longer has the characteristics of a sharp shooting type pain, but can be more constant and burning in quality. Some of the pain may be related to the partial nerve damage that has occurred as a result of the surgical procedure, but it could also have been present previously but remained masked.

Here is a description by a patient after her microvascular decompression:

"I have a consistent burning that never goes away around the incision and mouth. I have needle-like pains in my gums and aching through my whole right side. I get jackhammer-like headaches that bring me to my knees. There is still an aching burn towards the back of my jaw and the front of the ear area."

Some of these types of pains do respond to tricyclic antidepressant drugs and psychological methods. Many of the patients who have sent in their histories describe these types of pain. Examples include:

* *"constant tingling, burning, throbbing. Occasionally at the beginning of the increased pain, there will be a hot flash that lasts a couple of minutes."*
* *"experienced a dull, aching, continuous pain in my lower jaw at the location of a molar that had a gold cap. This pain would appear about one in every 10 days. It was always at a manageable level."*

It is important to realize that if this type of pain predominates, then surgery will not improve it.

Oral Problems

After any of the ablative procedures, patients may develop problems with eating. This is made worse because it is often associated with sensory loss. Patients cannot chew on the affected side and food tends to dribble out of the corner of the mouth. If sufferers have dentures, these can become more difficult to wear. In a post-operative survey that I did, I found that up to 34 % of patients may have problems with eating initially. However, with time this does improve and so new dentures should not be obtained in the immediate post-operative period because numbness will affect the inside of the mouth, preventing the correct fitting of the new denture.

Cheek biting and ulcers can occur without these causing considerable pain. It is therefore important that patients see a dentist regularly who understands the effects the surgery has had on the mouth and who may notice any changes that the patient is no longer aware of.

Eye Problems

Eye problems do occur in patients who have reduced, or absence of, sensation in the eye. Relatively few people develop these problems, as shown in the previous chapter. However, if the eye is numb, it is very important to wear protective glasses, especially when outside or in an environment where dust particles or other foreign bodies can enter the eye. Daily inspection of the eye for signs of redness is crucial. If any redness or increased weeping occurs, then it is vital to obtain an ophthalmologist's opinion. Some eye problems arise because of damage to the nerve activating the muscles that move the eye. These can result in double vision or a dropping upper eyelid. Most of these are transient and resolve over a period of a few months.

Hearing Problems

Patients, particularly those who have undergone microvascular decompression, are at risk of developing hearing problems. Some of these are temporary hearing impairments related to local operative changes in the **mastoid** air cells. In other instances, hearing loss is due to damage to the auditory nerve itself. This nerve lies close to the trigeminal nerve and can be bruised or injured by the procedure. This damage often results in permanent hearing loss.

Patients who have undergone ablative surgery may also complain of blowing noises or ringing in the ears, which can result from damage to the small nerves that open and close the Eustachian tube. Most of these are transient and will improve with time.

Psychological problems

Patients who have severe recurrences or develop severe complications are likely to get depressed, and this needs to be treated. Support groups provide these patients with much needed understanding and sympathy. Antidepressant drugs may be necessary, otherwise psychological methods such as mentioned in Chapter 7 may be most helpful.

MRS. G CASE STUDY
Mrs. G had a very successful MVD and was pain free and off all medications for two years. One day while eating a hard apple, she suddenly gets a sharp stab of pain. She thinks nothing of it, but it happens again at supper time. Within a week her pain is severe enough for her to go and get her old medication again.
What should Mrs. G be doing now to manage her pain?
Re-analyze the pain to determine whether it really is the trigeminal neuralgia rather then a dental pain or some other form of facial pain. Review the medical history and if Mrs. G is still on warfarin, she should re-start the oxcarbazepine. Mrs. G must keep a diary to monitor response to treatment. If the pain responds well to this medication, continue on it and once pain free for over a month, slowly reduce it. If the pain is initially controlled, but does not settle, then further surgery is indicated. If still using the warfarin, Mrs. G may want to consider game knife surgery. Any other surgery would necessitate change in her warfarin levels.

Management of trigeminal neuralgia

A simplified flow chart of overall management is shown below. A more detailed chart can be found in my book, **Assessment and Management of Orofacial Pain.**

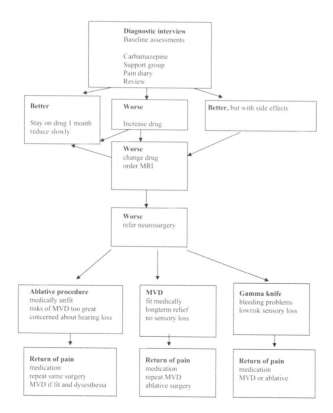

5. WHAT RESEARCH IS NEEDED?

There is very little data on complications and recurrence. Patients need to know not just which complications occur and how often they are likely to happen, but also how quickly they resolve and how they can be managed. Some questions that need addressing include:

- What are the recurrence rates after repeat surgery and why do they appear to be less satisfactory than after primary surgery?
- Do the complications improve with time or do they continue to affect quality of life?
- Are there any ways in which these complications can be predicted or are there certain individuals who are at higher risk of developing them?
- Can outcome be improved using stricter diagnostic criteria?
- How can patients with anesthesia dolorosa be best managed?

SUMMARY

- Medications result in side effects that can affect quality of life and are best dealt with by a reduction in the total dose.
- Pain recurrences occur after all forms of surgery and are a great disappointment.
- It is crucial to determine whether the pain is trigeminal neuralgia or some other form of pain.
- Recurrences can be treated with medication or repeat surgery, which may not be as successful the second time.
- Complications after surgery reduce quality of life and are not easy to manage. The patient may need psychological treatment and antidepressant medicine.

FURTHER READING AND REFERENCES

Books

Weigel, G, Casey K.F. (2004) **Striking Back! The Trigeminal Neuralgia and Face Pain Handbook.** Trigeminal Neuralgia Association, Gainesville, Florida-patient handbook ISBN 0-9672393-2-X

Zakrzewska JM. Trigeminal neuralgia in Zakrzewska JM & Harrison SD (Ed) **Assessment and management of orofacial pain.** Elsevier Vol 14 in Series on Pain Research and Clinical Management 2002 chapter 15 ISBN 0444509844

References

Barker FG2, Jannetta P J, Bissonette DJ, Larkins MV and Jho HD (1996) The Long-Term Outcome of Microvascular Decompression for Trigeminal Neuralgia. *N Engl J Med* **334**:1077-1083.

Latchaw JP, Jr., Hardy R W, Jr., Forsythe SB and Cook AF (1983) Trigeminal Neuralgia Treated by Radiofrequency Coagulation. *J Neurosurg* **59**:479-484.

Oturai AB, Jensen K, Eriksen J and Madsen F (1996) Neurosurgery for Trigeminal Neuralgia: Comparison of Alcohol Block, Neurectomy, and Radiofrequency Coagulation. *Clin J Pain* **12**:311-315.

Zakrzewska JM, Jassim S and Bulman JS (1999) A Prospective, Longitudinal Study on Patients With Trigeminal Neuralgia Who Underwent Radiofrequency Thermocoagulation of the Gasserian Ganglion. *Pain* **79**:51-58.

Zakrzewska JM and Nally FF (1988) The Role of Cryotherapy (Cryoanalgesia) in the Management of Paroxysmal Trigeminal Neuralgia: a SixYear Experience. *Br J Oral Maxillofac Surg* **26**:18-25.

CHAPTER 11

SUPPORT GROUPS

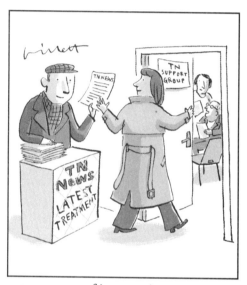

Support groups are of immense importance, especially
for individuals coping with rare diseases.

Take courage my friend
As many others have found

That getting together
At least once a month
Helps those who want info
To get a whole bunch.

So don't get discouraged
Keep faith for today.
Maybe soon a cure will be found
To take it away.

By V. J. Van Hoven

1. How did support groups arise?

It is becoming increasing obvious that the explosion in medical knowledge over the last few decades is making it impossible for doctors to keep up to date in all areas. On the other hand, a patient with only one disease is likely to be able to keep up to date and thus soon become more expert than most doctors.

Only the super specialist will be able to compete with the patient, who will need the specialist to be the knowledge manager and partner in decision making. As patients develop critical appraisal skills (outlined in Chapter 5), they will become equally competent at assessing the material they have found. With this also comes increasing responsibility for their own health care as discussed in Chapter 5.

Programs to help patients have been set up in the US, for example by Stanford University, and, in the UK, has led to the Expert Patient Programme. The UK program aims to "provide opportunities to people who live with long-term chronic conditions to develop new skills to manage their condition better on a day-to-day basis." After undergoing one of their programs, it is anticipated that "expert patients" will:
- feel confident and in control of their lives
- aim to manage their condition and its treatment in partnership with health care professionals
- communicate effectively with professionals and be willing to share responsibility on treatment
- become realistic about the impact of their disease on themselves and their family
- use their skills and knowledge to lead full lives

A UK trigeminal neuralgia sufferer, who completed the training to become an expert patient, describes her experience in the UK support group newsletter of Spring 2005. There is no doubt that some sufferers with trigeminal neuralgia have become expert patients and can teach many health care professionals a thing or two. Here are a couple of patients' comments:
- *"I reckon because we talk to more people than most neurologists do, we know more about the way people react to this situation and this pain."*
- *"We have the kind of information they need in order to take a step forward and take care of their own problems so that they can actually take some responsibility for how they deal with their situation."*

In the epilepsy field, a recent study has shown how insufficient the patients found the information provided by specialists, although this was due in part to a lack of specialists (Prinjha et al 2005).

The role of these expert patients has been increasing recognized, and they are now invited to participate in working groups organized by governments or organizations. The Cochrane Collaboration has an active consumer section, and all reviews are now summarized in jargon-free language. The UK government has set up a commission for Patient and Public Involvement in Health, which is "responsible for ensuring that all sectors of the community are involved in decision-making about health and health services in England."

The National Institutes of Health (NIH) in the United States secures input on priorities for funding research projects through public hearings, patient advocacy committees and testimonies presented by patients to committees of the United States Congress. The NIH also provides support for scientific meetings/patient conferences to promote the sharing of the most current information on specific disorders for both patients and medical clinicians. Clinical trials are also conducted by NIH to determine the effectiveness of medications and to assist in the development of new measures in the treatment of pain. The NIH provided a grant for the 5th TNA conference in the US in 2004.

Up until the last twenty years, patients on the whole were lone agents as compared to doctors, who are supported by numerous organizations and societies. The growth of support groups for patients, however, now means patients are also better organized and this opens up the means for an equal partnership between doctors and patients. Some of the support groups for common diseases are large and well funded, whereas those for rare diseases are small and self-funded through members. Most have good support from specialist doctors.

It is therefore no surprise that support groups for trigeminal neuralgia exist and that they are gradually increasing in number. Claire Patterson founded the first one in the US in 1990. Officially named the Trigeminal Neuralgia Association, it is based in Gainesville, Fl. and has a membership of 32,000 across the whole of the US, and 75 regional support groups and another 80 contact telephone numbers in regions where there are no support groups. The UK group is now five years old and has had over 1,000 contacts. Members come and go, depending on their needs. The TNA has the following objectives as shown on its Web site at www.TNA-SUPPORT.org:

- **Provide information, support and encouragement to TN patients and their families and reduce the isolation of those affected by the disorder**

- Act as a liaison between patients and qualified medical and dental practitioners, physicians, and treatment centers that diagnose and treat TN
- Facilitate a network of support groups in regions throughout the country
- Promote greater visibility, awareness and understanding of the disorder within the medical profession and broader public arena;
- Coordinate a centralized database of TN patients and other information about medical advancements in the treatment of this disorder
- Advocate for medical research needed to determine the cause, treatment options, and cure for TN

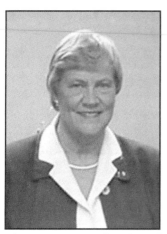

Claire Patterson, founder of the TNA support groups.

The TNA is closely linked with many other groups throughout the world, especially the UK and Australian organizations that have modelled themselves after the US group. Their Web sites, given at the end of the chapter, provide a wealth of information for those who can access the Internet. Sufferers need to remember that access to the Internet is often provided in libraries, community centers and increasingly in health care settings such as doctors' offices and hospitals. The NHS strategy on e-learning has stated its commitment to improve access to those who have not learned how to use the Internet. Elderly sufferers may want to ask their younger family members to access the Internet for them.

2. WHAT DO SUPPORT GROUPS OFFER?

Here are Claire Patterson's views (founder of TNA):

"One of the most valuable benefits a TN patient derives from contact with a support group, another TN patient or a call to the national office is the validation of their feelings. If one has been coping for months or even years in isolation, a great deal of self-doubt develops and many "head games" take place. The patient feels that the pain couldn't possibly be this severe so they must have a very low pain threshold; pain this severe could only be part of a fatal illness; if the pain is really this acute, why do they look so well when the pain is not there? Why does it come and

go... what did they do to bring it on - it must be their fault! Some individuals' religious background will create the feeling of being punished for their "sins." The validation of these feelings is a key factor in creating the special bond that develops between TN patients and support group members. This validation process is critical in one's achieving some control and management of their TN. Support groups are not essential to provide for the "Misery loves company," but really provide the unique opportunity for validating the feelings and emotions that only another TN patient has also experienced."

Support groups offer a wide range of benefits, which are summarized in Table 1 below.

Table 1: Key Facts

WHAT BENEFITS SUPPORT GROUPS OFFER AND HOW IS IT DONE
Benefits of support groups include: • education • sense of belonging • opportunities to meet people who understand what you're going through • exchange of advice • opportunities to make new friends
These benefits are achieved through a variety of ways: • face-to-face meetings in groups • larger national meetings • Internet sites virtual bulletin boards • chat rooms and e-mail • telephone contact • newsletters • books, information leaflets

Today's patient with trigeminal neuralgia, compared to one 10 years ago, has many sources of information, ranging from locally produced leaflets to national and international booklets and a book titled **Striking Back! The Trigeminal Neuralgia and Face Pain Handbook**, written by a TN patient in partnership with a neurosurgeon.

It is a major task to write information for patients, and often it can be too medically centered, even when done by expert patients. Written information produced by the support group should be tailored to members' expressed needs and also be based on their experiences so that they help in self management.

Just as the health care professionals can provide inadequate information, the same can be true of patient-prepared material; thus ideally the information should be evaluated by different groups of sufferers to ensure it answers all their needs and especially their experiences with the condition. There is currently no good evidence to show that patient education leaflets in general improve compliance with treatment. They also need to be evaluated, especially looking at whether they address sufferers' beliefs about factors such as cause, consequences, timeline, and cure-control.

The Internet remains a very important source of information, and both the US and the UK support groups have their own Web sites, which are linked to other sites that they consider may be of value. There is a vast amount of information at these sites, much of which can be downloaded and printed. It is crucial to be critical of all information that is found. Chapter 8 provides details of how the quality of Internet sites can be assessed.

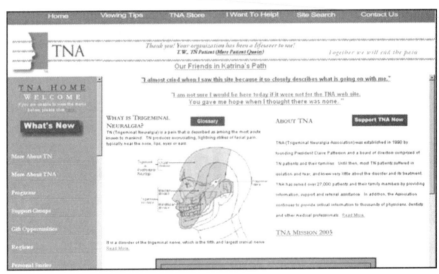

This is the opening page of the US TNA Web site.

A vital means of communication, particularly for the elderly or infirm sufferers who may not be able to travel to regional meetings, is a newsletter. This will usually provide information also available through the Internet such as:
- the make-up of the TNA group's Board of Directors or Executive Committee
- its mission statement and future strategy

- its forthcoming plans and proposals with regard to the running of the group
- its medical advisory board and any changes that may have taken place
- annual financial reports
- recent publicity about TN or the TNA
- up-to-date medical developments
- information about new drugs on the market
- information about surgical procedures and any new advances
- complementary and alternative medicines/therapies
- government or national health proposals
- useful Web sites or medical literature
- reports of recent TNA conferences, locally and abroad
- news about forthcoming meetings or conferences, locally and abroad
- news about TNA regional group activities
- fundraising events
- suggestions on nutrition and dietary supplements
- recommendations on diet, together with recipe suggestions
- advice and tips from members on how to cope
- letters and stories (and sometimes poems and pictures) from contributors
- useful products on the market such as weather protection for eyes/balaclava, etc.

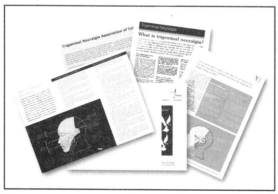

The support groups produce a wide range of leaflets for patients and health care providers.

Support groups offer more than just information and education, and it is here that their strength lies. These groups enable patients to link up with each other and also with health care professionals. This can be done through a wide variety of ways, including chat rooms, e-mail, telephone, letters, newsletters and meetings. These avenues of communication facilitate the sharing of information and the provision of emotional support.

Here are some comments from TN sufferers who are members of a support group:

- *"The local support group that I found online is fabulous. What a treat to be able to sit in a group of total strangers and know that I'm not alone. We all have some type of debilitating facial pain and we all know what each is experiencing. That's been the biggest gift to me in this whole mess patient, kind and lovely people who feel my pain."*
- *"It is precisely that rareness* (of trigeminal neuralgia*) which makes our seeking communion with other sufferers so vital."*
- *"Many of the stories that I have read regarding this condition have helped me to not give up my hope, to keep trying to find a way to deal with this."*
- *"Those friendships are very valuable to me because they know what I'm talking about - they understand because they have been there too."*
- *"A friend sent me the book* Striking Back, *which saved my life."*

It is important to remember that support groups may not be suitable for everyone and some may not be as beneficial as anticipated, sometimes leaving sufferers even more depressed. They complement medical care, but should not be used to replace it.

3. WHAT DO YOU NEED TO FIND OUT ABOUT A SUPPORT GROUP?

The following questions taken from the Mayo Clinic Web site are relevant to trigeminal neuralgia patients groups:

- Is it geared toward a specific condition?
- Is the location convenient enough to attend regularly?
- What time does it meet and for how long?
- How often does it meet?
- How long has the group existed?
- Is there a facilitator or moderator?
- What are the confidentiality guarantees?
- Does it have established ground rules?
- Is it sponsored by a reputable health care facility or organization?
- Does it avoid false promises of quick cures?

- Does it encourage you to continue your regular medical care and treatment?
- What is the mix of participants, such as gender and age?
- How many people usually attend?
- What is a typical meeting like?
- Does it charge reasonable fees, if any?

Members of a support group change over time and thus these evaluations may need to be done at regular intervals. Sufferers may want to try going to several group meetings before committing themselves to membership, since they may feel hesitant to share their personal experiences with people they do not know. Some may initially just want to listen rather than take an active role.

4. WHAT DO ATTENDEES THINK OF SUPPORT GROUP MEETINGS/CONFERENCES?

Support group leaders appreciate the need for face-to-face contact and the importance of networking. Therefore, many of them organize national or local meetings of sufferers. At these meetings sufferers can not only meet fellow sufferers to exchange news, but also meet health care specialists in an environment that is different from the office. Not only do the specialists provide information; their views and reports can be challenged by the consumers.

I have found it extremely useful to attend meetings run by patients, since it gives me real insight into what the patients are facing and helps us to treat patients in a biopsychosocial way as compared to a biomedical way. These meetings are an excellent forum for exchange of ideas and for surveys. It was at such a meeting that I conducted a survey of patients' views of treatment (Zakrzewska 2001). These conferences also provide an opportunity for health care professionals with a common interest in a condition to meet and discuss a variety of issues among themselves.

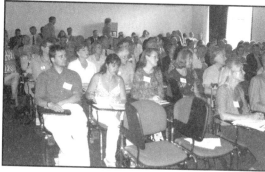

Sufferers and their spouses listening to a talk being given by a health care professional.

But do we really know what the sufferers are looking for when they come to such a conference, and do they find it? At the 5th TNA national conference in Florida in 2004, I attempted to answer this question by conducting a survey among the sufferers who attended. They were part of a larger group as shown in Table 2

Table 2

PARTICIPANTS IN THE SURVEY CONDUCTED AT THE 5TH TNA CONFERENCE IN 2004 IN FLORIDA	
Patients	130
Support group or telephone support leaders	60 (55 patients)
Healthcare workers	71
Supporters/spouses	120
Exhibitors	12
TNA staff & others	12
Questionnaire one taken	144 replied 110 (76%)
Questionnaire 2 returned	74 (67%)
TOTAL participants	405

Table 3 shows the **demographic** details of the sufferers attending the conference and their diagnoses. The sufferers who had undergone surgery tended to be older and to have had trigeminal neuralgia for a longer time. At the time of the conference, 81 % of the patients who had not had surgery were in pain, compared to 71 % of post-surgical patients. This seems to indicate that those likely to attend such a meeting are those still seeking treatment. They are not representative of the total trigeminal neuralgia population in which a larger percentage would be expected to be pain free based on the statistical data shown in the previous chapter.

Sufferers were asked to complete a two-page survey at the start of the conference and then hand in another one-page questionnaire at the end. The results (Table 4) show that sufferers come with a wide range of expectations and that the conference does appear to be able to fulfil them in the majority of instances.

Table 3

DETAILS OF SUFFERERS ATTENDING THE 5TH TNA NATIONAL CONFERENCE	
Questionnaire responders	110
Age	59.3 years (SD=10.2; range 35-77 yrs)
Gender	74 % female
Mean pain duration of sufferers	10.9 yrs (SD=8.5 yrs)
Pain at time of conference	25 %
Classic trigeminal neuralgia	69 %
Atypical trigeminal neuralgia	22 %
Other types of facial pain	9 %
No surgery	49 %
Radiofrequency thermocoagulation	2.6 %
Glycerol rhizotomy	2.6 %
Microcompression	3.9 %
Microvascular decompression	24.7 %
Posterior sensory rhizotomy	2.6 %
Gamma knife	11.7 %
Other procedures	2.6 %

SD = standard deviation

Table 4

SUFFERERS' ASSESSMENT OF THE 5TH TNA NATIONAL CONFERENCE		
Pre conference scale 0 - 10		
	Mean (sd)	Range
Meeting other facial pain sufferers	7.7 (2.6)	0-10
Improving my knowledge about trigeminal neuralgia / facial pain	9.6 (0.9)	5-10
Meeting doctors who are experts in trigeminal neuralgia / facial pain	9.1 (1.3)	4-10
Being better able to make a decision about my own treatment in the future	9.3 (2.0)	0-10
Finding out about new treatments	9.6 (1.1)	0-10
Helping me feel more in control of my condition	8.5 (2.4)	0-10
Finding ways of improving my quality of life	8.6 (2.3)	0-10
Finding more effective ways of explaining my pain to others	6.7 (3.0)	0-10
Finding ways of helping others with facial pain	8.3 (2.3)	0-10
Post conference		
How well did the conference fulfil your expectations? (0=not at all, 10=all fulfilled)	8.8 (1.3)	3-10
Did you find it useful to meet fellow sufferers (0=not at all useful, 10=very useful)	9.4 (1.2)	3-10
Did you find it useful to meet expert doctors (0=not at all, 10=very useful)	9.5 (1.1)	3-10
Has this conference improved your confidence in dealing with your pain (0=not at all, 10=greatly improved)	8.0 (2.3)	3-10

SD = standard deviation

Here are some comments added to the survey questionnaires by attendees:

- "*I wanted to take this opportunity to let you all know how very worthwhile I found the conference to be. I learned a lot, although now am more confused than ever as to what my next course of action will be regarding treatment of my trigeminal neuralgia. I found it extremely beneficial to be able to talk to so many patients and get their perspectives on the treatments they had done, as well as their histories with the disorder. I was also able to hook up with some people who, I am sure, will be able to offer me help in the future. I was extremely impressed with the physicians who spoke. The best patient is a well informed patient, and I will be able to meet with my neurologist from now on armed with a more thorough knowledge of TN. One suggestion I'd like to make is to supply newcomers like me with a vocabulary list of words used frequently by the session leaders and moderators. Finally, most of all, I appreciate the hard work it took to organize and pull off this conference. There was a lot of behind the scenes work preparing for this event. It did not go unnoticed. It is comforting to know that we who suffer have a group that is so supportive and professional as the TNA.*"

- "*I am reminded again how enlightening and empowering it is to discover that the suppressive fear of TN can be replaced with real hope! Thank you and the staff for delivering that message in such a professional yet personal and inclusive manner.*"

- "*Staff, organizers, Board members, volunteers, and physicians, I want to thank all of you for a most impressive conference. Before going to this event, I was unsure what to expect; I needed answers and reassurance; and both of these were met. My husband was also more comfortable after learning so much more about TN.*"

- "*There was an epiphany for me at the conference in that up to the conference, pain and fear were the driving forces behind my attempts to find a permanent solution to this pain that has become an unwelcome visitor in my head. There is a need for me to do more research, process all the information, and to carefully choose the method that is best for me. This is undoubtedly the most important idea that resonated with me.*"

- "*It was interesting for me personally to sit with a group of people who were bombarding the neurosurgeon with questions – nearly everyone came up with a question that had not occurred to others within the group and they were grateful to be able to listen to the answer. It is a wonderful way of increasing knowledge about TN.*"

- *"I wanted to say how beneficial it is to sufferers to speak to a neurosurgeon in a relaxed, informal atmosphere, instead of across a desk in a clinical environment in a patient/doctor relationship."*

During this conference I also held some focus groups with sufferers to determine their views on a variety of topics. One of the questions I posed was, "When you think of support groups, what do you think of?" These were the answers: *"sharing, compassion, owning condition, feedback, commonality, help, knowledge and information, I am not alone, creating relationship between patients and medical groups, sharing information, understanding, crying for help, special friends."*

The next question was, "What do your families want from support groups? The answers were: *"Encouragement, information, backup plan, knowledge, information, support, cure, hope, end of isolation, feeling better able to help someone, lower anxiety levels, backup for spouse."*

Although as yet not formally assessed, the trigeminal neuralgia support groups appear to provide a wealth of information, enable sufferers to meet each other without the need for a health-care professional and can influence national research institutes. The NIH provided some funding for this conference. Similar results have been obtained from surveys at National conferences in the UK and Australia and this data will be published.

Table 5: Key Facts

WHAT NATIONAL SUPPORT GROUP MEETINGS OFFER PARTICIPANTS
• Provide more information in a variety of formats
• Encourage face-to-face communication between fellow sufferers
• Provide a means of sufferers meeting health care professionals outside their usual setting
• Provide health care professionals from many disciplines the ability to network and evaluate each other's work
• Improve confidence in dealing with the condition and making decisions
• Provide support group leaders with help

5. WHAT DO THE LEADERS OF TNA SUPPORT GROUPS THINK OF THE WORK THAT IS BEING DONE BY THEIR GROUPS?

Since there is no literature currently about how the TNA support groups are used and who runs them, I met with the executive committee of the UK TNA support group and conducted an interview with them using some of the questions on the following page.

Who contacts the trigeminal neuralgia support groups?

- people who are looking for information and advice about symptoms, potentially a diagnosis – may or may not have trigeminal neuralgia
- newly diagnosed sufferers who want information about the condition
- sufferers who are overwhelmed by the information they have found on the Internet and who want someone to direct them further
- sufferers who have not been able to take in everything that has been said by the doctors and want detailed information, e.g. this patient's comment: *"They sometimes come back with the most extraordinary visions of surgery like he's going to operate through my ear."*
- sufferers who feel isolated and need reassurance, as indicated by this patient: *"We can say it's okay to be worried and concerned, but we're here; we can talk it through with you; you can talk to us at any time and they know that there is a lifeline and it's on an informal level, they don't have to be scared of us."*
- sufferers want to meet someone with the same problem, as these patients stated:
  - *"There is no doubt that the buddy system is something of great importance as nobody can appreciate the severity of the pain unless they have had it themselves. This therefore makes anything the support group leaders say to the contacting client of such value and improves credibility."*
  - *"helps to know that someone else truly knows what having trigeminal neuralgia is like. On down days is when I search for that support when a stranger becomes an unmet friend."*
- sufferers who want to discuss a wide range of topics, often straying off the topic of trigeminal neuralgia
- those who want to meet someone else with the condition, as this patient expressed: "to be able to pick up the phone or send an e-mail or meet someone face to face who suffers from the same thing and is therefore sympathetic."
- those who want information about which doctor to see or hospital to go to. The UK TNA view is, *"I never say I recommend. These are the hospitals nearest to you that can offer the full range of treatments and these are the leaders."* The UK TNA has a list, which states very clearly "if the name is in bold type, it means this is a hospital that offers all treatments for TN, and if the name has a star next to it, this has been recommended by another patient."

- sufferers whose treatment has not worked and are looking for alternative treatments
- relatives or friends of sufferers who are helping sufferers
- how to explain their condition to others One patient wrote, *"I would like to know how to explain it to employers and people you have to interface with who don't understand that something is wrong."* Another patient wanted to know *"how to explain trigeminal neuralgia and keep it simple when you are still learning about it yourself."*

The needs of these people are varied and there are probably four main categories of members. There are those who will only dip into the support groups, get what they want and leave (often "cured"). Others have ongoing problems and so remain in the group, and still others are relatives or friends of sufferers who want to help. The fourth group includes the members the associations need most. These are the sufferers who want to share what they have gained with others to improve the future experience of sufferers. This means that the membership of these associations is continually changing and this new influx enriches the support groups.

When I asked sufferers attending a conference what they wanted support groups to be doing, these were the answers:
- provide an ear to listen
- information
- understanding and continuous support
- support family members
- suggest suitable referrals to dentists and doctors locally
- reach out to new patients
- provide contact details of other sufferers
- provide details of good speakers
- increase the publics awareness
- reduce isolation, psychosocial

The following are the expectations for assistance from the main TNA organization:
- public relations
- help with publicity
- provide network lists
- guidelines on how to lead and conduct support groups
- referral lists
- lobby NIH for research
- access to Web site chat rooms, news items, bulletin boards, ask a doctor

- guidelines for press releases, topics for discussion at meetings
- raise funds for research
- education for health care professionals

How do sufferers contact support groups?

- telephone
- e-mail "extremely helpful as patients with severe pain do not want to talk or find it too painful, whereas communicating by e-mail provides support and help. It can, however, be very time consuming and potentially expensive."
- letter —- least commonly used
- vast majority of contacts are through the Internet; even though the sufferers may not be able to use the Internet themselves, their relatives will often find out for them
- through their health care provider

What do support group leaders do?

Support group leaders' roles are very far ranging. Some run groups in their own localities, while others are part of the executive committees of their national organizations. The latter decide on the aims and objectives of the organization and try to find the means to fulfil those. Ample details are provided on the Internet sites, which even have special sections for support group leaders to give them the necessary resources.

Running such a large organization, often over a wide geographic area, is a full-time task in itself and requires many staff members and increasingly large premises. One leader explains:

"If you have a support group that just meets for a cup of tea and a moan, it will probably last for about three or four sessions, but if you give them a program to work through, things to work toward, objectives to achieve, then the group will function."

One sufferer describes her support leader as *"the lay-neurologist-on-call. Through the years, he has collected information, and through his fantastic support network, he makes people, literature, facts, you name it, all available for the asking."*

Below is a list of tasks a support group may do with the help of a team:

- Be sure to give information and not advice
- Make sure that all information distributed has been checked by the TNA's medical advisory board
- Make notes on anything that may be useful to pass on to group members

- Get in touch with new members
- Keep in touch with members regularly
- Find guest speakers for meetings
- Structure the meetings; for example, plan sessions on dealing with a flare-up of pain, coping with anxiety and fear, relaxation and distraction, the pain/stress cycle
- Arrange meeting venues, provide refreshments
- Gather and record feedback from group members about their experiences
- Keep a list of specialists who have been helpful (and otherwise)
- Make a list of questions to ask the doctor and keep this as a master list to give to new members as they join
- Maintain a supply of hand-outs that contain useful information for members – booklets, copies of articles, etc.
- Be prepared to research answers to members' questions
- Write progress reports for the TNA board, executive committee and newsletter
- Maintain contact with other organizations
- Encourage members to publicize the TNA wherever possible
- Organize funding for the group to cover general expenses, maintain records of expenses and submit expense accounts on a regular basis

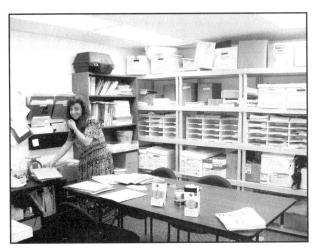

Sending out information is a major task for support groups. This is the mailing room of the TNA US headquarters in Gainesville, FL.

What do you as support group leaders find difficult about talking to sufferers?

- not having enough knowledge is always a problem when first beginning

    One leader's comment: *"You feel quite often that you're bumbling along on your own unless you have someone medically experienced and qualified to back you up."*

- diagnosing a recurrence

    Leader's comment: *"I think the hardest thing is telling them that it's actually likely to come back."*

- The diagnosis has changed and the patient does have trigeminal neuralgia

    Leader's comment: *"They come to me to talk about it and there's not much I can do to help them other than to try and direct them towards pain-management programs, to help them simply by talking to them to come to terms with the fact that this is something they have to live with and it's a very difficult thing to say, you've got to say it very carefully indeed. I try always to stress the positives rather than the negatives."*

- understanding the variations of the condition

    Leader's comment: *"There remains a very wide range of presentations and descriptions of trigeminal neuralgia, and everyone is always surprised at the amount of variability that is noted."*

- sometimes when you are feeling unwell yourself, it's very difficult to talk to others and provide support

- talking to patients who are depressed for a variety of reasons due to the diagnosis, the drugs, their situation, having to give up their job, changes in their lives

    Leader's comment: *"For whatever reason they're depressed, I think is very hard because that's draining."*

- being used for support, it is very difficult to cope with patients who latch onto a person on whom they can unburden, and sometimes the information they want is not within the expertise of the support group

    Leader's comment: *"As one gains more experience, it is easier to tell the patient where to stop and where they must go to get help."*

What do you find most rewarding about talking to sufferers?

- being told that you have helped

  Leader's comment: *"It's great when somebody has phoned you in tears and at the end of half an hour says, 'I can't tell you how good it's been to be able to talk to you,' and you know it has all been worthwhile."*

- being able to give people information

  Leader's comment: *"Having somebody say 'I understand, that's fine, now I'll try it' and then writing perhaps a little later and saying they're feeling better. It is shepherding people through a process, not necessarily finding a complete cure, but a process of finding a way of managing and explaining it in their language."*

- providing sufferers with hope

  Leader's comment: *"A lot of people just don't have any hope, they don't see a light at the end of the tunnel because a lot of their specialists or their GP's say 'oh well you know this is something you're going to have to live with.'…..It's great to be able to say to someone 'oh no, there's plenty of things that can be done, okay so you're allergic to Tegretol, try something else' – 'oh is there something else?' because their GP doesn't always know. 'Ask him for a referral to a neurologist, he can sort out a cocktail of drugs' – 'oh, oh I didn't know that.' It's that that gives you a tremendous sense of satisfaction."*

- putting patients in contact with each other

  Leader's comment: *"One woman said she was so pleased she'd received a letter from someone who'd contacted her through the contact list and saying how she'd helped this particular patient."*

- finding that information that has been linked to other Internet sites that potential sufferers access does bring them into contact with the support group

  Leader's comment: *"GP's are going into NHS Direct and then coming to us. I've had quite a few like that."*

Why do sufferers become involved in running support groups?

"There is plenty that needs to be done in the organization, and many people from broad backgrounds are needed to help realize the aims of the organization. It is important to continue to canvas for new members to join the organization and help, since burn-out can occur and people will need to leave the organization from time to time."

- To ensure that fewer people are in the position of having no information

  Leader's comment: *"I wish I'd have known a bit more about it when I first was suffering."*

- To decrease the isolation

  Leaders' comments*: "I think because we've all had it and probably felt a bit isolated ourselves." "Reaching out and trying to help others is rewarding. To see so many people in pain and still not have answers is depressing at times, but at least we are in it together."*

- to provide reassurance and hope

  Leader's comment*: "I was terrified because nothing was working. I was taking more and more and more of the pills and I wanted to kill myself. I got to the point where I had so little quality of life. Had I been able to talk to somebody else, I would have been perhaps given some hope because I didn't have any hope."*

- to provide a buddy system when the sufferer finds it difficult to talk with a health care professional

  Leader's comment: *"It's very difficult to explain to someone medical sitting opposite a desk from you, who is matter-of-factly saying, 'well this is what you need to take and this is what you need to do' and you're sitting there thinking I am terrified and I can't explain that to this person because I don't think he'll be able to understand. You can see that same fear in other people when you talk to them, you can tell, they mentioned that they thought of committing suicide and they have been really, really frightened. I think that it's very important to be able to understand when somebody else is frightened. You can say 'yes I know, I do understand, I've been there, I understand that.'"*

- to be sure help is there should the pain return
- to provide quick access to accurate information and instant communication about any new developments
- to help others as a way of saying thank you

  Leader's comment: *"I wanted to give something back because I could see what was going on, I can see how much effort was going into it and I wanted to be able to help in return."*

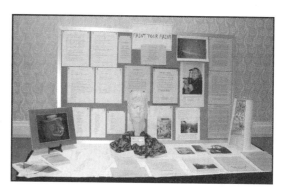

An example of a stand made by patients with their materials at the 5th TNA US conference in 2004.

What qualities do support group leaders need?

Many of these are discussed on the Internet sites and in the material available from the support groups. Here are just a few of them:
- dedication and time
  Leader's comment: *"You have to have a level of dedication because it takes an enormous chunk out of your life and it can be very draining."*
- being prepared to look for and understand more information than just for your own personal use
  Leader's comment: *"people who are prepared to do a bit of homework. Reading around and getting to know more than what you personally need; it's having a much broader brush. I've got to be able to explain in simple words how the nervous system works as far as I can. I'm not a neurologist, but I have got to be able to understand that and I think we all have put it in layman's language."*
- empathy
- patience

What makes these organizations effective?

- being professional and maintaining high standards
  Leader's comment: *"People's impression of the organization when they first come to it are very important and this will effect whether they would be prepared to help the organization."*
- very quick with responses
- efficient
- sets itself objectives for each year in order to make sure that progress is being made

- responsive to members' needs
- being considered as partners with health care professionals and invited to participate in events

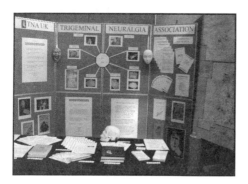

Example of the TNA UK exhibit at the British Pain Society meeting.

MRS. G CASE STUDY

After Mrs. G left the specialist for the first time, she was horrified to find that she could not remember everything she had been told. She decided to ask some friends, but no one had heard of trigeminal neuralgia, and this made her feel very lonely. She had also forgotten to ask how long the condition would last this time, since she had previously had a short episode. This time things seemed more serious and there had also been some mention of surgery.

What was Mrs. G to do?

Discussion

Mrs. G needs to write down all her questions so when she goes back for her review appointment, she at least will know what to ask. Access to the Internet is her best solution. She can get access through a Cybernet café at the local hospital, library or a commercial place. It could be she has some friends who can help her. Having found access to the Internet, Mrs. G uses a search engine like "Google" to type in the words trigeminal neuralgia. The first hits are the support groups. She then checks out the quality of the sites using the information in Chapter 8. Having established that the trigeminal neuralgia support groups are genuine organizations, she then contacts them for more information and may contact fellow sufferers. She finds high quality information, a local support group she can attend and a list of fellow sufferers.

This process made Mrs. G feel much less isolated and fearful, and she was feeling much more positive about her return to the specialist. She still felt she had a vast amount of information, but not sure what to do with it.

6. What evaluation of the impact of support groups is needed?

Although intrinsically it would seem that support groups are essential and meet important needs of sufferers, there are still questions that need to be answered.

- How do the objectives of support groups match up with the needs and experiences of the users?
- How well are the objectives of the support groups being realized?
- How does membership in a support group affect the relationship with health care practitioners (Hart et al 2004)?
- Support groups now make full use of the Internet. How does the information they provide compare to that on other Internet sites, especially those that do not adhere to quality guidelines?
- How is the information provided by support groups used by patients to improve their outcomes?
- Have the support groups had an impact on health care practitioners and if so, in what way?
- Do the support groups reduce the use of health care services by sufferers and increase self management?
- What types of meetings are most useful, cost effective and why, e.g. local, national, international?
- How important is it for uniformity of information between the different support groups or does this add to confusion, especially for the first-time user?

SUMMARY

- The increasing number of support groups provides some evidence that these types of organizations have a role to play, probably in supplementing formal health care and reducing the use of health care services.
- TNA support groups provide more than just information through a variety of different ways.
- The psychosocial support, especially the "buddy system," is highly valued by all sufferers.
- The US has the largest TNA national organization but the UK, Australia and Canada also have national groups with growing networks of local support groups .
- Conferences and meetings provide face-to-face contacts not only with health sufferers, but also with health care professionals.
- Leaders of these support groups need to be dedicated individuals, since demands on their time and psychological support is great. They do not necessarily need to be TN sufferers themselves.
- Research is needed into how best they can fulfil their roles.

FURTHER READING AND REFERENCES

Web sites
Checked April 2005

A very full list of Web sites can be found in the book, **Striking Back! The Trigeminal Neuralgia and Face Pain Handbook**, or on the Web sites of the support groups. These are some key Web sites:

Web site of the US TNA group http://www.tna-support.org/

Web site of the UK TNA support group http://www.tna.org.uk/

Web site of the Australian TNA group http://www.tnaaustralia.org.au/

Web site of the Canadian TNA support group http://www.tnac.org/

Details on the expert patient program
http://www.expertpatients.nhs.uk/index.shtml

DIPEx shows you a wide variety of personal experiences of health and illness. You can watch, listen to or read their interviews, find reliable information on treatment choices and where to find support. It includes one on chronic pain, specifically trigeminal neuralgia
http://www.dipex.org/main.asp

The American Chronic Pain Association http://www.theacpa.org/#

Pain Relief Foundation, based in Liverpool UK, provides detailed information on a series of pain topics, including trigeminal neuralgia
http://www.painrelieffoundation.org.uk/paininfo.html

The Neuropathy Trust Support group for anyone with neuropathic pain www.neurocentre.com

Health on the Net (HON) guides health care consumers and providers on the World Wide Web to sound, reliable medical information and expertise. In this way, HON seeks to contribute to better, more accessible and cost-effective health care. It aims to improve the quality of medical information http://www.hon.ch/

Books and Booklets

The Brain and Spine Foundation publishes a leaflet on facial pain and MRI scans, also available on their Web site: http://www.brainandspine.org.uk/

Muir Gray, JA (2002) **The Resourceful Patient** eRosetta Press Oxford UK ISBN 1-904202-00-4 This is also a Internet based book and tool-kit for those wishing to address the problems of health care in the 21st century. Visit this Web site: http://www.resourcefulpatient.org/

Weigel G and Casey K F. (2004) **Striking Back! The Trigeminal Neuralgia and Face Pain Handbook.** the Trigeminal Neuralgia Association. Florida ISBN 0-9672393-2-X patient handbook

References

Hart A, Henwood F and Wyatt S. (2004) The role of the Internet in patient-practitioner relationships: findings from a qualitative research study. *J Med Internet Res.* **30**;6(3):e36.- this is a free, open access electronic journal that contains many other articles of similar topics.

Prinjha S, Chapple A, Herxheimer A, and McPherson A. (2005) Many people with epilepsy want to know more: a qualitative study. *Fam Pract.* **4**: 435-41

Zakrzewska JM (2001) Consumers' views on management of trigeminal neuralgia. *Headache* **41**:369-376

CHAPTER 12

RESEARCH QUESTIONS

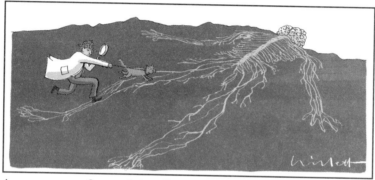

A vast amount of research is still needed before trigeminal neuralgia can be fully controlled.

Trigeminal neuralgia, one of the world's most excruciatingly painful human disorders, is associated with a huge vocabulary used to define variations of the nerve problem and its progression, and to describe the various approaches used to diagnose and treat it. Key words and phrases in this lexicon are provided in the following acronym:

Trigger Points
Rare Nerve Disorder
Information – Trigeminal Neuralgia Association
Gamma Knife Stereotactic Radiosurgery
Exacerbations and Remissions
Magnetic Resonance Imaging
Invasive Microvascular Decompression
Non-Invasive Balloon Compression
Anti-Convulsant Medication – Tegretol
Lightning – Shock-like Attacks

Neurologists-Neurosurgeon
E-Mail
Utilize Computer TNA "Home Page"
Radiofrequency Rhizotomy
Alternative Therapies
Lancilating Pain
Glycerol Rhizotomy
Internet Worldwide Web http://neurosurgery, mgh.edu/tna/#services
Artery and Vein Compression

1. What research questions do sufferers have?

During one of the focus group meetings we held with TN sufferers, we asked them to tell us what research questions they had and these are the answers:

- Could it be passed on to your kids? Or can it skip a generation?
- Is there a relationship between season and TN?
- Is it an infectious element that triggers it?
- Are there certain risk factors?
- I want to solve the MS and trigeminal neuralgia link; are they linked?
- Does diet play a role, especially Vitamin B?
- We need to get into the mode of researching the chemistry of the pain.
- What causes a case of trigeminal neuralgia to go atypical, and will it go back again?
- What causes stress-related pain and how we are going to treat that pain?
- Why does the pain get worse?
- Does it always continue to get worse as we get older?

- Are different treatments better depending on what pattern of pain you have?
- What medications work best in most people?
- How do the drugs take effect?
- What operations work best in most people?
- Why does the pain come back after a microvascular decompression?
- 75 % of people who have MVD get improvement, but I think there should be more research on the other 25 %. Why are the other 25 % still suffering?
- I'd like more research into the cause of the atypical form and why don't we respond to treatment in the same way?
- I would like to know how to explain it to employers and people you have to interface with, who don't understand that something is wrong.
- Just how do you cope with it?

2. HOW ARE RESEARCHERS TRYING TO ANSWER THESE QUESTIONS?

In September 1999 the National Institute of Neurological Disorders and Stroke (NINDS) and the National Institute of Dental and Craniofacial Research (NIDCR) sponsored a workshop on trigeminal neuralgia. It brought together people from a wide range of backgrounds: basic scientists, clinicians, epidemiologists, and patients' advocates. Several research questions were identified, and these were published in Pain in 2000, (Kitt et al 2000). Early in 2004 the Special Interest Group in Orofacial of the International Association for the Study of Pain held a two-day meeting on the topic of trigeminal neuropathic pain and its findings were then reported in the winter edition of the Journal of Orofacial Pain in 2004. Progress is being made in a wide range of fields, but there are still many unanswered questions.

One of the major hindrances to research is the lack of large multi-center grants that would enable dedicated research staff to be engaged. Virtually all areas need support, but probably one of the key issues is that of how common is this condition, since this will dictate the scale of resources needed for the other projects.

Funding is needed to set up national databases of all patients with trigeminal neuralgia, who can then be followed up on an annual basis. In addition, research projects, preferably multi-center studies that are also multidisciplinary, should be centrally registered so patients can enroll in them to ensure that they are completed as quickly as possible

with the optimum number of patients. Ideally, every trigeminal neuralgia sufferer should become a research patient in order to contribute to
the common goal of ending the pain of trigeminal neuralgia, which will
only be achieved after more research.

This chapter will re-assess the questions raised in Kitt et al's document in the light of the newest evidence available and which has been
highlighted in each chapter. It needs to be borne in mind that research
attempting to answer one question often results in the generation of even
more questions.

This chapter will look specifically at research issues in trigeminal neuralgia, but research in the field of **neuropathic pain** and even pain itself
will often be applicable to patients with trigeminal neuralgia and may be
easier to obtain funding for, since they include a larger group of patients.

3. WHAT RESEARCH IS NEEDED IN THE AREA OF EPIDEMIOLOGY AND POPULATION STUDIES?

There has been little new literature in this area, and the publications
that have been added to those available in 1999 make relatively little
impact and still do not answer the most important question of all —
"How many patients have trigeminal neuralgia?"

Any **epidemiological** studies of trigeminal neuralgia must use very
clear **diagnostic** criteria to ensure that the same group of patients are
being included. Population studies on trigeminal neuralgia alone would
be too expensive, given the rarity of the condition; thus they need to be
embedded in other studies of facial pain or utilize large databases used
for all diseases.

The most comprehensive data so far has been derived from the Mayo
Clinic based in Rochester, Minn. It may be of value to revisit this database and see if changes have occurred over time. Data is now also collected by large insurance companies in the US, and these could also be uti-
lized to gain basic data on the distribution of trigeminal neuralgia
throughout the US. Other institutions may also keep databases using
clear diagnostic criteria.

Epidemiological studies could provide answers to some of the following questions:

- What is the **prevalence** of trigeminal neuralgia and how does it
  relate to gender, age, education, socio-economic status, ethnicity?
- Is there a specific geographical, racial distribution that may provide
  a clue about causality?
- What is the role of heredity and genetics?

- What are the risk factors, e.g. dental treatment, trauma to the head (including mouth), blood pressure, infections, diet, Vitamin B12, weather, radiation and skull shape, psychological factors?
- Are there particular risk groups, e.g. those who have had herpes infections?
- What is the natural history of the condition?
- What are the predictors for progression?
- What is the cost of this disease to the individual and society as a whole?

4. What research is needed in the area of diagnosis?

In theory, it seems that the diagnostic criteria for trigeminal neuralgia have been clearly defined, but in clinical practice this is not the case. The current criteria have not been tested for their accuracy and ability to distinguish between trigeminal neuralgia, its variants, and other forms of facial pain.

Objective tests are needed to prove that the history and examination obtained from the sufferer really equates with a diagnosis of trigeminal neuralgia. Is trigeminal neuralgia made up a several variants, all due to different causes, or are the varying presentations of trigeminal neuralgia most often labelled as atypical or type 2 really just representative of the degree of nerve damage?

Research in the area of diagnosis could provide answers to the following questions:

- What are the key features of classical trigeminal neuralgia and its variants?
- What is the importance of the different characteristics of the pain and would the management of patients change depending on the major characteristics of the pain, e.g. burning or just shooting, paroxysmal or continuous?
- Would a well-validated questionnaire make it easier to consistently make the correct diagnosis and also establish the effect the pain has on quality of life?
- Would such a questionnaire be sensitive to change?
- How do cultural, social and psychological factors affect trigeminal neuralgia?

5. WHAT RESEARCH IS NEEDED TO DETERMINE THE CAUSE OF TRIGEMINAL NEURALGIA AND THE MECHANISMS INVOLVED IN PAIN GENERATION?

Until we know more about the causes of the disease and the functioning of the trigeminal nerve, it will be impossible to provide effective treatments. This is one of the areas that requires a vast amount of research at all levels, but principally at the molecular level. There are still no completely satisfactory animal models of trigeminal neuralgia, which would facilitate research. Neuroscientists must work closely with clinicians, since both sides need to contribute to the generation of hypothesis, which then can be tested.

Questions that need answering in broad terms include:

- What is the molecular basis for neuropathic pain and, in particular, trigeminal neuralgia, including identification and functional studies of the neurotransmitters, **neuromodulators** and intracellular messengers involved?
- Is there a genetic basis? What are the gene and protein networks implicated in the initiation and persistence of facial pain? Does the inheritance of specific gene **polymorphisms** predispose an individual to particular orofacial pain conditions?
- Is chronic orofacial pain a disease in its own right and is it possible to identify individuals more likely to develop chronic orofacial pain? Are sex differences in pain response and susceptibility to specific pain conditions genetically determined?
- What is the role of the immune system?
- What is the role of dental, infective and compression factors in the generation of trigeminal neuralgia?
- How do psychological factors affect pain perception?
- Would a tissue bank from sufferers with trigeminal neuralgia help to answer some of these questions?

6. WHAT RESEARCH IS NEEDED IN ASSESSMENT AND INVESTIGATION OF TRIGEMINAL NEURALGIA?

Perhaps one of the most exciting new areas of research is neuroimaging using functional magnetic resonance imaging (ƒMRI). This technology may provide answers to the causation of trigeminal neuralgia and factors that affect it. See Chapter 4 for more details.

Research in the area of assessment could provide answers to the following questions:

- Is there a neuropathic scale that is objective and usable for evaluation of treatment outcomes, or does one need to be developed?
- What is the role of qualitative sensory testing (QST) and laser-evoked potentials in providing details on the functioning of the trigeminal nerve?
- Is the **MRI** sensitive enough to predict the presence of vascular compression in all patients who have trigeminal neuralgia, or do some individuals have nerve compression with no symptoms of trigeminal neuralgia?
- What is the role of magnetic resonance tomographic angiography (MRTA) and how does it compare to magnetic resonance imaging (MRI)?
- What can *f*MRI tell us about trigeminal neuralgia both in terms of structure and function, and how this is affected by treatment and other factors?

7. WHAT RESEARCH IS NEEDED IN GENERAL MANAGEMENT OF TRIGEMINAL NEURALGIA?

The following are some research questions that are common to all treatment modalities that need to be addressed:

- How do the various types of treatments compare when using the same measurements in randomized controlled trials?
- What outcomes for treatment are considered effective by health care workers, sufferers and other stakeholders?
- What effect does provision of information and sharing of experiences with other sufferers have on treatment expectations and outcomes?
- Does patient-centered care for patients with trigeminal neuralgia improve outcomes?

8. WHAT RESEARCH IS NEEDED TO IMPROVE OUTCOMES FOR PATIENTS BEING TREATED WITH DIFFERENT DRUGS?

This area requires input from several specialists. Basic scientists working in the area of pharmacology need to look at mechanisms of drug action to target specific sites of action in order to increase effectiveness and reduce side effects. This then needs to be rapidly translated into drugs that can be used in treating patients.

Any new drugs being considered for use in trigeminal neuralgia should first be evaluated in a small **open-label trial** and, if showing promise, should be the subject of a powerful randomized controlled trial. These may need to be carried out in several centers to ensure that the number of patients recruited is large enough to show a difference.

Questions that need answering include:

- Why are there individual variations in patients' responses to drugs; does it have a genetic basis?
- Can a generic template be designed to be used in the potential evaluation of any new drugs so that results are comparable?
- Which drugs or class of drugs provide the best pain relief with the fewest side effects?
- Is there merit in using a combination of drugs, including the use of antidepressants and opioids?
- Are there ways of delivering drugs to their site of action other than orally?
- Would the use of internationally approved guidelines improve outcomes for patients?

9. WHAT RESEARCH IS NEEDED TO DETERMINE WHETHER ADDITIONAL TREATMENTS ARE EFFECTIVE?

The use of complementary and alternative medicine in trigeminal neuralgia remains controversial. Although pain management courses have been shown to be effective in relieving chronic pain, especially in improving quality of life, none have been developed specifically to use in patients with neuropathic and/or facial pain.

The following research questions still need answering:

- Would pain management programs be beneficial for patients with trigeminal neuralgia?
- Do physicians and surgeons need training in order to adopt a more **biopsychosocial** approach to the care of patients with trigeminal neuralgia?
- Would the use of art and narrative, in pain diagnosis and management, open up new avenues of communication both with health care workers and with the family and the wider public?
- How can complementary and alternative medicine help sufferers with trigeminal neuralgia? Researchers need to evaluate the roles of acupuncturists and chiropractors and the role of vitamins and in particular vitamin B12 on a large multi-center basis.

10. WHAT RESEARCH IS NEEDED TO ENABLE PATIENTS TO MAKE DECISIONS ABOUT THEIR TREATMENT?

The whole process of shared decision making for trigeminal neuralgia is hampered by the lack of high quality information that would provide the facts on which decisions are made. There is also a lack of tools for risk assessment, which is an integral part of decision making. If this data is to be obtained, then it is essential that:

- more high quality trials are performed, especially of the **randomized controlled** type. They should be registered so that duplication is avoided, and details of results can be obtained quickly. Patients can ask to be enrolled in them if they are taking place near where they live.
- the data on treatment outcomes, trade-offs, etc., that are needed for the decision-making template are nationally, if not internationally, agreed upon so that patients get exactly the same information.
- the quality standards Zakrzewska and Lopez (2003) have suggested for reporting of surgical results should be adhered to, and editors of journals can do much to enforce this standard.

To achieve these aims, consensus meetings of experts, patients and other stakeholders are necessary to evaluate the evidence available so that treatment guidelines can be drawn up to help patients make decisions.

- reliable patient experiences would be a great advantage and add a further dimension to the information-gathering process. Funding would be needed to work with an organization like DIPEx (see Chapter 8 for more details) to generate videos, interviews and reading materials on trigeminal neuralgia.

The whole area of risk assessment needs considerable research, which includes:

- What innovative methods of training for doctors in risk management, including communication, can be developed?
- What types of visual aids can be developed to describe risk of complications after surgery and how can their validity be tested?
- How do culture, age, gender and education affect the perception of risk?
- What are the effects of shared decision making on patient outcomes, both in terms of satisfaction and quality of life?

health care workers and patients need uniform high quality information and so the following are needed:

- assessments of Internet sites that may be a value to trigeminal neuralgia sufferers, using specially developed toolkits

• development of more high-standard material in a wide variety of formats that have been awarded kite marks (see Chapter 8 for further details), so they can be easily identified

Once all this data is available, it should be possible to develop Decision Aids for patients with trigeminal neuralgia, which could be done with an organization such as the Foundation for Informed Medical Decision Making.

11. WHAT RESEARCH IS NEEDED TO EVALUATE SURGICAL MANAGEMENT?

The current data on surgical outcomes is very disparate and difficult to compare, since different criteria are being used for patient enrollment and for reporting outcomes of treatment.

Surgical treatments for trigeminal neuralgia need to be audited using the same principles that other surgical specialities use. These include both the process of care and the outcome. The standards need to be set by consensus and then independently audited by external observers. Robust objective measures, which are sensitive to change, need to be used. If this data is collected on an annual basis and sent to one center, then a **meta-analysis** of the results could be done. The large numbers would enable meaningful analysis to be done and may enable answers to be obtained to some of these questions:

• Why do surgical treatments fail and why does this happen, especially in the first two years? Could these be due to technical errors and, if so, can they be reduced?

• How do the different ablative procedures compare in terms of recurrence rates, complications, quality of life?

• Are there any prognostic factors that could aid in selection of patients for surgery?

• What are the long-term effects of gamma knife treatments?

• What are the economic costs of each of these treatments compared to long-term medical care?

• What are the psychological costs of treating patients surgically compared to medically?

Any new surgical treatments that may be proposed must be the subject of a randomized controlled trial, which can take into account patient and surgeon preferences.

Surgical information leaflets attached to consent forms should be prepared for national use, which are written together with patients and then trailed as suggested by Ross (2004).

12. WHAT RESEARCH IS NEEDED IN PATIENTS WHO HAVE A RECURRENCE OF PAIN OR DEVELOPED COMPLICATIONS AS A RESULT OF TREATMENT?

There is very little data on complications and recurrence. Patients need to know not just which complications and how often they are likely to occur, but also how quickly they resolve and how they can be managed. A centralized database would quickly provide answers to questions such as these:

- Does tolerance to drugs occur and so lead to increasing poor pain control?
- What are the recurrence rates after repeat surgery and why do they appear to be less satisfactory than after primary surgery?
- How do the complications of surgery impinge on the quality of life of patients?
- Are there any ways in which these complications can be predicted or are there certain individuals who are at higher risk of developing them?
- Can outcome be improved using stricter diagnostic criteria?
- How can patients with anesthesia dolorosa be best managed?

13. WHAT RESEARCH IS NEEDED ON THE ROLE OF SUPPORT GROUPS?

Although intrinsically it would seem that support groups are essential and fill much-needed roles, there are still questions that need to be answered.

- How do the objectives of support groups match up with the needs and experiences of the users?
- How well are the objectives of the support groups being realized?
- How does membership of a support group affect the relationship with health care practitioners?
- Support groups now make full use of the Internet. How does the information they provide compare to that on other Internet sites, especially those that do not adhere to quality guidelines?
- How is the information provided by support groups used by patients to improve their outcomes?
- Have the support groups had an impact on healthcare practitioners and, if so, in what way?
- Do the support groups reduce the use of health care services by sufferers and increase self-management?
- What types of meetings are most useful, cost-effective and why?

• How important is uniformity of information among the different support groups?

Not only does the research need to be done, but the results need to be rapidly disseminated so they enter everyday medical practice. This is a much faster process than previously and it may be even faster if expert patients are used to help find the information and share it with their health care providers.

SUMMARY

Research on trigeminal neuralgia is needed in all areas, from basic science through clinical studies to public health issues, and this cannot be carried out without substantial funding. Funding is difficult to obtain for rare diseases and costs are often high, since national and international collaborations are needed.

FURTHER READING AND REFERENCES

Web sites

The DIPEx Web site shows you a wide variety of personal experiences of health and illness, including chronic pain. You can watch, listen to or read their interviews, find reliable information on treatment choices and where to find help http://www.dipex.org

References

Kitt CA, Gruber K, Davis M, Woolf CJ and Levine JD (2000) Trigeminal neuralgia: opportunities for research and treatment. *Pain* **85**:3-7.

Ross N. (2004) Improving surgical consent *Lancet* **364**:812-3.

Zakrzewska JM and Lopez BC. (2003) Quality of papers reporting outcomes after surgical management of trigeminal neuralgia: Recommendations for future reports Neurosurgery **53**:110-122

Journal Orofacial Pain 2004 Issue 4 contains a series of articles on research in the field of neuropathic trigeminal pain.

APPENDIX

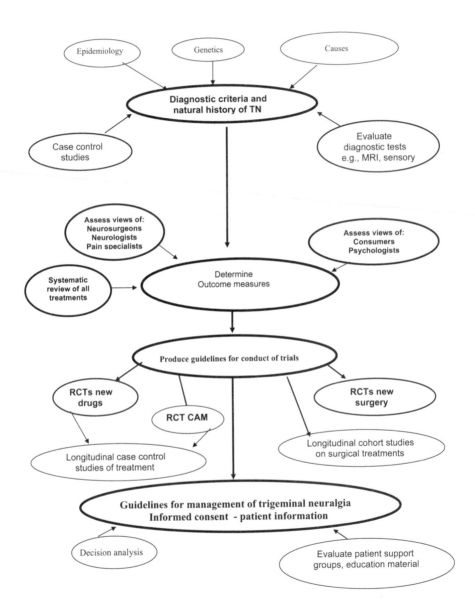

GLOSSARY

Based on the glossary in the book, **Striking Back! The Trigeminal Neuralgia and Face Pain Handbook** by Weigel and Casey, and **Dorland Illustrated Medical Dictionary**

Ablative - removal, separation or cutting of a structure

Acoustic neuroma - a tumor growing on the acoustic or hearing nerve. This can sometimes cause TN when the nearby tumor pushes a blood vessel onto the trigeminal nerve

Acromegaly - a condition caused by increased secretion of the growth hormone

Adhesions - fibrous growths similar to scar tissue that form at the site of tissue damage.

Aetiology - cause of disease

Allele - one of two or more contrasting characters transmitted by genes

Allodynia - pain due to a stimulus which does not normally provoke pain

Analgesics - medications that relieve pain

Anesthesia dolorosa - a combination of pain and numbness

Anesthetic - an agent used to abolish pain

Aneurysm - weakness in a blood vessel that allows vessel to bulge and possibly rupture

Anhydrous - dry

Anterior - front

Anticonvulsant - medication that prevents convulsions or seizures

Anxiety - feeling very troubled by worries or fears. Often associated with physical symptoms such as dry mouth, rapid beating of the heart, diffculty breathing and a feeling of tenseness

Aplastic anemia - potentially fatal blood disorder caused by damage to bone marrow. Rare but potential side effect of some anticonvulsant medications

Asymptomatic - no symtoms or complaints

Aseptic - not due to an infection

Arachnoid, arachnoiditis - a membrane of the brain. When abnormally thickened, it is a potential cause of compression on the trigeminal nerve and is then termed arachnoiditis.

Arteriovenous malformation (AVM) - an abnormal growth of blood vessels that sometimes rupture without warning. These vessels can cause TN if they grow near and compress the trigeminal nerve.

Atlas - The top-most bone of the spine.

Ataxia - inability to walk straight

Atrophic - wasted, smaller than usual

Atypical - irregular, not conforming to the type

Atypical face pain - facial pain with mixed symptoms and of unknown origin. More recently termed chronic facial pain to reflect its unkown cause

Atypical odontalgia - pain in the tooth-bearing area, which is not due to dental causes.

Atypical trigeminal neuralgia - a type of facial pain that may have some of the characteristics of classic TN (i.e. sharp stabs and trigger points) but also symptoms that are not common to classic TN (i.e. constant, aching or burning pain in addition to the stabs).

Avulsion - tearing away of a structure, as in removing or cutting away a section of nerve.

Axon - process of a nerve cell by which impulses travel away from the cell body

Auditory - hearing

Balloon compression - also called microcompression. Is a technique performed at the level of Gasserian ganglion, which is aimed at pressing the nerve against some bony tissue and, in so doing, damage it enough to stop transmission of painful stimuli. (See Chapter 9 for further details).

Baseline - at the start

Bilateral - referring to both sides. Bilateral TN means pain on both sides of the face.

Biofeedback - a technique in which people learn to control body functions such as breathing rate, blood pressure and body temperature by responding to feedback from electrodes that monitor changing body conditions

Biomedical model of care - a model in which he doctor makes a diagnosis and then treats the condition or disease using medicines or surgery

Biopsychosocial model of care - the doctor makes a diagnosis and then provides treatment based not just on medicines and surgery, but also taking into account the patients' social circumstances and their psychological approach to the illness.

Blinded - the investigator and /or the patient involved in a clinical study do not know what is being administered or looked for, which is done to reduce bias

Botox - a purified form of the botulinum toxin that, when injected, can partially paralyze muscles. Usually used in tightening wrinkled skin, it also is being being tried as a temporary TN pain-relief measure. It is used for treatment of hemifacial spasm.

Bradycardia - slowing of the heartbeat

Buccal - inside the cheek

Burning mouth syndrome - sensation of burning, especially of the tongue, but can include all of the mouth. Often associated with altered taste, dryness, and is considered a neuropathic pain.

CT scan - an internal picture of the body constructed by a computer by piecing together a series of X-ray images. Sometimes used in detecting tumors (CT stands for *"computed tomography)*

Capsaicin - the chemical that makes hot peppers hot. Used in a topical cream, it sometimes is used to treat TN.

Case control study - a study of a particular disease or factor in which there is a control group of individuals who do not have the disease or factor being studied

Catastrophizing - tendency to think the worst about situations

Cause - that which brings about a condition or produces an effect

Causal - pertaining to a cause, directed against a cause

Causalgia - an old term for Complex Regional Pain Syndrome Reflex Sympathetic Dystrophy.

Cauterize - to seal off, as in sealing off sections of blood vessels to stop or prevent bleeding

Catheter - a hollow tube used to drain fluids from the body, to introduce liquids to the body, or in the case of TN, to allow passage of a balloon to the site of the trigeminal nerve.

Cerebellum - part of the brain that controls movements

Cerebral cortex - part of the brain that analyzes nerve signals and sends out responses

Cerebrospinal fluid (CSF) - a fluid composed mostly of water, glucose, salt and proteins that surrounds, cushions and provides nutrients to the brain and spinal cord

Cervix - the top vertebrae of the spine where the trigeminal nerve originates and through which the spinal cord passes to connect to the brain stem

Cistern - space around a structure; in the case of the trigeminal nerve, it is the area around the Gasserian ganglion

Cisternography - closed space filled with fluid so it can be seen on X-ray films; in the case of trigeminal neuralgia, the Gasserian ganglion

Clinical trial - special medical study in volunteer human participants (see Chapter 5)

Cluster headache - searing, boring, come-and-go pain in the face or forehead thought to be caused by dilation of the blood vessels in the skull. Sometimes confused with trigeminal neuralgia

Cluster tic syndrome - combination of cluster headaches and trigeminal neuralgia

Cohort - a group of individuals with a particular disease or factor who are being followed up for a longer period of time – it is prospective if planned in advance and retrospective if the data was collected before the study was planned

Cognitive - process by which we become aware of objects of thought or perceptions, including all aspects of perceiving, thinking and remembering

Cognitive behavior therapy (CBT) - a psychological treatment that helps people examine the way they think and respond to situations. Treatment aims at learning more helpful ways of responding

Complex Regional Pain Syndrome/Reflex Sympathetic Dystrophy - chronic pain condition. The key symptom of CRPS is continuous, intense progressive pain out of proportion to the severity of the injury, which most often affects one of the arms, legs, hands or feet.

Compounding - a pharmacy technique in which medications are custom-pre-
pared to meet specific needs of individual customers. Those who offer
this service are called "compounding pharmacists."

Computer tomography CT - sophisticated X-ray imaging technology that which
produces pictures of layers of the body at any depth

Conjunctiva - thin lining of the eylelids and the exposed sclera of the eye

Contrast medium - a liquid solution that can be seen on X-ray films

Control - a standard against which experimental observations may be evaluated.
Matched control means that the experimental group only differs from
the control group by the one factor that is being studied, e.g. all groups
are the same in age, gender

Controlled prospective studies or cohort studies - studies that have been
planned in advance and follow patients for a longer period of time

Convulsants - see anticonvulsants.

Cornea - transparent part forming the front of the eye

Corneal reflex - eye closure reflex, protective mechanism to close the eye if it is
irritated

Coping strategies - thoughts and behaviors that are used to manage or cope with
stressful situations

CSF - cerebro spinal fluid this fluid – this serumlike fluid circulates through
parts of the the brain, the cavity of the spinal cord, and the subarachnoid space, functioning as a shock absorption.

Cranial nerves - twelve pairs of nerves that serve various areas and functions of
the head. The trigeminal nerve is one of these nerves, called the fifth.

Craniectomy - surgical opening in the skull necessary for brain surgery. The bone
is not replaced after surgery.

Craniotomy - surgical opening in the skull necessary for brain surgery. The bone
is replaced after surgery.

Cross sectional studies - look at measurements in a sample at a particular time
point

Cryotherapy - using cold agents to deaden or kill nerve fibers. Sometimes used
to treat TN.

Deafferentation pain - pain that occurs when parts of a nerve are injured to the
point where they're disabled. It's usually a constant, burning type of pain.

Deep brain stimulation - an experimental procedure in which surgeons insert a
thin electrode through a small opening in the skull into the thalamus, a
part of the brain where pain sensation occurs. A stimulation device
attached to the electrode delivers low-grade electrical signals in an
attempt to override pain signals.

Demyelination - the process of losing or destroying myelin, the protective sheath
around nerve fibers

Depression - a feeling of sadnss and lack of interest in life. If severe, can be considered an illness and needs treatment

Decision aid - a method to help people make a decision about treatment options that involves both information and assessment of risk

Diagnosis - the art of distinguishing one disease from another; clinical diagnosis is based on clinical signs and symptoms

Diagnostic - distinctive feature of a disease

Diplopia - seeing two images instead of one

Dura - the waterproof covering that surrounds the brain

Distally - further from the point of reference

DREZ - acronym for *"dorsal root entry zone,"* a surgical procedure done in the neck region to disable the origin of the trigeminal nerve in the upper spine

Dysesthesia - a numbness or abnormal sensation severe enough that a patient considers it disturbing. An <u>unpleasant</u> sensation, whether spontaneous or evoked

Edema - swelling

Electrode - small pointed tool used to deliver controlled charges of electricity or radiowaves

Electromyography - the recording and study of the electrical properties of muscles, either merely to determine whether a muscle is contracting or to make more scientific observations of electrical activity

Emboli - clot brought by the blood from another vessel and forced into a smaller one so obstructing blood flow

Endodontist - dentist who specializes in filling root canals of teeth

Endoscope - a new surgical instrument that uses a tiny camera to project brightened and magnified images from inside the body

Epidemiology - the study of disease as it occurs in groups of people or even other populations

Epilepsy - disorder of the nervous system marked by seizures and temporary losses of consciousness or concentration

Endorphins - pain-killing proteins produced naturally by the body

Ephaptic transmission - conduction across nerves at sites where it should not normally occur

Ethnicity - has many definitions, a group that perceives themselves to share social and cultural

Etiology - cause

Facial arthromyalgia - another name for TMD pain — see below.

Facial nerve - a cranial nerve that controls most of the muscles in the face. This is a separate nerve from the trigeminal nerve, which controls sensation in the face and some of the muscles that control chewing

Facial palsy - weakness of the muscles of facial expression

Fluoroscope - a fluorescent X-ray device that surgeons use to guide a needle or catheter to the right location in the body.

Folic acid - an essential vitamin found in green vegetables and red meat, which can be depleted by some anticonvulsant drugs.

Foramen ovale - the opening in the skull through which the trigeminal nerve passes on its way into the face **Fothergill's Disease** - another name for TN. Comes from 18th-century English physician John Fothergill. Seldom used anymore.

Gamma Knife - a non-incision surgical device that uses Gamma radiation to cause precisely aimed damage to targeted tissue. Used to create lesions on the root of the trigeminal nerve.

Ganglion - a cluster of nerve cells

Gangliolysis - A surgical procedure to create targeted damage to a ganglion, usually to stop pain signals from getting to the brain

Gasserian ganglion - the cluster of nerve cells where the trigeminal nerve branches out into its three divisions and exits the skull. Sometimes just called trigeminal ganglion.or semilunar ganglion.

Gate control - a theory to explain how pain is experienced (see Chapter 2)

Genetics - the study of heredity and in clinical genetics, it is the study of possible genetic factors that influence the occurrence of a disease

Glial cells - type of cells that the body uses to build myelin, the insulating sheath around nerves. Also see oligodendrocytes and Schwann cells.

Glossopharyngeal neuralgia - similar condition to TN, except that this pain is in the throat and neck. Causes are thought to be similar to TN, but involving the glossopharyngeal nerve.

Glycerol - an oily alcohol substance that damages nerve fibers when in direct contact with the fibers

Gold standard - the best possible treatment available at this time

Granulomas - abnormal growths as a result of irritation

Hematoma - bruise

Half life - the time it takes to eliminate one half of an ingested drug

Hemiplegic - paralysis of one side of the body

Hemostasis - arresting of bleeding

Herpes zoster - also known as shingles, this is a viral infection caused by the same virus that causes chickenpox. When it strikes the face, it can cause burning pain

Hypesthesia - medical term for numbness

Hyperalgesia - an increased response to a stimulus, which is normally painful

Hyper reflex - increased reflex

Hypertension - high blood pressure

Hyponatremia - abnormally low levels of blood sodium. Can be a side effect of some TN medications.

Hypothesis - a supposition that appears to explain a group phenomena

Iatroplacebogenesis - the effect that the doctor treating the patient can have on a patient in helping to remove symptoms

Idiopathic - refers to a disease or condition of unknown cause or origin

Incidence - number of new cases of a disease occurring during a certain period

Infarct - area of death of tissue due to reduced blood supply, which can be a vital area such as in the heart where it is called a heart attack

Inflammatory response - a series of responses of the body to damage, which results in swelling, redness, heat and pain

Intracellular messengers - chemical transmitting information within a cell

Intraoral - inside the mouth

Informed consent - a person's consent based on a shared decision between physician and patient, with the physician understanding the relevant values of the patient and the patient understanding the nature of the disease and intervention, including risks and benefits

Kaplan-Meier method (survival curves) - an analysis that accounts for subjects who fail treatment, as well as subjects who are censored (withdrawn either because of death or not having failed treatment. It enables the probability of an event occurring to be predicted. The data is most often shown as a graph.

Keratatis - inflammation of the cornea, transparent front lining of the eye

Lacrimal - pertaining to tears

Lesion - an area of tissue damage.

Leukopenia - a deficiency in white blood cells, which protect the body against disease-causing microorganisms. Can be a side effect of some TN medications.

Levetiracetam - anticonvulsant drug used to treat trigeminal neuralgia.

LILT - acronym for "low-intensity laser therapy," in which beams of highly focused laser light are delivered to an area of pain in order to provide pain-relief

LINAC - acronym for linear accelerator, a non-incision surgical device that uses high-energy X-rays to cause precisely aimed damage to targeted tissues. Often used for tumors, but sometimes for TN

Lumbar puncture - insertion of a needle into the back to tap out CSF for testing

Magnetic resonance imaging (MRI) - a device that creates computerized images of the body's interior. Instead of using radiation as in an X-ray, MRI involves a rapid series of pictures taken while the subject is inside a magnetized chamber. An MRI brain scan is painless and is useful in detecting multiple sclerosis and brain tumors.

Magnetic resonance tomographic angiography (MRTA) - a type of imaging similar to MRI that can pick up even very small blood vessels. Gadolinium dye is injected into the patient's bloodstream to enhance the image.

Mandibular - area referring to the lower jaw region of the face

Mastoid - part of the temporal bone that forms the skull

Master - one the muscles used in chewing

Maxillary - area referring to the upper jaw and cheek region of the face

McGill Pain Questionnaire - a questionnaire to assess pain character and severity

Mean - average

Meckel's cave - cavity inside the skull that is made up of dura mater (brain lining material) in which sits the trigeminal (Gasserian) ganglion and the divisions of the trigeminal nerve

Median - a statistical term referring to the value above which 50 % of the other values lie and below which 50 % of the values lie, or is the middle value in a series of values

Meningitis - an inflammation of the membrane that covers the brain and spinal cord. It is a potential complication of brain surgery. It can be bacterial, i.e due to an infection, or aseptic due to irritation.

Meningioma - a tumor of the meninges, the membrane that covers the brain and spinal cord. This can cause TN if the tumor pushes a blood vessel against the trigeminal nerve.

Meta analysis - see Chapter 5

Microcompression - see balloon compression

Microvascular decompression (MVD) - a type of brain surgery in which the aim is to lift a compressing blood vessel off the trigeminal nerve and insulate the two with a small cushion

Modality/ies - a specific sensory entity, e.g. taste, or a specifc type of treatment

Morbidity - a disease/ or side effect

Motor - muscle, nerve or center that affects or produces movement

Motor cortex stimulation - a surgical procedure in which one or two small contact plates – attached to an electrical stimulation device – are placed on the surface of the brain over the cortex region. Stimulating this region with low-grade electrical current reduces activity in the thalamus, where pain is felt.

Multiple sclerosis (MS) - a degenerative disease affecting the central nervous system. MS causes scarring of nerve fibers and leads to such symptoms as arm and leg weakness, numbness, double vision and impaired coordination and movement.

Myelin - the protective coating that surrounds nerve fibers. It's made out of a layer of proteins packed between two layers of lipids (fats).

Myofascial pain - dull, aching muscle pain of uncertain cause. When it occurs in the facial muscles, it's sometimes confused with TN because the pain can be triggered by touching the area.

Nasolabial - area down the side of the nose and the lips

Natural history of a disease - how the disease would run its course if no treatment was given

Nerve block - use of a drug, chemical or surgery to stop a nerve signal from getting through to the brain. In the case of TN, these can be used for temporary pain relief or as a way to diagnose the exact nature and location of a pain.

Nerve fiber - a strand of tissue made up of nerve cells that carry nerve impulses (biochemical signals to and from the brain)

Nervus intermedius - a branch of the facial nerve formed in the geniculate ganglion, provides fibers for taste to the front of the tongue and releases secretions for the salivary glands

Neurectomy - surgical removal of a nerve or nerve branch

Neuroaugmentation - attempting to block pain signals by overriding them with a competing signal generated by an implanted or attached electrical stimulation device

Neuroma - a tangle of poorly developed nerve endings that resprout following a nerve injury

Neuromodulators - substances that alter the way a nerve transmits (transmits what?)

Neuropathic pain - pain that originates in the nerve, usually due to injury or disease

Neuropathy - disturbance of function or pathological change in a sensory nerve causing numbness

Neurophysiological - the way that nerves function

Neurons - cells that send and receive electrical signals to and from parts of the body. These are the nerve cells that are stimulated to send impulses (messages) to and from the brain.

Neuroradiologists - medical doctors trained to interpret scans and MRIs; these specialists have a special interest in images related to neurological disease

Neurotransmitter - a body chemical that's used to transmit nerve impulses from one nerve cell to another. Sodium and calcium are two of the most common.

Neurovascular - nerve and blood vessel

Neutropenia - a diminished number of neutrophils, a type of white blood cell needed to fight infections. Can be a side effect of some TN medications

NICO - acronym for "neuralgia-inducing cavitational osteonecrosis," a controversial type of facial pain that may be confused with TN. Presumed cause is a chronic infection of bone in the jaw that can damage the nerve branches in the affected bone

Nociceptor - a type of nerve receptor that activate when there's a painful stimulus

Noxious insult - painful injury

Occipito-mental X-ray - an X-ray image of the skull taken from a particular angle to show up the sinuses

Oedema (also edema) - swelling

Oligodendrocyte - a specific type of glial cell that the body uses to build myelin in the central nervous system

Open label trial - a clinical trial in which patient and doctor are aware of the intervention being evaluated

Ophthalmic - area referring to the region of the face around the eyes.

Opioids - pain-killing agents that originate from the poppy flower and its product opium (Morphine and codeine were two of the earliest opioids).

Orofacial - area of the face around the mouth

Orthopontomogram (OPG) - an X-ray film showing both upper and lower jaws, as well as all the teeth

Otitis media - inflammation of the middle ear

Palsy - paralysis

Pain threshold - the point at which an applied, escalating sensory stimulus (heat, cold, pressure, pin-prick, etc.) is reported by a person as pain

Pain tolerance - the reaction of a person to reported pain after it has crossed the pain threshold

Pancytopenia - abnormal decrease in all types of blood cells. Can be a side effect of some TN medications.

Paratrigeminal neuralgia - throbbing headache-like pain in the upper branch of the trigeminal nerve, thought to be caused either by an inflammation or infection of the nerve. Also called "Raeder's syndrome."

Paresthesia - an unusual sensation that may be described as "tingling," "crawling" or "pins and needles." Often accompanies mild numbness. An abnormal sensation, whether spontaneous or evoked.

Pathogen - a disease-producing organism

Percutaneous - through the skin. When referring to percutaneous procedures in treating TN, it means a type of surgery in which the surgeon inserts a needle or electrode through the cheek as opposed to entering the skull.

Peripheral nerves - nerves outside the brain and spinal cord. In the case of TN, these include the many branches of the trigeminal nerve that serve the teeth, gums and other parts of the face.

Petrous - part of the skull bones that resemble a rock

Phenotype - entire physical, biochemical and phsysiological makeup of an individual as determined by genetics and environment

Polymorphism - the occurrence together in the same population of two or more genetically determined phenotypes in such proportions that the rarest of them cannot be maintained merely by recurrent mutation

Pons - part of the brain stem to which the trigeminal nerve is connected; posterior part lying between medulla and midbrain

Post-herpetic neuralgia - a type of facial pain caused by damage from the herpes zoster (chickenpox) virus. Can occur after a bout of shingles.

Posterior - anterior X-ray of the skull - a standard view of the skull

Posterior fossa - hollow in the back of the skull where the brain stem lies and area where the trigeminal nerve emerges from the brain

Post-traumatic neuralgia - a type of facial pain caused by physical damage to the trigeminal nerve and/or its branches

Preganglionic - situated proximal to the ganglion; in the trigeminal nerve, this refers to <u>before</u> the Gasserian ganglion

Pretrigeminal neuralgia - a precursor to TN marked by more of a constant ache than sharp, stabbing attacks that are triggered by light touches to the face

Prevalence - the total number of cases of a disease at a certain time in a particular place

Prognosis - forecast as to the probable outcome of a disease

Proprioception - position sense

Prostaglandins - hormones that kick into action to help fight infections, specifically by creating pain, inflammation and fever that causes us to reduce activity and allow our body's energy to focus on stopping the infection

Protocol - an experiment

Psychogenic - having a psychological component

Pulmonary - lung

Race - a group of people who share a set of physical charactertistics

Radiofrequency - the use of generated heat through an electrode to cause selected damage to tissue. One type of surgical treatment for TN

Radiographer - specialist trained to carry out scans and MRIs (Radiographers are not medical doctors)

Radiosurgery - the use of radiation devices to treat diseases and disorders without having to cut into tissue. Two examples of devices used in treating TN are Gamma Knife and Linac

Raeder's Syndrome - also known as Paratrigeminal Neuralgia, is a combination of pain, drooping eyelid and constricted pupil (See Chapter 1)

Random - purely by chance

Randomized controlled trial (RCT) - refers to a study that aims to reduce bias towards the new treatment being used by keeping both doctors and patients blinded as to which is the new treatment

Receptors - cells that are attached to nerve fibers that monitor the environment in, on and around the body for changes

Reflex Sympathetic Dystrophy/Complex Regional Pain Syndrome - see Complex Regional Syndrome

Refractory - does not respond

Remyelination - the process of rebuilding lost or damaged myelin, the protective sheath around nerve fibers

Retrospective studies or case series - those studies in which data is extracted from medical notes some time after they were first collected and then analyzed

Risk - the possibility of suffering harm or loss

Root canal - an oral surgical procedure in which the nerve is removed from an inflamed tooth

Root entry zone - the section of the trigeminal nerve near the brain stem at which point the myelin (covering) changes

Rhizotomy - a surgical procedure to cut or damage a nerve root so as to interfere with the transmission of pain signals to the brain

Schwann cell - a type of glial cell that the body uses to build myelin in nerves outside the central nervous system

Sensory - pertaining to sensation

Shared Decision Making - presents patients with evidence-based, unbiased views of their health care options, and encourages patients to work with their doctors to choose the health care options that are right for them

Sluder's neuralgia - pain around eye and sinuses in association with nasal congestion produced by lesions of the sphenopalatine ganglion; redness of the eye and excessive tearing may occur

Sociodemographic - includes the details of individuals' social circumstances

Somatosensory - senations of the body

Stylet - small needle

Suprathreshold stimulation - above the normal threshold at which it would be stimulated

Surrogate outcomes - measuring outcomes indirectly

Survival curves - see Kaplan Meier

Systematic review - as the name implies, this is a rigorous process of finding every single clinical study on the given topic, and then critically appraising this data and only using the high quality studies to make observations in terms of treatment

Subluxation - chiropractic term that means one or more vertebrae are out of their proper alignment

Stereotactic - Guided by X-ray imaging or similar scanning devices. A way for TN surgeons to be guided to precise, three-dimensional locations in the skull and face.

SUNCT - acronym for "short-lasting, unilateral, neuralgiform headaches with conjunctival injection and tearing." Sometimes confused with TN, it's a sharp, come-and-go pain centering around the eye, along with a red eye, tearing and a runny nose. Believed to be caused by an inflammation of blood vessels around the eye.

Symptomatic - any subjective evidence of disease perceived by a patient, which indicates some bodily or mental state

Symptomatic trigeminal neuralgia - trigeminal nerve pain that occurs as a result of another condition, such as multiple sclerosis or a tumor.

Synapse - gaps between nerve fibers that nerve impulses must jump to continue on.

Systemic - whole body

Tarsorrhaphy - an operation for suturing together a part or all of the upper and lower eyelids to protect the cornea

Temporomandibular joint disorder - see TMJ/TMD

Temporal arteritis - aching, throbbing and sometimes burning pain in the temple area caused by an inflamed artery in that area. Sometimes confused with TN.

TENS unit - a device that delivers regular, low-grade electrical signals that distract or override pain signals. TENS stands for "transcutaneous electrical stimulation."

Thermocoagulation - a procedure using heat to create tissue injury. It's the technique applied in the radiofrequency lesioning surgery used to treat TN.

Thalamus - the part of the brain that relays messages between various parts of the body and the appropriate other part of the brain. It functions as the brain's "central switching station."

Thin-cut MRI - see MRI. Words "thin cut" relate to the special technique used to enhance visibility of the trigeminal nerve and vessels.

Thrombocytopenia - abnormally low blood platelets, which are needed for clotting; can be a side effect of some TN medications

Tic douloureux - another name for trigeminal neuralgia. (means "painful spasm" in French)

Tinnitus - ringing in the ears

TMJ/TMD - pain in the jaw joint sometimes confused with TN. The jaw joint is the temporomandibular joint.

Tolosa Hunt Syndrome - pain around the eye, double vision due to inflammation, which responds to steroid therapy

Topirimate - anticonvulsant drug that may be useful for trigeminal neuralgia (See Chapter 6)

Transconjunctival therapy - medicine that's delivered by drops or creams in the eye. The conjunctiva is the tissue around the eye

Trigeminal autonomic cephalgia - refers to a group of facial pains that are all associated with over activity of the trigeminal nerve. Includes conditions such as cluster headaches. Tolosa Hunt (See Chapter 1)

Trigeminal neuritis - an inflammation of the trigeminal nerve and/or its branches

Trigeminal nucleus - the origin of the trigeminal nerve in the top three bones of the spinal column (the upper-cervical spine)

Trigger point - the site, often at the end of a nerve, which, if touched, results in pain

Trismus - spasm of the muscles opening the mouth

Tumor - abnormal growth of tissue; if uncontrolled and progressive, called malignant; if under control, called benign

Vertigo - illusion of movement and a feeling that the outside world is rotating round, not the same as dizziness

Visceral - any large internal organ